DENTAL INSTRUMENTS

A POCKET GUIDE

EDITION **7**

LINDA R. BARTOLOMUCCI BOYD, RDA, BA

Emeritus Professor, Registered Dental Assisting Program

Diablo Valley College

Pleasant Hill, California

ELSEVIER

3251 Riverport Lane
St. Louis, Missouri 63043

ISBN: 978-0-323-67243-6

Notices

Knowledge and best practice in this field are constantly changing. As new research and experience broaden our understanding, changes in research methods, professional practices, or medical treatment may become necessary.

Practitioners and researchers must always rely on their own experience and knowledge in evaluating and using any information, methods, compounds, or experiments described herein. In using such information or methods they should be mindful of their own safety and the safety of others, including parties for whom they have a professional responsibility.

With respect to any drug or pharmaceutical products identified, readers are advised to check the most current information provided (i) on procedures featured or (ii) by the manufacturer of each product to be administered, to verify the recommended dose or formula, the method and duration of administration, and contraindications. It is the responsibility of practitioners, relying on their own experience and knowledge of their patients, to make diagnoses, to determine dosages and the best treatment for each individual patient, and to take all appropriate safety precautions.

To the fullest extent of the law, neither the Publisher nor the authors, contributors, or editors, assume any liability for any injury and/or damage to persons or property as a matter of products liability, negligence or otherwise, or from any use or operation of any methods, products, instructions, or ideas contained in the material herein.

ISBN: 978-0-323-67243-6

Senior Content Strategist: Joslyn Dumas
Publishing Services Manager: Deepthi Unni
Senior Content Development Manager: Luke Held
Senior Project Manager: Manchu Mohan
Senior Book Designer: Amy Buxton

Printed in China

Last digit is the print number: 9 8 7 6 5 4 3 2 1

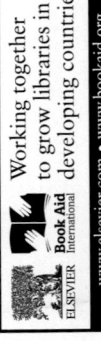

Ann Marie Gorcyzca, DMD, MPH, MS

Thank you,

for your words of praise and encouragement in the ongoing process of publishing.

To all of my professional affiliations that support the profession of dentistry especially the National organization; The American Dental Assistants Association!

Preface

It is extremely exciting to publish the seventh edition of *Dental Instruments: A Pocket Guide.*

Several new additions have been added to this text. First, the Sterilization Notes on each written page have more detailed information on how to correctly process instruments. Second, many new photos were taken to enhance and identify the working end in greater detail as well as the entire instrument for clarity. Third, on the text page, many new photos are inserted to demonstrate how the instrument is commonly used. This is referred to as the "In Use" photos. Also, new technology equipment has been added, as well as new/current models of technology that already existed in the previous editions.

This text is designed to help all dental students; dental assistants, dental hygienists, students in dental school as well as practicing professionals to master the identification and use of common and specialty dental instruments and equipment as well as following sterilization guidelines for possessing instruments. Whereas certain chapters focus on the instruments used in all dental practices, such as components of the basic tray setup, the anesthetic syringe and its parts, evacuation devices, and so on, other chapters are designed around various routine dental procedures, such as the instruments used in hygiene, amalgam, and composite procedures. The dental specialty chapters include instruments used in prosthodontics, orthodontics, endodontics, and periodontics. Three chapters focus on oral surgery—one addresses the general surgical instruments used in oral and periodontal surgery, and the other two focus on surgical extractions and implants. The third focuses on periodontal instruments. Significant advances in detection of oral cancer equipment have been added to this text as well. There are also chapters devoted to dental material equipment.

Additionally, in keeping with the concept of total patient care, the chapter called "Patient Assessment and Emergency Equipment" focuses on the equipment used to monitor patients for routine dental treatment as well as treatment of sedated patients. At the end of most chapters, there are examples of tray setups, enhancing the reader's ability to set up trays and use the instruments in the correct sequence, depending on the procedure.

In the 21st century, dentistry has certainly evolved with technology. It is more important than ever for students and clinicians to have an excellent understanding of the instruments and equipment they will encounter in practice. This seventh edition will help students and the clinicians stay current with the quickly changing technology of dentistry, as well as more detailed information on some instruments in the text pages. However, although basic dental instruments and equipment have remained relatively unchanged throughout the years, there have also been new advances that accommodate new technology in the dental field. These include, but are not limited to, the development of heat-resistant metals, synthetic material used for dental instruments, and new equipment. Examples can be seen in the special coatings available on some instruments, such as the titanium coating found on composite instruments that allow these instruments to be adapted to the different types of materials, as well as new designs of instruments.

I am confident that this text will assist you to more easily learn the dental instruments, dental equipment, and tray setups that clinicians use in dental practices. It is imperative that all students begin their careers with a thorough knowledge of dental instruments and equipment and that they expand their knowledge throughout their careers. Certainly, this text will help you achieve these goals. I wish you all success in the field of dentistry. I know you will be a great asset to the dental profession!

Linda R. Bartolomucci Boyd

New to This Edition

- **Several new photos** in many chapters, including both a full-instrument view and specifically more precise close-up views to better view the working ends of the instruments to assist in easier identification

- Additional **"In Use"** photos and illustrations of instruments and equipment to enhance the understanding of the function in specific procedures

- **Sequence of instruments** in the chapters continue to give a better understanding of method of use for procedures.

- Addition of specific identification **of parts of instruments and equipment have** been added.

FEATURES OF THIS TEXT

- **Flashcard format** makes it easy to quiz yourself on dental instruments and their uses.

- **More than 700 high-quality photographs and illustrations** enhance your ability to quickly and accurately identify dental instruments. These new photos include: full instruments, close up photos of the working end and many "In Use" photos.

- Convenient **spiral-bound design** helps you easily access key information at a glance as well as use the pages as a **flash card technique** for studying.

- **Clear, consistent organization** helps you master basic instruments before introducing more complicated instruments.

- **Tray setups** (Note: The tray setups usually only have an example of instruments for the designated procedure; they do not include any axillary items needed for that particular procedure, such as cotton rolls or 2 × 2 gauze, etc.)

Each written page has information on each individual instrument including:

- Name of the instrument
- Main function of the instrument
- Characteristics of the instrument: Information on other uses for the instrument
- Practice Note: Possible tray setups for the instrument
- Sterilization Note:
- In addition to the Sterilization Note on each written page, it should be noted that instruments and items used during dental procedures are categorized as **critical, semicritical, or noncritical.** Below are excerpts from the *Guidelines for Infection Control in Dental Health-Care Settings—2003* that explain the categories.

- "Patient-care items (dental instruments, devices, and equipment) are categorized as critical, semicritical, or noncritical, depending on the potential risk for infection associated with their intended use. . . . **Critical** items used to penetrate soft tissue or bone have the greatest risk of transmitting infection and should be sterilized by heat. **Semicritical** items touch mucous membranes or nonintact skin and have a lower risk of transmission; because the majority of semicritical items in dentistry are heat-tolerant, they also should be sterilized by using heat. If a semicritical item is heat-sensitive, it should, at a minimum, be processed with high-level disinfection. . . .

- "**Noncritical** patient-care items pose the least risk of transmission of infection, contacting only intact skin, which can serve as an effective barrier to microorganisms. In the majority of cases, cleaning, or if visibly soiled, cleaning followed by disinfection with an EPA-registered hospital disinfectant is adequate. When the item is visibly contaminated with blood or OPIM, an EPA-registered hospital disinfectant with a tuberculocidal claim (i.e., intermediate-level disinfectant) should be used. . . . Cleaning or disinfection of certain noncritical patient-care items can be difficult or damage the surfaces; therefore, use of disposable barrier protection of these surfaces might be a preferred alternative."

- For detailed information regarding guidelines for infection control in a dental setting please refer to *Guidelines for Infection Control in Dental Health-Care Settings—2003* at http://www.cdc.gov/mmwr/index.html.

EVOLVE

For the Student ▶ Chapter Quizzes • Drag-and-Drop Tray Setup Exercises • Tray Setup Quizzes

For the Instructor ▶ Image Collection for Power Point Presentation and Testing • Test Bank

Acknowledgments

My deepest appreciation is to acknowledge all of my colleagues, dentist affiliations, professors, and my dearest family and friends for all of their insight, support, love, and prayers during the writing of this seventh edition. Of course, I value and appreciate each and every student as their zest and enthusiasm for learning gives me such encouragement to write a text that enhances their desire to learn.

Two people have played an incredible role in making this text such a great learning tool with the availability of the instruments and the creative skill in photography. First and foremost, I have the greatest respect for Jeff McMillian in his ability to photograph dental instruments. Jeff's artistic ability and incredible photography skills have enhanced this text with clearer and more precise photographs, especially the close-up working ends of dental instruments and the all-new photographs of the instruments "In Use". Second, these photographs would not be possible without Andrew Hartzell, former president and owner of G. Hartzell & Son, Inc., now DentMat™ who allowed me to borrow most of the instruments to photograph. Thank you, Andy!

Kristin Wilhelm, I value and thank you for your expertise as Director, Private Sector Education Content, in overseeing and publishing this seventh edition.

I am absolutely grateful to Luke Held, Senior Content Development Manager and Laurie Gower, Director, Content Development Manager. I continue to be thankful to Courtney Sprehe as she was my senior content development specialist from the second edition to the sixth edition.

I continue to express my gratitude to **Joyce M. Litch, RDH, DDS, MSD,** for her expertise as a consultant to the book, who assisted in developing the periodontal and hygiene chapters. I thank you for always being there for me! The bur chapter would not be as comprehensive without the consultation from **Wayne Joseph, DDS.** His insight into this chapter has been appreciated from the first edition to the seventh. I am thankful and appreciate the experience I have received from Eugene Santucci, DDS during the years of working together as a dental team. My continued knowledge and encouragement from Timothy Farley is much appreciated.

I would like to express my deepest gratitude to **Cathy Clarke, RDA, CDA, BA,** for her continuous support and many hours of such quality consulting. Thank you for always being available to answer my questions at any time.

A very special thank you to Paul Charles Hans, BS, MBA, an author himself, for his ability in keeping my focus in the process of the photography as well as the research and creative technical writing of this text. Your love, support, and encouragement mean more to me than I can express.

I could not have written this seventh edition without the love, support, and prayers from my family: my sons, Michael and Matthew, who always gave me a nudge of encouragement; my cousin Elaine Strizzi, for her gentle and loving ways of support; and my brother and sister-in-law, Ray and Meri, for the nourishment of my body and soul during this process. Also, the concept my parents taught me, **"To honor the dream inside of me,"** constantly resonates in my mind. Last, but certainly not least, are the wonderful, refreshing moments with my grandchildren, Christian, Collin, Liberty Rae, Alexis, Jaxson, Maxwell, and Jaylin who teach me the simplicity, enthusiasm, and zest for learning that encourages my writing. Ti Amo!

Linda R. Bartolomucci Boyd

For information about the author or to ask questions about the text, please contact
Linda@Dentalpocketguide.com.

Contents

Photo/Illustration Credits

Photo/Illustration Credits (Manufacturers)

Photos on the following pages are courtesy of:

3M ESPE: p. 640 [www.3m.com]

3M Littmann Stethoscopes. p. 722 [www.littmann.com]

Acteon North America: p. 102 [www.acteonusa.com]

A-dec Inc.: pp. 72 (right), 74, 76, 78, 80, 108, 112 [www.a-dec.com]

Air Techniques, Inc.: pp. 394, 690, 710 [www.airtechniques.com]

Align Technology, Inc. (Invisalign clear aligners): pp. 466 (right), 467 (bottom) [www.aligntech.com]

Alfa Medical: p. 620 [www.alfa-medical.com]

Carestream Health, Inc.: pp. 668, 712 [www.carestreamdental.com]

Coltène/Whaledent, Inc.: p. 312 [www.coltene.com]

Criticare Technologies Inc.: 730, 732 [www.criticareusa.com]

Dentsply Sirona: pp. 90, 92, 94, 98, 100, 106, 110, 116, 120, 122, 124, 126, 128, 130, 132, 134, 136, 138, 140, 142, 194, 268, 270, 466 (left), 467 (top), 686, 694, 696, 698, 700, 702, 704, 705, 706, 714 [www.dentsplysirona.com]

DynaFlex: pp. 404, 408 (right), 444, 445 [www.dynaflex.com]

Garrison Dental Solutions: p. 232 [www.garrisondental.com]

GE Healthcare: p. 728 [www.gehealthcare.com]

GettyImages.com: p. 586 [www.gettyimages.com]

Fehrenbach MJ, Herring SW: Illustrated anatomy of the head and neck, ed 5, St. Louis, 2017, Elsevier—illustration on page 39 (Photo courtesy Margaret Fehrenbach)

Freedman G: Contemporary esthetic dentistry, St. Louis, 2012, Mosby—illustration on page 388

Garg AK: Implant dentistry, ed 2, St. Louis, 2010, Mosby—illustration on page 549

Graber TM, Vanarsdall RL, Vig KWL: Orthodontics: current principles and techniques, ed 4, St. Louis, 2006, Mosby—illustration on page 418

Graber LW, Vanarsdall RL, Vig KWL, et al: Orthodontics: current principles and techniques, ed 6, St. Louis, 2017, Elsevier—illustration on page 459

Gutmann JL, Lowdahl PE: Problem solving in endodontics: prevention, identification and management, ed 5, St. Louis, 2011, Mosby—illustrations on pages 485, 497

Hargreaves KM, Berman LH: Cohen's pathways of the pulp, Expert Consult, ed 11, St. Louis, 2016, Elsevier—illustrations on pages 287, 313, 317, 321

Hatrick CD, Eakle WS, Bird WF: Dental materials: clinical applications for dental assistants and dental hygienists, St. Louis, 2003, Saunders—illustration on page 354

Hatrick CD, Eakle WS, Bird WF: Dental materials: clinical applications for dental assistants and dental hygieners, ed 3, St. Louis, 2016, Elsevier—illustrations on pages 153, 245, 249, 641, 643, 659

Heymann HO, Swift EJ, Ritter AV: Strudevant's art and science of operative dentistry, ed 6, St. Louis, 2013, Mosby—illustration on page 31

Hupp JR, Ellis E, Tucker MR: Contemporary oral and maxillofacial surgery, ed 6, St. Louis, 2014, Mosby—illustrations on pages 495, 535, 555, 606, 681

Iannucci J, Howerton LJ: Dental radiography: principles and techniques, ed 5, St. Louis, 2017, Elsevier—illustrations on pages 688, 692 (adapted)

Malamed SF: Handbook of local anesthesia, ed 6, St. Louis, 2013, Mosby—illustration on page 45

Malamed SF: Sedation: a guide to patient management, ed 5, St. Louis, 2010, Mosby—illustration on page 481

Newman MG, Takei H, Klokkevold PR, Carranza FA: Carranza's clinical periodontology, ed 11, St. Louis, 2012, Saunders—illustrations on pages 343, 345, 372, 373, 511, 517

Papadopoulos MA, Tarawneh F: The use of ministcrew implants for temporary skeletal anchorage in orthodontics: a comprehensive review. *Oral Surgery, Oral Medicine, Oral Pathology, Oral Radiology, and Endodontology,* 103(5): e6-e15, 2007—illustration on page 468 (left)

Perry DA, Beemsterboer PL: Periodontology for the dental hygienist, ed 4, St. Louis, 2014, Saunders—illustrations on pages 355, 513, 572

Proctor DB, Young-Adams AP: Kinn's the medical assistant: an applied learning approach, ed 13, St. Louis, 2017, Elsevier—illustrations on pages 724, 729

Proffit WR, Fields HW, Sarver DM: Contemporary orthodontics, ed 5, St. Louis, 2013, Mosby—illustrations on pages 405, 407, 419, 439, 441, 461

Robinson DS, Bird DL: Essentials of dental assisting, ed 5, St. Louis, 2013, Saunders—illustration on page 118

Rose LF, Mealey BL, Genco RJ, Cohen W: Periodontics: medicine, surgery and implants, St. Louis, 2004, Mosby—illustrations on pages 503, 519

Rosenstiel SF, Land MF, Fujimoto J: Contemporary fixed prosthodontics, ed 4, St. Louis, 2006, Mosby—illustration on page 155

Rosenstiel SF, Land MF, Fujimoto J: Contemporary fixed prosthodontics, ed 5, St. Louis, 2016, Elsevier—illustrations on pages 137, 143, 155, 273, 307, 315

Singh PP, Cranin AN: Atlas of oral implantology, ed 3, St. Louis, 2010, Mosby—illustrations on pages 293, 489, 491, 545

White SC, Pharoah MJ: Oral radiology: principles and interpretation, ed 7, St. Louis, 2014, Mosby—illustration on page 684 (adapted)

1

Basic Dental Instruments

1

2

2

Mouth Mirror

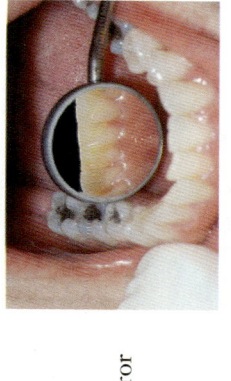

Functions ▶

To provide indirect vision

To retract lips, cheeks, and tongue

To reflect light into the mouth

Characteristics ▶

1 Front surface mirrors—Accurate, distortion-free image

2 Double-sided mirrors—Used to retract tongue or cheek and view intraoral cavity simultaneously

Flat surface mirrors—Used in disposable mirrors

Concave mirrors—Magnify image

Range of sizes

Commonly used sizes: 4 and 5; refer to diameter of mirror

Single ended

Different mirror handles available (see p. 8)

Practice Notes ▶

Mouth Mirror is used on most tray setups.

Sterilization Notes ▶

Mouth Mirror must be precleaned. Then, place in a sterilizing pouch with an internal process indicator, seal, then sterilize. OR, wrap with an internal process indicator inside and secure on the outside with process indicator tape, then sterilize. Verify appropriate color change has been achieved in external process indicator immediately after removal from sterilizer. Check internal process indicator before treatment. Refer to state regulations for any additional state requirements.

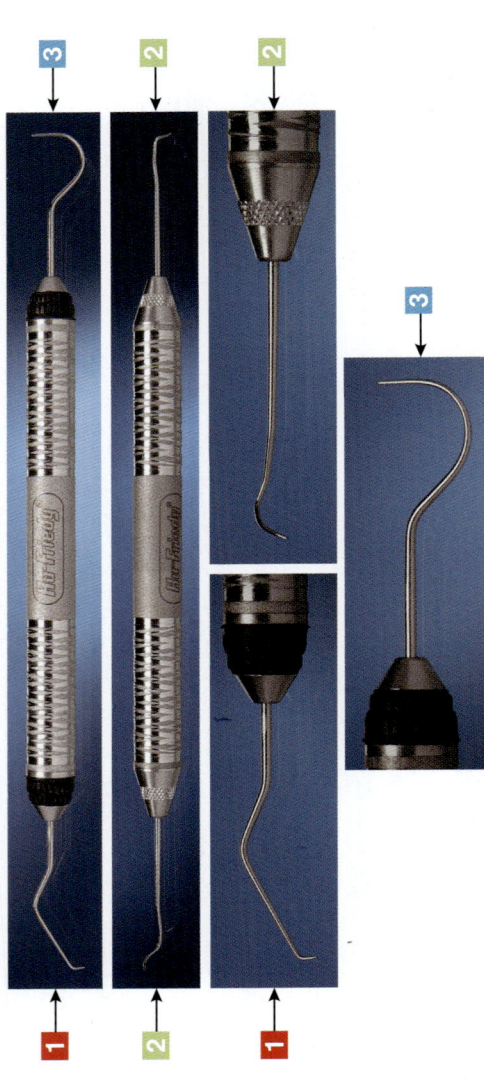

Explorers

Function ▶ To examine teeth for decay (caries), calculus, furcations, or other abnormalities

Characteristics ▶ Pointed tips; sharp, thin, flexible

Single or double ended

- Double-ended instruments—May have the same style on working ends or different styles of working ends; may also have explorer on one end and periodontal probe on the other end (for periodontal probe, see Chapter 16).

Variety of sizes and types:

1 Orban
2 Pigtail
3 Shepherd's hook

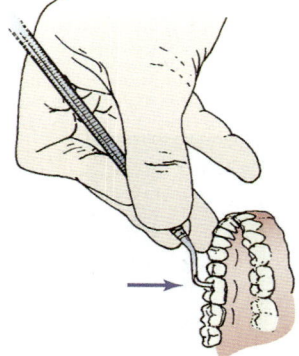

Practice Notes ▶ Explorer is used on most tray setups.

Sterilization Notes ▶ Explorer must be precleaned. Then, place in a sterilizing pouch with an internal process indicator, seal, then sterilize. OR, wrap with an internal process indicator inside and secure on the outside with process indicator tape, then sterilize. Verify appropriate color change has been achieved in external process indicator immediately after removal from sterilizer. Check internal process indicator before treatment. Refer to state regulations for any additional state requirements.

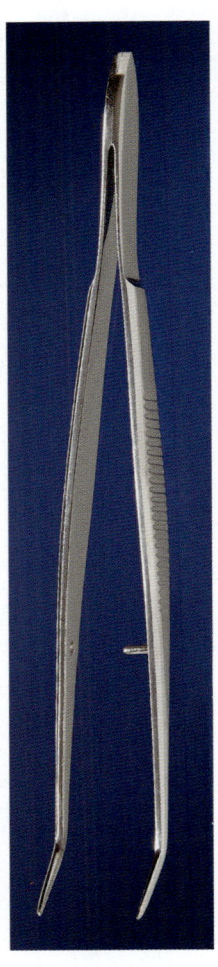

■ INSTRUMENT

Cotton Forceps (Pliers)

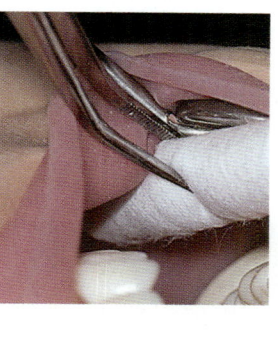

Function ▸ To grasp or transfer items and/or material into and out of the oral cavity

Characteristics ▸ Plain or serrated tips
Pointed or rounded tips
Thin or thick tips
Locking forceps (see Chapter 11)
Range of sizes available

Practice Notes ▸ Cotton Forceps is used on most tray setups.

Sterilization Notes ▸ Cotton Forceps must be precleaned open and unlocked. Then, place in an open and unlocked position in a sterilizing pouch with an internal process indicator, seal, then sterilize. OR, wrap with an internal process indicator inside and secure on the outside with process indicator tape, then sterilize. Verify appropriate color change has been achieved in external process indicator immediately after removal from sterilizer. Check internal process indicator before treatment. Refer to state regulations for any additional state requirements.

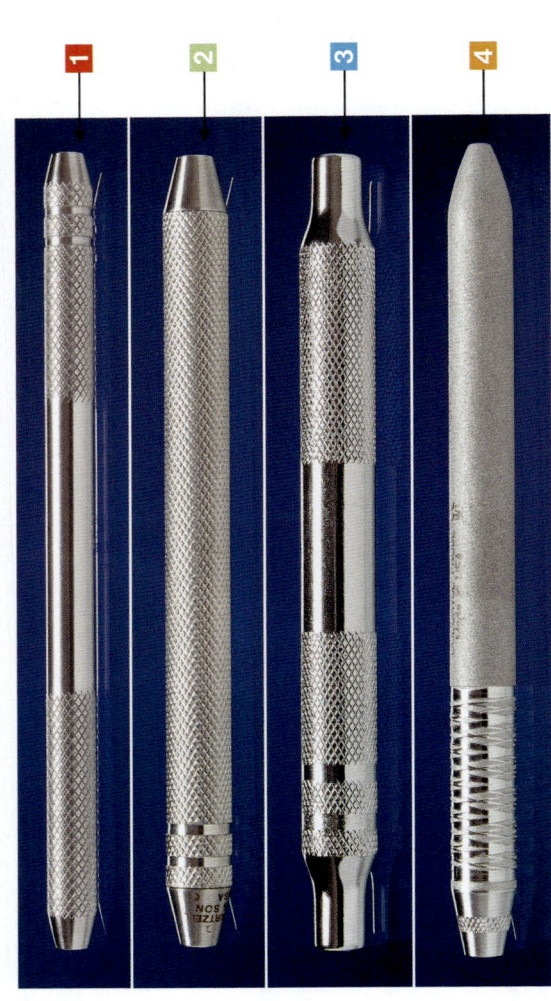

■ INSTRUMENT

Instrument Handles

Function ▶ To hold (grasp) instrument

Characteristics ▶ Single or double ended

Removable working ends (replaceable and interchangeable) attach to handle

Examples: Mouth mirror, scaler

Nonremovable working ends also available (commonly used)

Larger diameter models—Help lighten grasp and maximize control

Alternating diameter models—Lessen stress associated with carpal tunnel syndrome

Lighter weight models—Minimize fatigue

Variety of sizes, styles, and textures:

1. Small, round ¼-inch stainless steel
2. Standard, hollow ⁵⁄₁₆-inch stainless steel
3. Lightweight, ³⁄₈-inch slip-resistant pattern
4. Satin steel model—Lightweight, ergonomically designed

Sterilization Notes ▶ Instrument Handles must be precleaned. Then, place in a sterilizing pouch with an internal process indicator, seal, then sterilize. OR, wrap with an internal process indicator inside and secure on the outside with process indicator tape, then sterilize. Verify appropriate color change has been achieved in external process indicator immediately after removal from sterilizer. Check internal process indicator before treatment. Refer to state regulations for any additional state requirements.

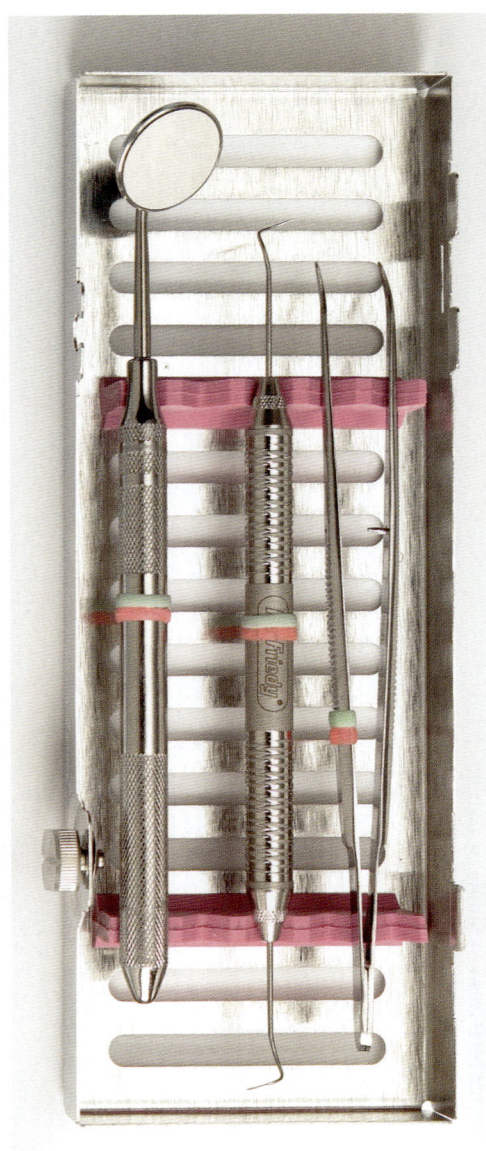

Basic

Mouth mirror, explorer (pigtail explorer pictured), cotton forceps—Example of color-coded instruments in cassette

Practice Notes ▸ Basic Setup is found on almost all dental tray setups.

Sterilization Notes ▸ Basic Setup instruments with Cassette must be precleaned. Then, place in a sterilizing pouch with an internal process indicator, seal, then sterilize. OR, wrap with an internal process indicator inside and secure on the outside with process indicator tape, then sterilize. Verify appropriate color change has been achieved in external process indicator immediately after removal from sterilizer. Check internal process indicator before treatment. Refer to state regulations for any additional state requirements.

11

2

Enamel-Cutting Instruments

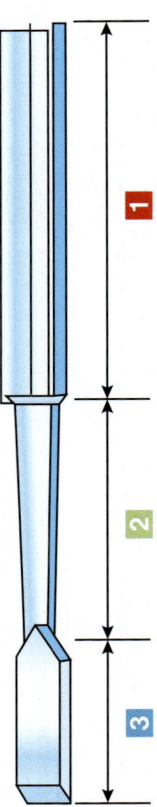

■ INSTRUMENT

Parts of an Instrument

1 Handle ▸ Grasping end of instrument
Variety of sizes and styles
Handle styles (refer to pp. 8 & 9)

2 Shank ▸ Connects handle to working end of instrument
May be straight or may have one or more angles to accommodate specific areas of the mouth

3 Working End ▸ May have cutting edge, blade, bevel, point, nib, or beaks

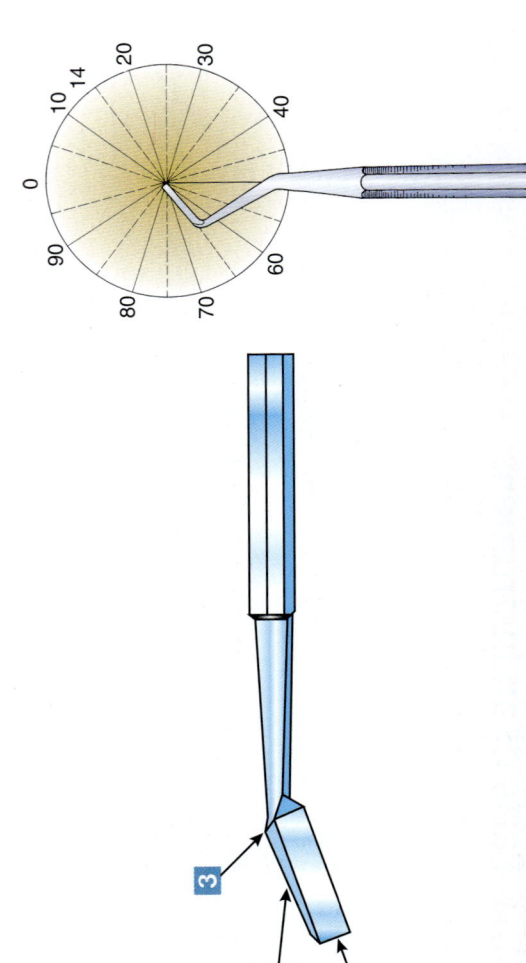

■ INSTRUMENT

Three-Numbered Instrument*

Function ▶ Numbers on handle indicate width, length, and angle of blade.

1 Indicates width of blade in tenths of millimeters
Example: 20 indicates a width of 2 mm

2 Indicates length of blade in millimeters
Example: 8 indicates a length of 8 mm

3 Indicates angle of blade from long axis of shaft
Example: 12 indicates an angle of 12 degrees

The designation for the instrument described above is 20-8-12; the number of instrument size is indicated on the handle.
Examples of three-numbered instruments: Enamel Hatchet, Enamel Hoe, Wedelstaedt

*The instrument number formula was designed by Dr. G.V. Black, Northwestern University.

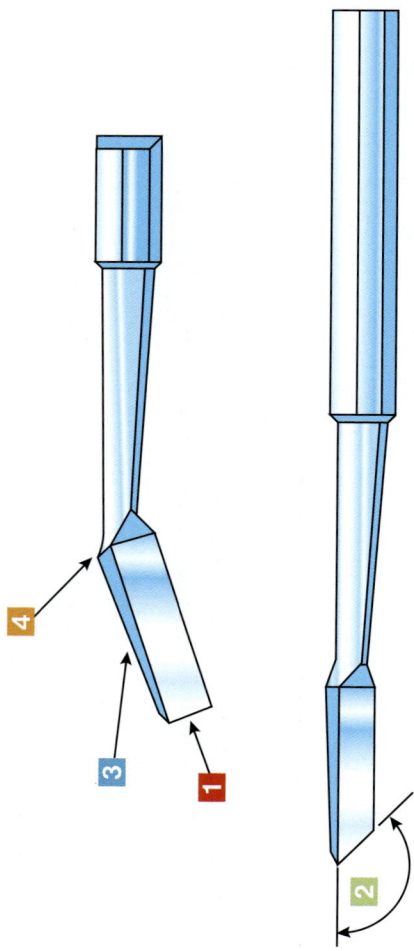

Four-Numbered Instrument*

Function ▸ Numbers on handle indicate width of blade, angle of cutting edge, length of blade, and angle of blade.

1 Indicates width of blade in tenths of millimeters
Example: 20 indicates a width of 2 mm

2 Indicates angle of cutting edge of blade in relation to handle
Example: 95 indicates a cutting edge angle of 95 degrees

3 Indicates length of blade in millimeters
Example: 8 indicates a length of 8 mm

4 Indicates angle of blade from long axis of shaft
Example: 12 indicates a blade angle of 12 degrees

The designation for the instrument described above is 20-95-8-12; the number of instrument size is indicated on the handle.

Examples of four-numbered instruments: Angle Former, Gingival Margin Trimmers—Mesial and Distal

*The instrument number formula was designed by Dr. G.V. Black, Northwestern University.

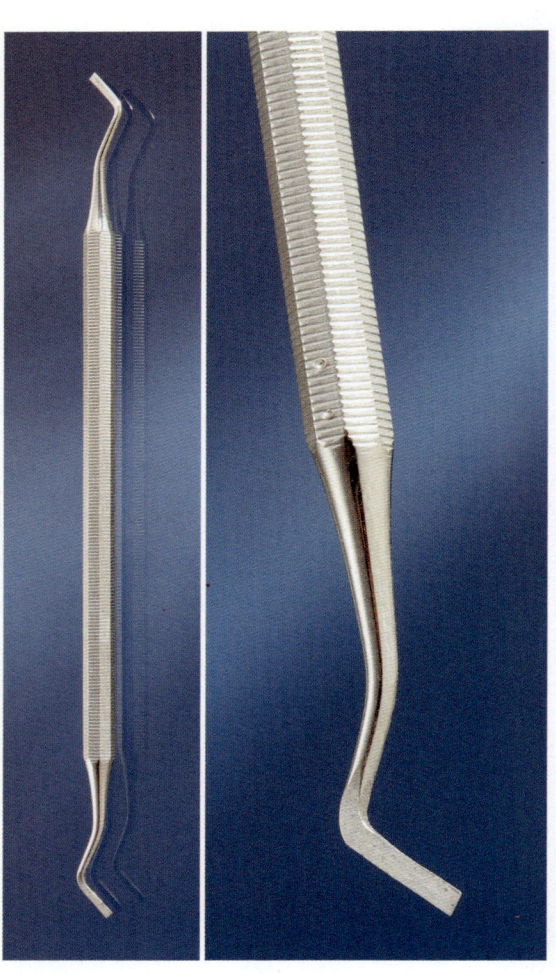

INSTRUMENT

Enamel Hatchet

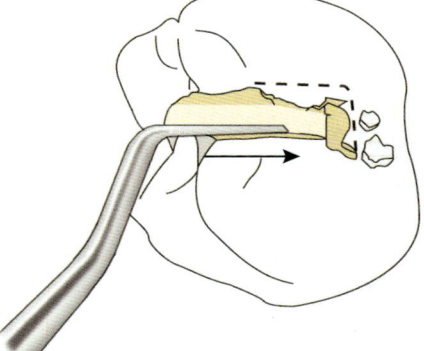

Functions ▸ To cut, clean, and smooth walls in cavity preparation

To remove enamel not supported by dentin

Characteristics ▸ Used with push motion

Cutting edge on same plane as handle

Single or double ended

Is a three-numbered instrument

Examples of instrument numbers:

20-9-14

15-8-14

15-8-12

Practice Notes ▸ Enamel Hatchet is used on restorative tray setups.

Sterilization Notes ▸ Enamel Hatchet must be precleaned. Then, place in a sterilizing pouch with an internal process indicator, seal, then sterilize. OR, wrap with an internal process indicator inside and secure on the outside with process indicator tape, then sterilize. Verify appropriate color change has been achieved in external process indicator immediately after removal from sterilizer. Check internal process indicator before treatment. Refer to state regulations for any additional state requirements.

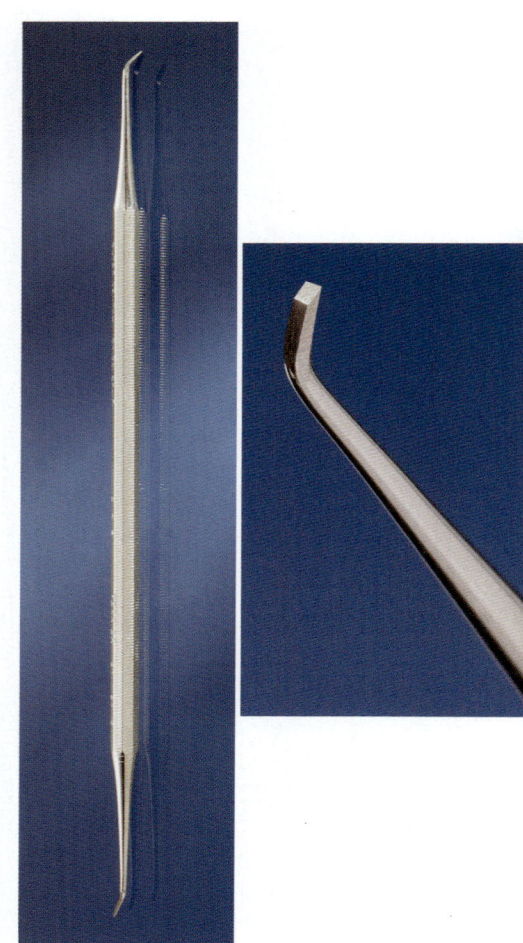

■ INSTRUMENT

Enamel Hoe

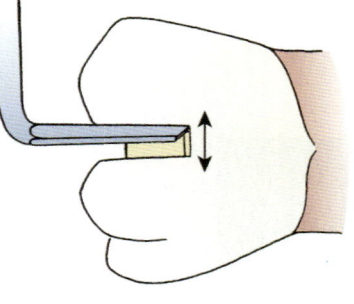

Function ▶ To clean and smooth floor and walls in cavity preparation

Characteristics ▶ Used with pulling motion

Cutting edge or blade nearly perpendicular to handle

Is a three-numbered instrument

Examples of instrument numbers:

10-4-8
10-4-14

Practice Notes ▶ Enamel Hoe is used on restorative tray setups.

Sterilization Notes ▶ Enamel Hoe must be precleaned. Then, place in a sterilizing pouch with an internal process indicator, seal, then sterilize. OR, wrap with an internal process indicator inside and secure on the outside with process indicator tape, then sterilize. Verify appropriate color change has been achieved in external process indicator immediately after removal from sterilizer. Check internal process indicator before treatment. Refer to state regulations for any additional state requirements.

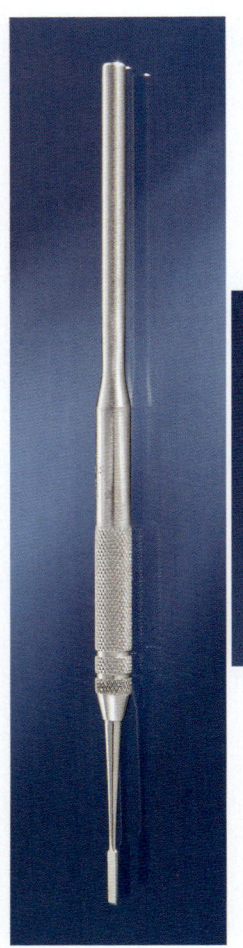

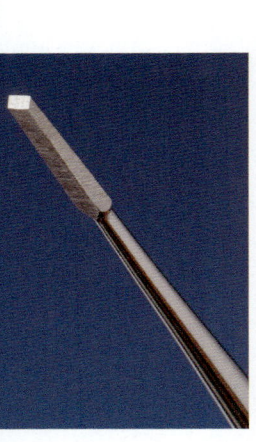

Straight Chisel

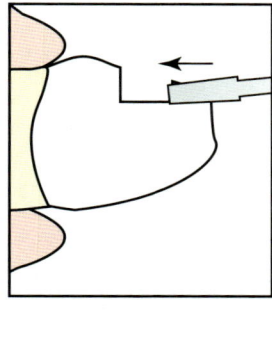

Function ▸ To plane and cleave enamel in cavity preparation

Characteristics ▸ Used with push motion
Single-bevel cutting edge
Single or double ended

Examples of instrument numbers:

15
20

Practice Notes ▸ Straight Chisel is used on restorative tray setups.

Sterilization Notes ▸ Straight Chisel must be precleaned. Then, place in a sterilizing pouch with an internal process indicator, seal, then sterilize. OR, wrap with an internal process indicator inside and secure on the outside with process indicator tape, then sterilize. Verify appropriate color change has been achieved in external process indicator immediately after removal from sterilizer. Check internal process indicator before treatment. Refer to state regulations for any additional state requirements.

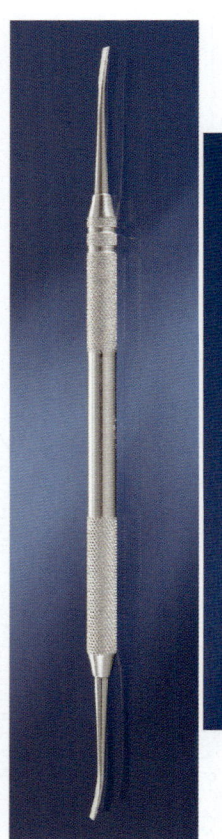

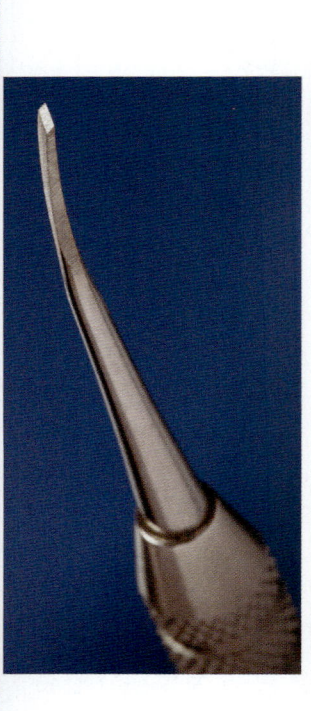

Wedelstaedt Chisel

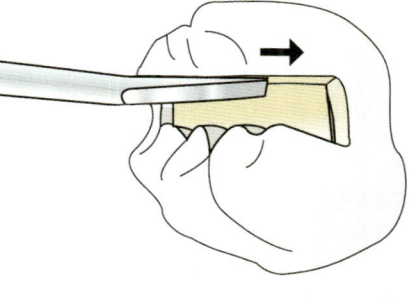

Function ▸ To plane and cleave enamel in cavity preparation

Characteristics ▸ Used with push motion
Curved blade on working end
Single-bevel cutting edge
Single or double ended
Is a three-numbered instrument

Examples of instrument numbers:

15-15-3
11.5-15-3

Practice Notes ▸ Wedelstaedt Chisel is used on restorative tray setups.

Sterilization Notes ▸ Wedelstaedt Chisel must be precleaned. Then, place in a sterilizing pouch with an internal process indicator, seal, then sterilize. OR, wrap with an internal process indicator inside and secure on the outside with process indicator tape, then sterilize. Verify appropriate color change has been achieved in external process indicator immediately after removal from sterilizer. Check internal process indicator before treatment. Refer to state regulations for any additional state requirements.

27

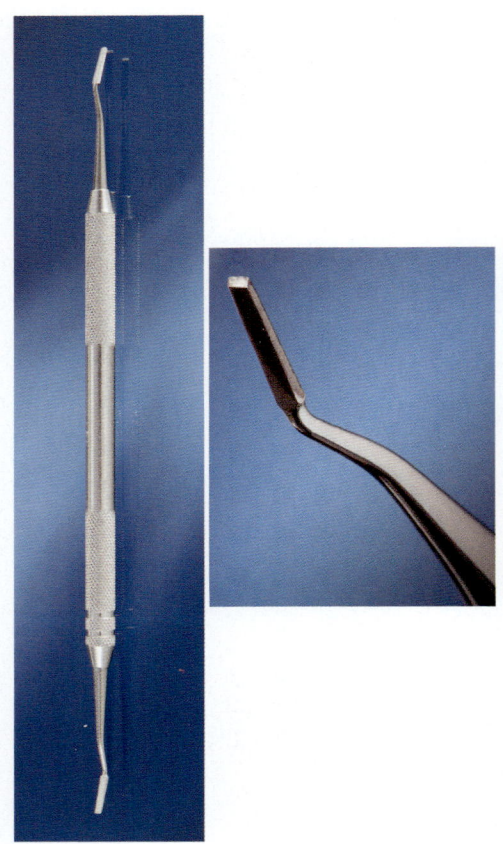

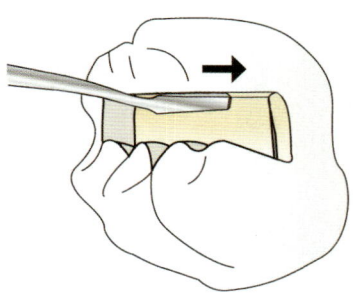

■ INSTRUMENT

Binangle Chisel

Function ▶ To plane and cleave enamel in cavity preparation

Characteristics ▶ Used with push motion

Two angles in the shank

Single or double ended

Is an example of three-numbered instrument

Examples of instrument numbers:

20-9-8

15-8-8

Practice Notes ▶ Binangle Chisel is used on restorative tray setups.

Sterilization Notes ▶ Binangle Chisel must be precleaned. Then, place in a sterilizing pouch with an internal process indicator, seal, then sterilize. OR, wrap with an internal process indicator inside and secure on the outside with process indicator tape, then sterilize. Verify appropriate color change has been achieved in external process indicator immediately after removal from sterilizer. Check internal process indicator before treatment. Refer to state regulations for any additional state requirements.

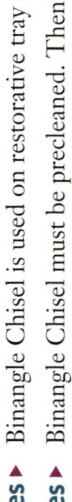

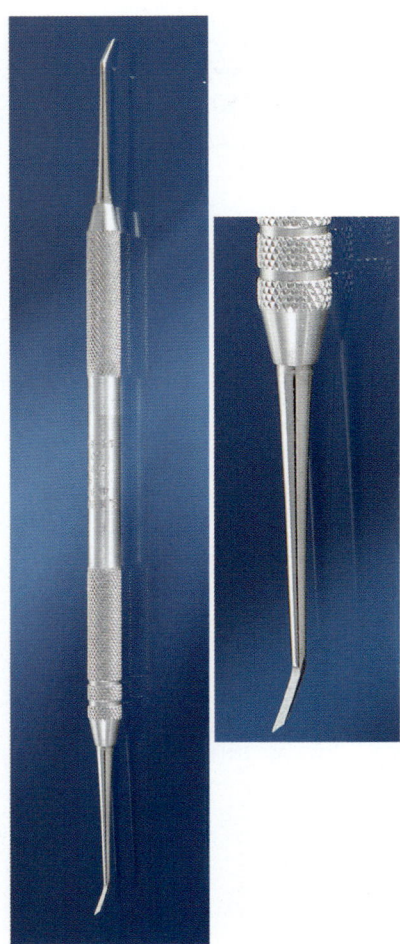

■ INSTRUMENT

Angle Former

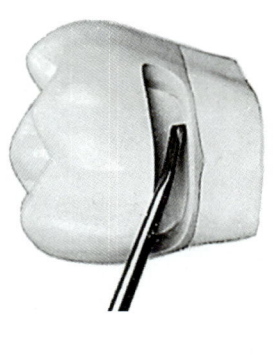

Function ▶ To accentuate line and point angles in internal outline and retention in cavity preparation

Characteristics ▶ Cutting edge at an angle
Single or double ended
Is a four-numbered instrument

Examples of instrument numbers:

12-80-5-8
9-80-4-8

Practice Notes ▶ Angle Former is used on restorative tray setups.

Sterilization Notes ▶ Angle Former must be precleaned. Then, place in a sterilizing pouch with an internal process indicator; seal, then sterilize. OR, wrap with an internal process indicator inside and secure on the outside with process indicator tape, then sterilize. Verify appropriate color change has been achieved in external process indicator immediately after removal from sterilizer. Check internal process indicator before treatment. Refer to state regulations for any additional state requirements.

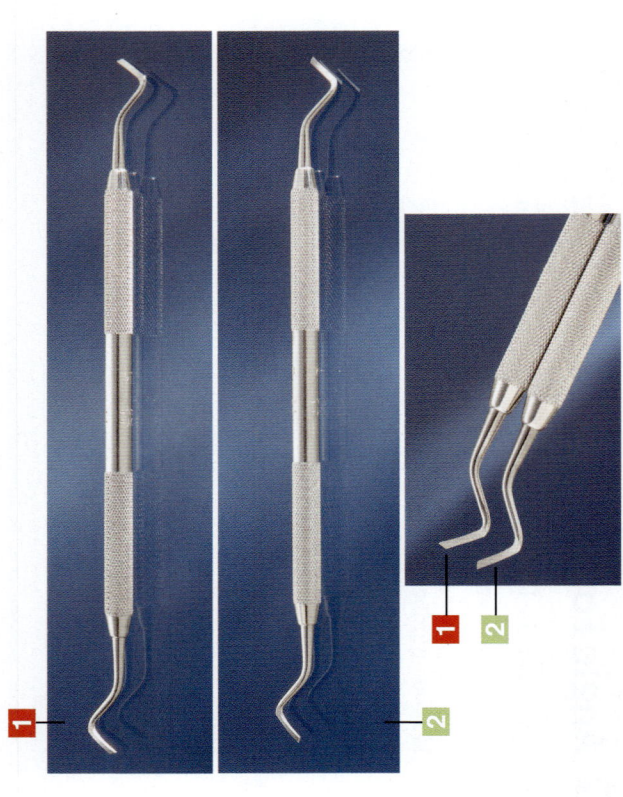

Gingival Margin Trimmer—Mesial and Distal

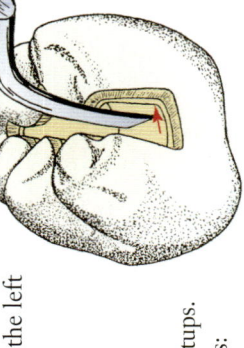

Function ▶ To bevel cervical walls of mesial and distal retention areas

Characteristics ▶
1 Mesial: To create bevels on the mesial cervical margin of the preparation
2 Distal: To create bevels on the distal cervical margin of the preparation

Curved blade—Cutting edge at angle to blade
Double ended—One end curves to the right; the other to the left
Is a four-numbered instrument

Examples of instrument numbers:

Mesial: 13–80–8–14 or 15–80–8–12
Distal: 13–95–8–14 or 15–95–8–12

Practice Notes ▶ Gingival Margin Trimmer is used on restorative tray setups.
Gingival Margin Trimmer is placed on tray setups in pairs: mesial and distal.
Refer to the amalgam tray setup in Chapter 8.

Sterilization Notes ▶ Gingival Margin Trimmer must be precleaned. Then, place in a sterilizing pouch with an internal process indicator, seal, then sterilize. OR, wrap with an internal process indicator inside and secure on the outside with process indicator tape, then sterilize. Verify appropriate color change has been achieved in external process indicator immediately after removal from sterilizer. Check internal process indicator before treatment. Refer to state regulations for any additional state requirements.

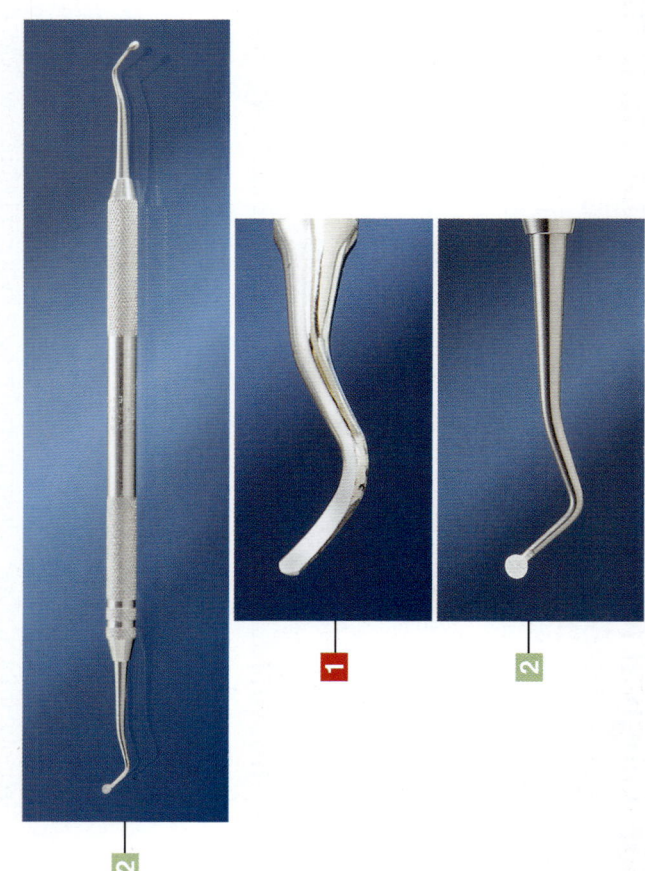

Spoon Excavators

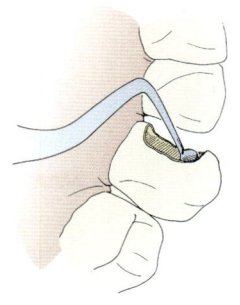

Function ▶

To remove carious dentin

Secondary functions:

To remove temporary crowns

To remove temporary cement in temporary restoration

To remove permanent crown during try-in

Characteristics ▶

Concave design, spoon-shaped with cutting edge

Range of sizes:

1. Large—Curved blade—also referred to as Black Spoon
2. Small—Round blade

Single or double ended

Practice Notes ▶

Spoon Excavator is used on restorative tray setups.

Refer to the amalgam tray setup (see Chapter 8), composite tray setups (see Chapter 9), and crown and bridge restorative tray setups (see Chapter 10).

Sterilization Notes ▶

Spoon Excavator must be precleaned. Then, place in a sterilizing pouch with an internal process indicator, seal, then sterilize. OR, wrap with an internal process indicator inside and secure on the outside with process indicator tape, then sterilize. Verify appropriate color change has been achieved in external process indicator immediately after removal from sterilizer. Check internal process indicator before treatment. Refer to state regulations for any additional state requirements.

3

Local Anesthetic Syringe/ Components and Nitrous Oxide Sedation

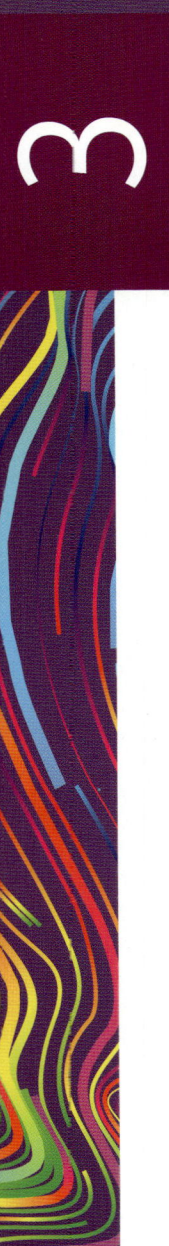

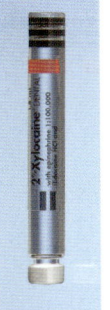

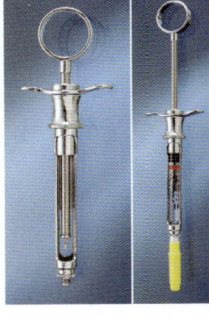

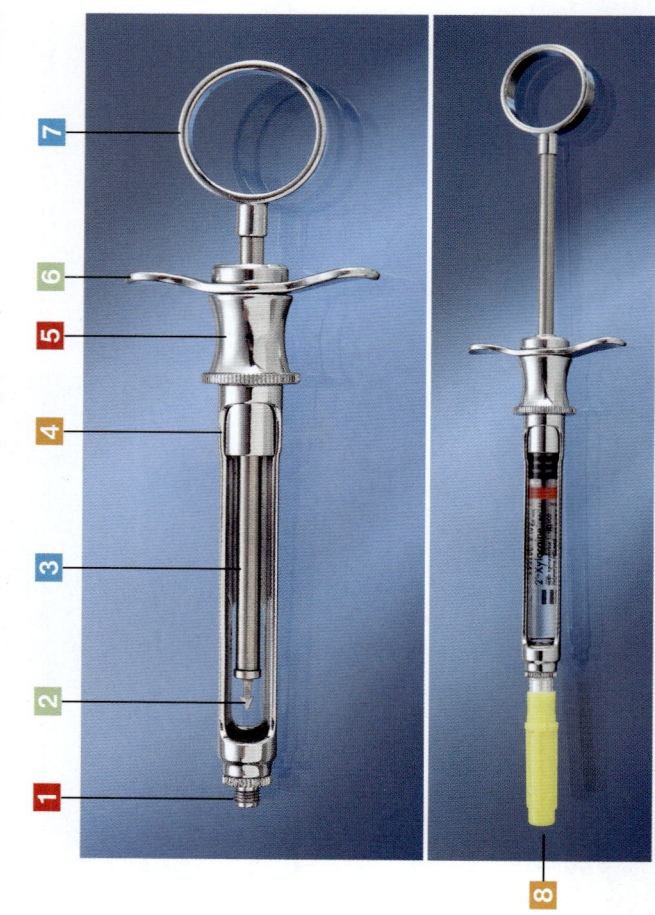

■ INSTRUMENT Anesthetic Aspirating Syringe

Function ▸ To administer a local anesthetic

Characteristics ▸ Parts:

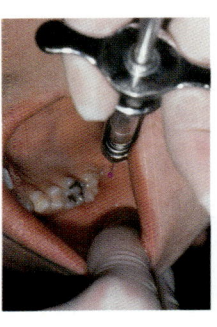

1 Threaded tip		**2** Harpoon	
3 Piston rod		**4** Barrel of syringe	
5 Finger grip		**6** Finger bar	
7 Thumb ring		**8** Syringe assembled with needle and anesthetic cartridge	

Practice Notes ▸ Syringes with harpoons are considered aspirating syringes. Disposable syringes equipped with needles and preloaded with anesthetic are available. Anesthetic Aspirating Syringe is used on most tray setups.

Sterilization Notes ▸ Anesthetic Aspirating Syringe must be precleaned. Then, place in a sterilizing pouch with an internal process indicator, seal, then sterilize. OR, wrap with an internal process indicator inside and secure on the outside with process indicator tape, then sterilize. Verify appropriate color change has been achieved in external process indicator immediately after removal from sterilizer. Check internal process indicator before treatment. Refer to state regulations for any additional state requirements. Disposable preloaded syringes with needle must be disposed of in a sharps container. Anesthetic cartridge and needle must be disposed of in a sharps container. Refer to local and state recommendations for disposal of anesthetic cartridge.

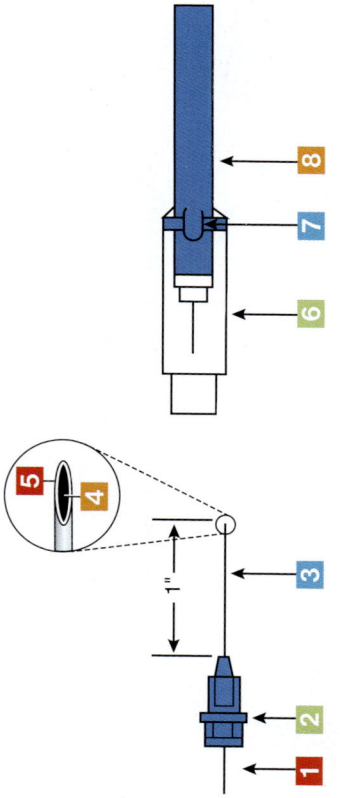

■ INSTRUMENT

Short Needle

Function ▶ To administer anesthetic by infiltration injection on maxillary arch

Characteristics ▶ Parts:

1 Cartridge end of needle	**2** Needle hub
3 Injection end of needle	**4** Lumen of the needle
5 Bevel of the needle	**6** Protective cap
7 Seal on cap	**8** Needle guard

1 inch long for infiltration injection

1 End of needle inserts into the anesthetic cartridge

4 Anesthetic solution is ejected through the lumen of the needle

Variety of gauges:

- Gauge number—Identifies diameter (thickness) of needle
- Larger gauge number—Indicates thinner needle (e.g., 30 gauge is thinner than 25 gauge)

Practice Notes ▶ Local anesthetic syringe setup is used on most tray setups

Sterilization Notes ▶ Short Needle must be disposed of in a sharps container. Single use only.

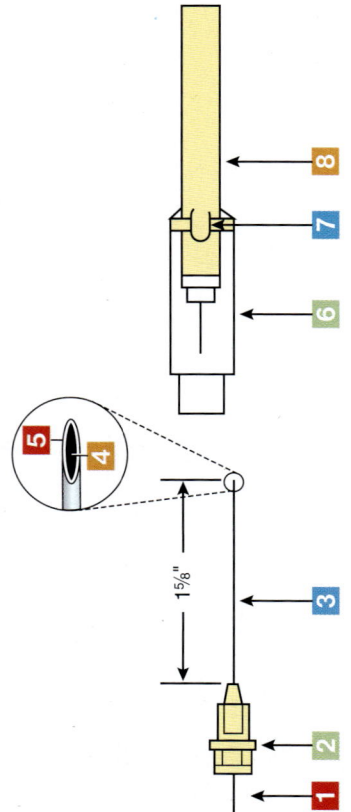

1⅝"

■ INSTRUMENT

Long Needle

Function ▶ To administer anesthetic by block injection on mandibular arch

Characteristics ▶ Parts:

1 Cartridge end of needle   **2** Needle hub
3 Injection end of needle   **4** Lumen of the needle
5 Bevel of the needle   **6** Protective cap
7 Seal on cap   **8** Needle guard

$1\frac{5}{8}$ inches long for block injection

1 End of needle inserts into the anesthetic cartridge
4 Anesthetic solution is ejected through the lumen of the needle

Variety of gauges:

- Gauge number—Identifies diameter (thickness) of needle
- Larger gauge number—Indicates thinner needle (e.g., 30 gauge is thinner than 25 gauge)

Practice Notes ▶ Local anesthetic syringe setup is used on most tray setups.

Sterilization Notes ▶ Long Needle must be disposed of in a sharps container. Single use only.

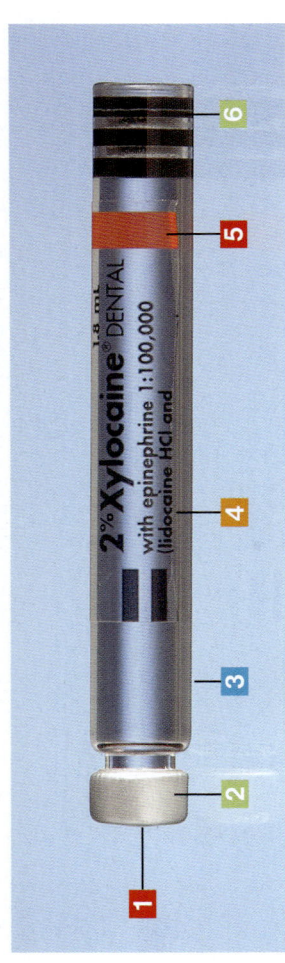

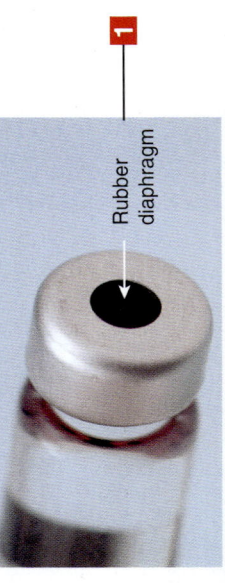

Rubber diaphragm

Anesthetic Cartridge

Function ▸ To hold liquid anesthetic for local injection in the oral cavity

Characteristics ▸ Parts:

1 Rubber diaphragm—Syringe needle is inserted into the diaphragm to penetrate into the cartridge.

2 Aluminum cap holds the rubber diaphragm in place.

3 Glass cartridge (also referred to as a carpule)

4 Indicates type of anesthesia

5 Color-coded band indicating type of anesthetic (required by the American Dental Association, June 2003)

6 Silicon rubber plunger—Harpoon of syringe inserts into silicon rubber plunger.

Composition of solution in cartridge—Contains 1.7 to 1.8 mL of anesthetic solution

Plunger slightly indented from rim of glass

Practice Notes ▸ Type of anesthetic used depends on patient's health history and dental procedure performed. Local anesthetic syringe setup is used on most tray setups.

Sterilization Notes ▸ Anesthetic Cartridge must be disposed of in a sharps container. Refer to local and state recommendations for disposal of cartridge. Single use only.

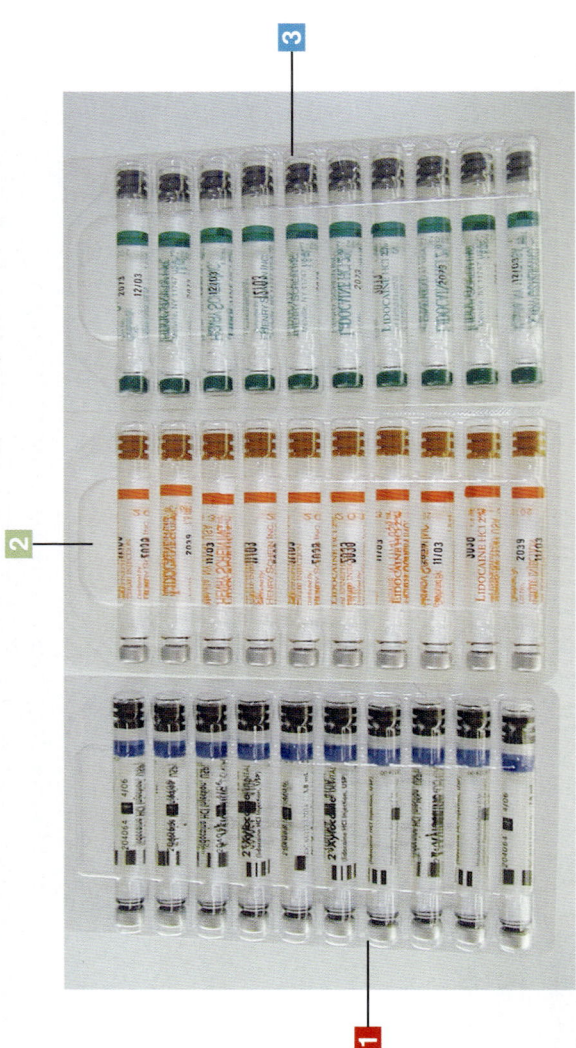

Anesthetic Cartridges/Blister Packs

Function ▲ To hold liquid anesthetic for injection

Characteristics ▲ Several types of anesthetic solutions available

Each cartridge is labeled.

Color code system on cartridge—Identifies type of anesthetic (required by the American Dental Association, June 2003). Color band on each cartridge indicates type of anesthetic solution. Type of anesthetic used depends on patient's health history and dental procedure performed:

1 Anesthetic is available without a vasoconstrictor.

2 Ratio of epinephrine: the lower the second number, the higher the percentage of vasoconstrictor. Information printed on cartridge. Example of common anesthetic for routine dental procedures 1:100,000.

3 Longer lasting anesthetic has a higher percentage of vasoconstrictor. Example: 1:50,000.

Practice Notes ▲ Remove each cartridge from blister pack as needed for each procedure and place cartridge on tray setup.

Local anesthetic syringe setup is used on most tray setups.

Sterilization Notes ▲ Anesthetic Cartridge must be disposed of in a sharps container. Refer to local and state recommendations for disposal of cartridge. Each anesthetic cartridge for single use only.

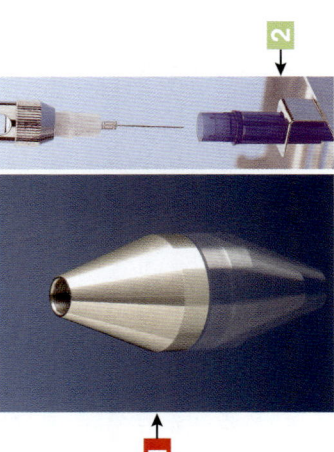

■ INSTRUMENT

Recapping Device

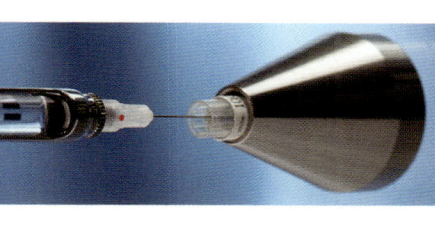

Function ▸ To hold needle sheath for one-hand recapping after injection

Characteristics ▸
1 Jenker—Low center of gravity for stability in recapping
2 Needle Cap Holder attached to cassette

Helps prevent needle stick accidents
Different styles of needle stick protectors available

Practice Notes ▸ Needle Stick Protector is used on most tray setups.
Scoop Technique Procedure—Recap needle by scooping end of needle into needle guard (not shown).

Sterilization Notes ▸ Needle Stick Protector—Jenker or Needle Cap Holder must be precleaned. Then, place in a sterilizing pouch with an internal process indicator, seal, then sterilize. OR, wrap with an internal process indicator inside and secure on the outside with process indicator tape, then sterilize. Verify appropriate color change has been achieved in external process indicator immediately after removal from sterilizer.
Check internal process indicator before treatment. Refer to state regulations for any additional state requirements. Disposable preloaded syringes with needle must be disposed of in a sharps container. Anesthetic cartridge and needle must be disposed of in a sharps container. Refer to local and state recommendations for disposal of anesthetic cartridge.

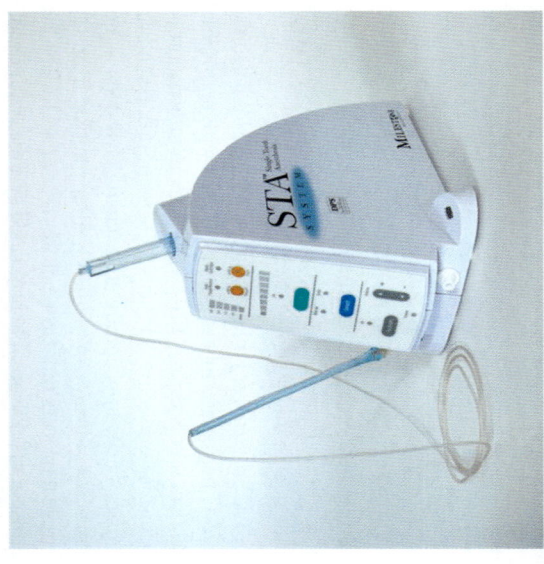

Computer-Controlled Local Anesthetic Delivery System (The Wand/STA Single Tooth Anesthesia System)

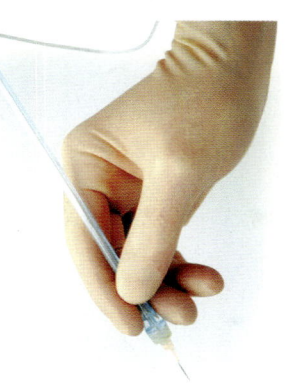
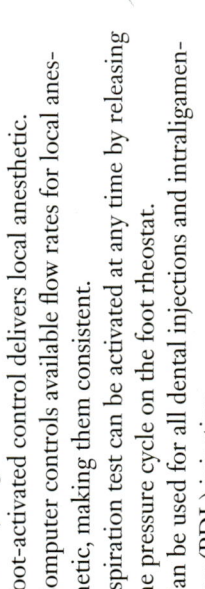
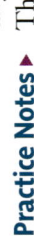

Functions ▸ To administer a local anesthetic

To improve ergonomics and precision of dental anesthetic delivery

Characteristics ▸ Lightweight wand handpiece held in a penlike grip.

Presterilized bonded handpiece—Not a traditional dental syringe

Foot-activated control delivers local anesthetic.

Computer controls available flow rates for local anesthetic, making them consistent.

Aspiration test can be activated at any time by releasing the pressure cycle on the foot rheostat.

Can be used for all dental injections and intraligamentary (PDL) injection

Practice Notes ▸ The operator focuses on needle insertion and positioning while the motor in the device administers the drug at a preprogrammed rate of flow.

Increased tactile control and ergonomics decreases patient discomfort.

Sterilization Notes ▸ Anesthetic cartridge must be disposed of in a biohazard container. Refer to local and state recommendations for disposal of cartridge. Single use only. Needle must be disposed of in a sharps container. Single use only. Tubing must be disposed of in garbage. One time use only. Refer to manufacturer's recommendation for disinfection of unit.

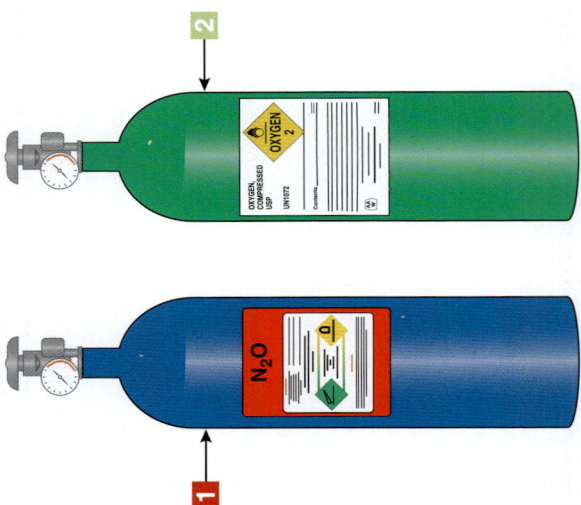

Nitrous Oxide and Analgesic Tanks

Function ▶ To use as an analgesic to relax patients for dental procedures
To be inhaled through a mask placed over the nose

Characteristic ▶
1 Blue tank is N_2O
2 Green tank is O_2

Nitrous oxide is a chemical compound with the formula N_2O. It is an oxide of nitrogen. Room temperature, N_2O is a colorless, nonflammable gas, with a slightly sweet odor and taste. Nose piece has tubing attached to a scavenger system that evacuates excess N_2O that patient does not breath.

Practice Notes ▶ Nitrous oxide is used for apprehensive patients for all types of dental procedures.
Oxygen must be given to patient before dismissing from the dental chair.
Fail-safe system:

All N_2O and O_2 systems used in dentistry have a fail-safe system.
Sufficient amount of O_2 gas must be present in the tank while system is functioning or the system will shut down.

Sterilization Notes ▶ Nitrous Oxide Tanks and Oxygen Tanks—Refer to manufacturer's recommendation for disinfection.

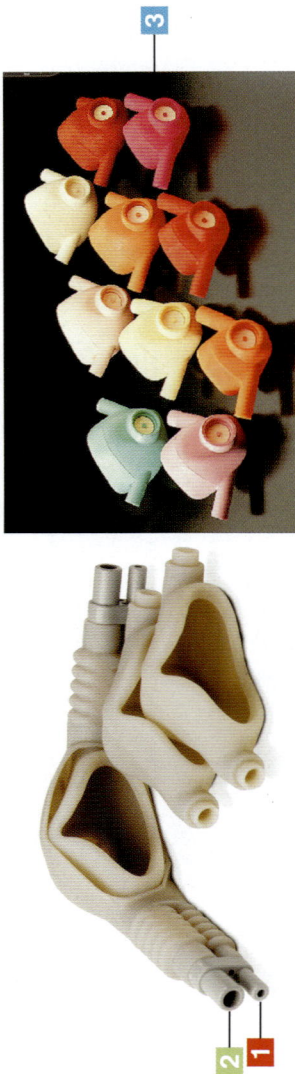

Nitrous Oxide Nasal Mask

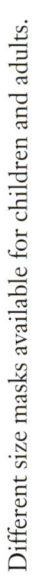

Functions ▶

To place mask over the patient's nose for the delivery of N_2O

To evacuate excess N_2O that is not breathed in by the patient

Characteristics ▶

1 Tubing for N_2O

2 Tubing for scavenger system to evacuate excess N_2O

3 Disposable masks available in different scents

Refer to Protocol for administering N_2O and O_2

Different size masks available for children and adults.

Practice Notes ▶

Gauze is placed under mask for patient comfort. N_2O is used for apprehensive patients for all types of dental procedures.

Oxygen must be given to the patient before dismissing the patient from the dental chair.

Sterilization Notes ▶

N_2O Masks refer to manufacturer's recommendation for sterilization. Disposable masks single use only. Dispose of in the garbage.

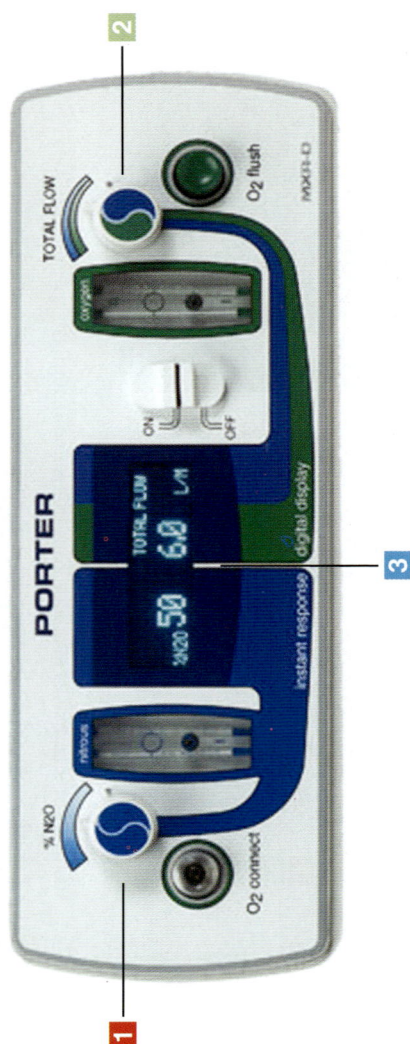

■ INSTRUMENT Nitrous Oxide and Oxygen Flowmeters

Function ▶ To monitor the N_2O and O_2 that is administered to the patient

Characteristics ▶

1 % N_2O adjustment knob: Controls the % of N_2O

2 Total flow adjustment knob: Controls the combined flow of O_2 and N_2O or O_2 flow only when the % of N_2O knob is set to zero

3 Digital display readout of N_2O and O_2 using knobs for adjustment of gas flow

Tubing from the tanks go to flowmeters and tubing from flowmeters go to the face mask that delivers the gases to the patient.

All masks have tubing attached to a scavenger system: An appropriate evacuation/HVE system that evacuates the excess gas that the patient does not inhale.

Practice Notes ▶ N_2O is used for apprehensive patients for all types of dental procedures. Oxygen must be given to the patient before dismissing from the dental chair. Refer to Protocol for administering N_2O and O_2.

Sterilization Notes ▶ Flowmeters refer to manufacturer's recommendation for disinfection.

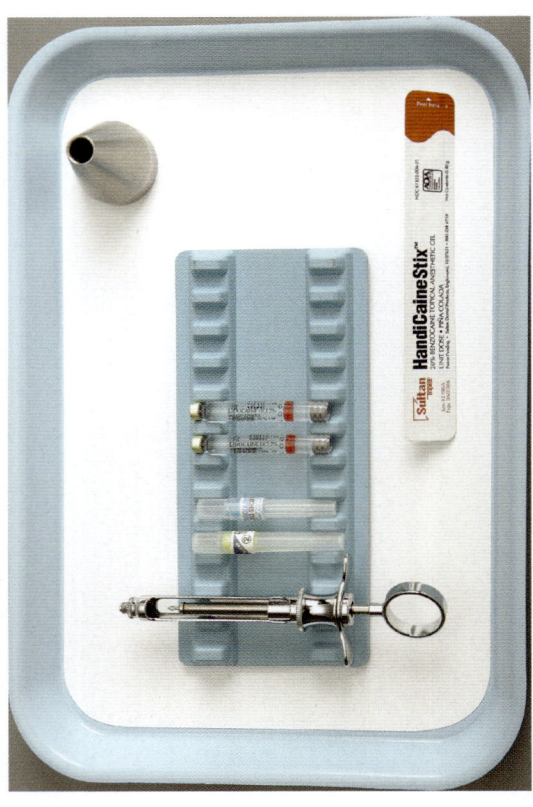

Local Anesthetic Syringe

From Left to Right ▶ Anesthetic aspirating syringe, long needle, short needle, anesthetic cartridges, needle stick protector (Jenker) (top right), individually packed topical anesthetic (bottom right)

Practice Notes ▶ Local Anesthetic Syringe setup is found on most tray setups.

Sterilization Notes ▶ Anesthetic Syringe and Needle Stick Protector Jenker must be precleaned. Then, place in a sterilizing pouch with an internal process indicator, seal, then sterilize. OR, wrap with an internal process indicator inside and secure on the outside with process indicator tape, then sterilize. Verify appropriate color change has been achieved in external process indicator immediately after removal from sterilizer. Check internal process indicator before treatment. Refer to state regulations for any additional state requirements. Anesthetic cartridge and needle must be disposed of in a sharps container. Refer to local and state recommendations for disposal of anesthetic cartridge. Dispose of topical in garbage. Single use only.

4

Evacuation Devices, Air/Water Syringe Tip, and Dental Unit

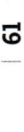

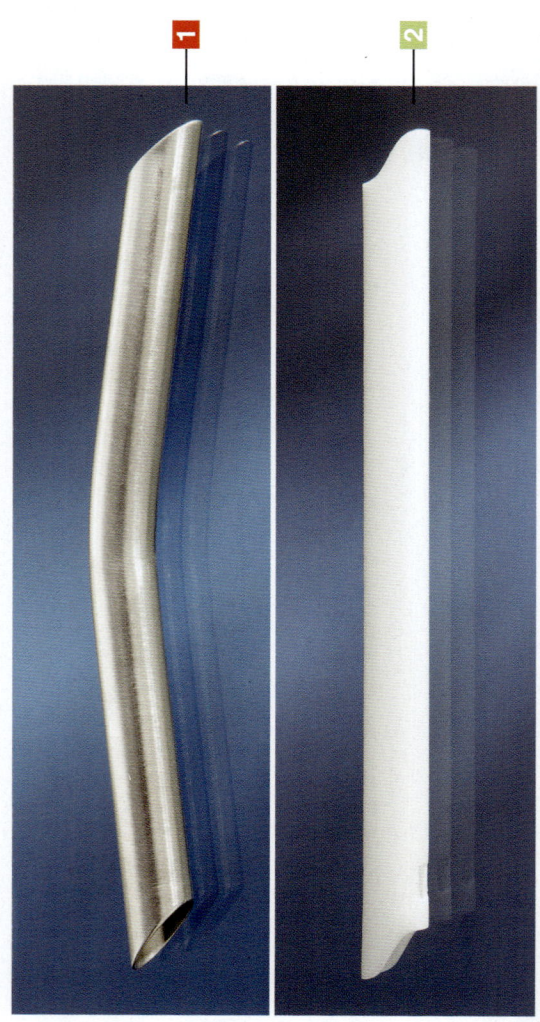

▪ INSTRUMENT

High-Volume (Velocity) Evacuator (HVE) Tip

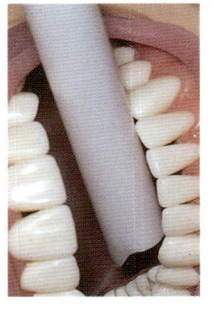

Function ▸ To evacuate large volumes of fluid and debris from the oral cavity

Characteristics ▸
1. Stainless steel evacuator tip
2. Plastic evacuator tip—Disposable plastic

Straight or slightly angled at one or both ends
Also available in plastic that may be sterilized

Practice Notes ▸ Evacuator Tip attaches to high-velocity tubing on dental unit.
HVE Tip is used on most tray setups.

Sterilization Notes ▸ HVE Tip must be precleaned. Then, place in a sterilizing pouch with an internal process indicator, seal, then sterilize. OR, wrap with an internal process indicator inside and secure on the outside with process indicator tape, then sterilize. Verify appropriate color change has been achieved in external process indicator immediately after removal from sterilizer. Check internal process indicator before treatment. Refer to state regulations for any additional state requirements. Disposable plastic HVE tip should be disposed of in the garbage.

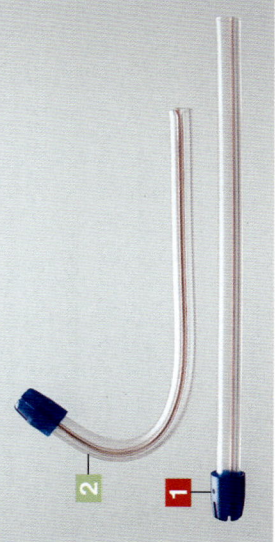

INSTRUMENT

Low-Volume (Velocity) Saliva Ejector Tip

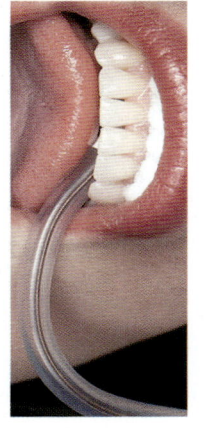

Function ▶ To evacuate smaller volumes of fluid from the oral cavity

Characteristics ▶
1. Disposable plastic for single use only
2. Can be bent for placement under tongue and in other areas of mouth or can be used straight

Variety of styles

SAFE-FLO® Saliva Ejector one-way valve attachment, also available, provides a barrier that prevents saliva backflow

Practice Notes ▶ Attaches to low-velocity tubing on dental unit Saliva Ejector Tip is used on most tray setups.

Sterilization Notes ▶ Disposable Saliva Ejector Tip and SAFE-FLO® valve, not shown, should be disposed of in the garbage. Single use only. Refer to the Centers for Disease Control and Prevention (CDC) guidelines regarding possible backflow from low-volume saliva ejectors.

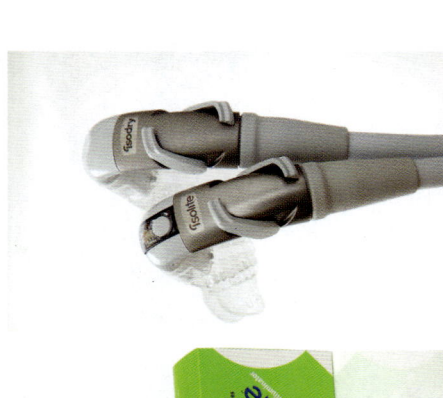

Isolite®—Illuminated Dental Isolation System

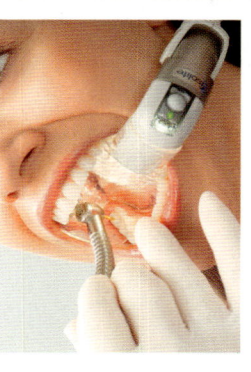

Functions ▶

To retract tongue and evacuate fluid from patient's mouth
To provide light to the working area of the mouth
To gently hold patient's mouth open during use
To serve as a barrier to the airway, protecting the patient from inadvertent aspiration of dental material

Characteristics ▶

Isolite is attached to high-velocity evacuation port of the vacuum system.
No special devices are required to operate system installed on the dental unit.

Practice Notes ▶

Isolates two quadrants at once on the same side
Used for maxillary and mandibular procedures
Light settings for light-sensitive curing material

Sterilization Notes ▶

Please follow manufacturer's instructions for cleaning and sterilization. Applicable components must be precleaned. Then, place in a sterilizing pouch with an internal process indicator, seal, then sterilize. OR, wrap with an internal process indicator inside and secure on the outside with process indicator tape, then sterilize. Verify appropriate color change has been achieved in external process indicator immediately after removal from sterilizer. Check internal process indicator before treatment. Refer to state regulations for any additional state requirements. Disposable plastic should be disposed of in the garbage. Single use only. Refer to manufacturer's recommendation and the CDC guidelines.

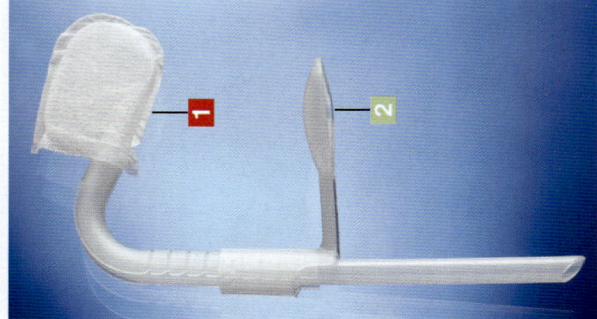

Low-Volume (Velocity) Mandibular Evacuator

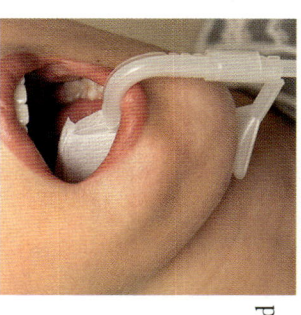

Functions ▶ To evacuate smaller volumes of fluid from the oral cavity

To use on mandibular arch

To retract tongue during evacuation

Characteristics ▶
1 Blade for retraction of tongue is covered for patient comfort

2 Adjustable device to place under patient's chin to hold evacuator in place

Disposable plastic for single use only (may be referred to as a Linqua-fix)

Also available in metal, referred to as a Svedopter, must be sterilized

Practice Notes ▶ Attaches to low-velocity tubing on dental unit

Disposable Low-Volume Mandibular Evacuator is used on sealant tray setups and on procedures for mandibular arch when operator is working without an assistant.

Sterilization Notes ▶ Disposable Low-Volume Mandibular Evacuator (pictured) should be disposed of in the garbage. Single use only. Svedopter (metal evacuator—not shown) must be precleaned. Then, place in a sterilizing pouch with an internal process indicator, seal, then sterilize. OR, wrap with an internal process indicator inside and secure on the outside with process indicator tape, then sterilize. Verify appropriate color change has been achieved in external process indicator immediately after removal from sterilizer. Check internal process indicator before treatment. Refer to state regulations for any additional state requirements.

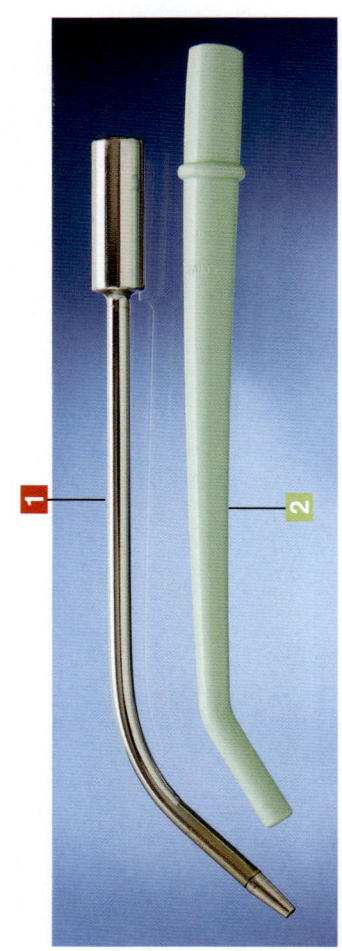

High-Volume (Velocity) Surgical Evacuation Tip

■ INSTRUMENT

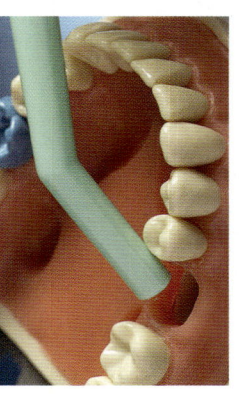

Function ▶ To evacuate fluid from oral cavity and surgical site

Characteristics ▶ Stainless steel, autoclavable plastic, disposable plastic:

1 Stainless steel evacuation tip

2 Plastic disposable tip

Narrowed tip accommodates surgical site.

Practice Notes ▶ Surgical Evacuation Tip attaches to high-velocity tubing on dental unit.

May require connecting tube for adaptation to Surgical Evacuation Tip

Some stainless steel surgical tips narrow at insertion of tubing; additional tubing is necessary to connect to high-velocity tubing on dental unit.

Surgical Evacuation Tip is used on most surgical tray setups.

Sterilization Notes ▶ Surgical (Metal) Evacuation Tips must be precleaned. Then, place in a sterilizing pouch with an internal process indicator, seal, then sterilize. OR, wrap with an internal process indicator inside and secure on the outside with process indicator tape, then sterilize. Verify appropriate color change has been achieved in external process indicator immediately after removal from sterilizer. Check internal process indicator before treatment. Refer to state regulations for any additional state requirements. Disposable Surgical Evacuation Tip should be disposed of in the garbage. Single use only.

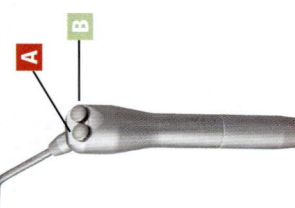

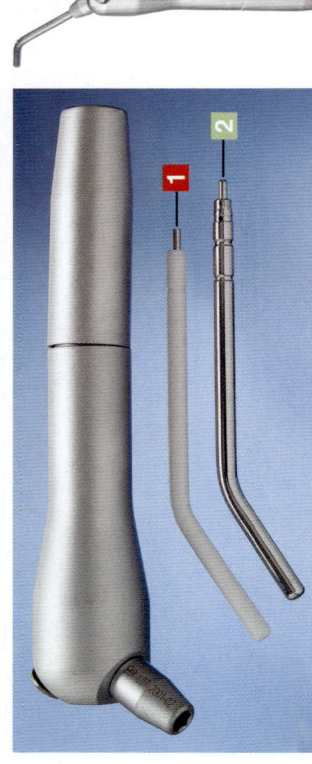

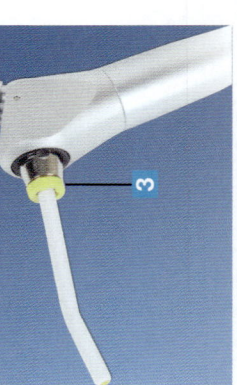

Air/Water Syringe with Removable Tip

Function ▶ To rinse and dry specific teeth or entire oral cavity

Characteristics ▶ Air/Water Syringe is also referred to as a three-way syringe. Characteristics of buttons on Air/Water Syringe: **A** Left button expels water only; **B** Right button expels air only; pressing both buttons at the same time will result in a spray by combining air and water.

Types of tips:

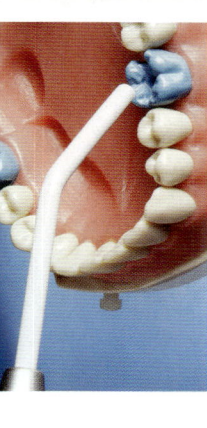

1 Disposable plastic syringe tip for single use

2 Metal syringe tip

3 Seal-Tight tip seals water passage from getting into the air passage of the tip

Practice Notes ▶ Syringe Tip—Attaches to Air/Water Syringe
Air/Water Syringe—Attaches to tubing on dental unit

Sterilization Notes ▶ Metal Air/Water Syringe Tip must be precleaned. Then, place in a sterilizing pouch with an internal process indicator, seal, then sterilize. OR, wrap with an internal process indicator inside and secure on the outside with process indicator tape, then sterilize. Verify appropriate color change has been achieved in external process indicator immediately after removal from sterilizer. Check internal process indicator before treatment. Refer to state regulations for any additional state requirements. Single use only. Air/Water Syringe that tip is attached to must be disinfected according to manufacturer's recommendation.

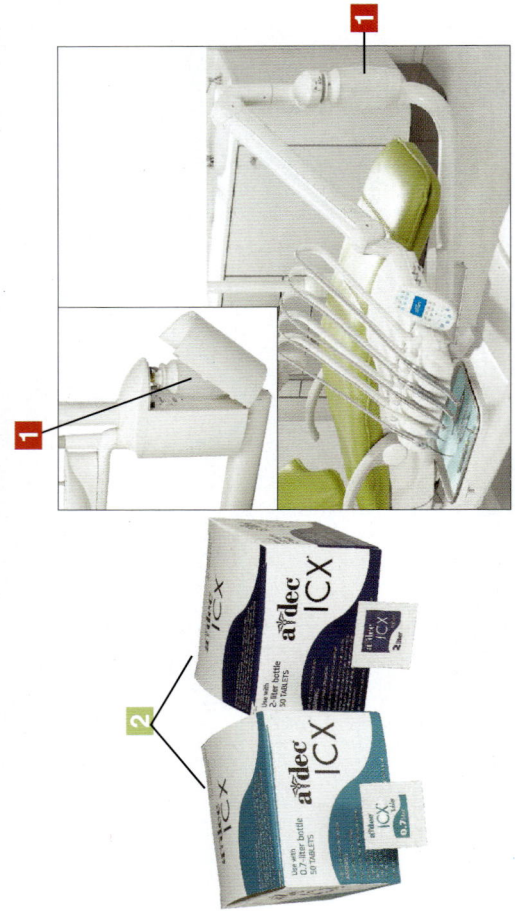

Self-Contained Water Unit and Waterline Treatment Tablets

Functions ▶ To assist in the quality of water entering the dental unit that supplies water to handpieces, air/water syringe, and cuspidor cupfill

To assist when there is a possibility of contamination to the water supply to the dental unit

Characteristics ▶ Water system may be mounted in different areas of the dental unit.

Different size bottles are available.

Example: 7 L or 2 L

1 Self-contained water bottle attached to dental unit

2 Tablets—Place tablets in each water bottle every time bottle is filled.

Sterisil Straw available instead of tablets.

Reduces accumulation of contaminants

Reduces accumulation of odor and foul-tasting bacteria

Practice Notes ▶ Follow manufacturer's recommendations for periodic shock treatment of water lines using special tablets; safety precautions while using tablets and filling bottles.

Sterilization Notes ▶ CDC recommends monitoring dental unit water regularly. Example: weekly testing of water either in office or commercial monitoring system (Guidelines for Infection Control in Dental Health Care Setting, 2003).

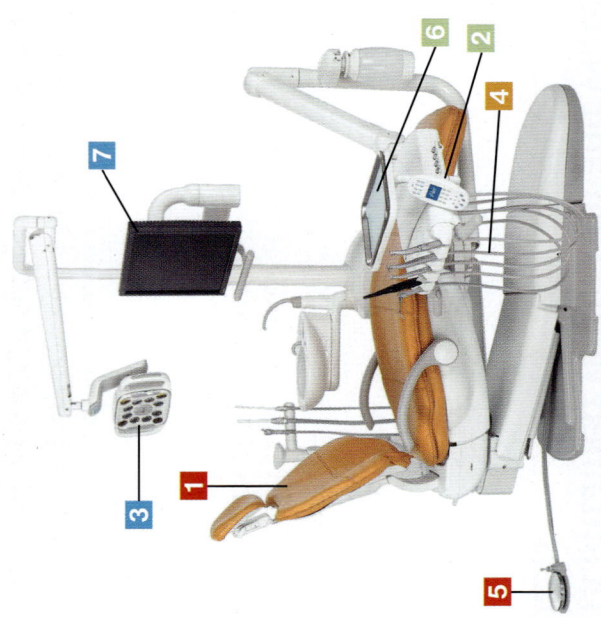

Dental Delivery System

Function ▶ To deliver dental care to patients

Characteristics ▶

1 Ergonomically structured chair for patient, operator, and assistant

2 Chair adjustment device for height and reclining patient

3 Light with adjustable intensity—LED light with curing option for composite restorations

4 Tubing for high and slow speed handpieces, air/water syringe, low- and high-velocity vacuum systems

5 Rheostat for running handpieces with water toggle switch option

6 Tray for placing instrument setups

7 Computer screen available for patient information and digital images

Practice Notes ▶

Many different designs of dental delivery systems available

Air/water syringes available on one or both sides of operator or assistant's side

Evacuation tubing on assistant's side of patient chair

Tubing for handpieces available on operator or assistant's side of patient chair

Sterilization Notes ▶ Refer to manufacturing and CDC guidelines on purging dental lines, tubing, disinfecting chair, tubing, and dental unit.

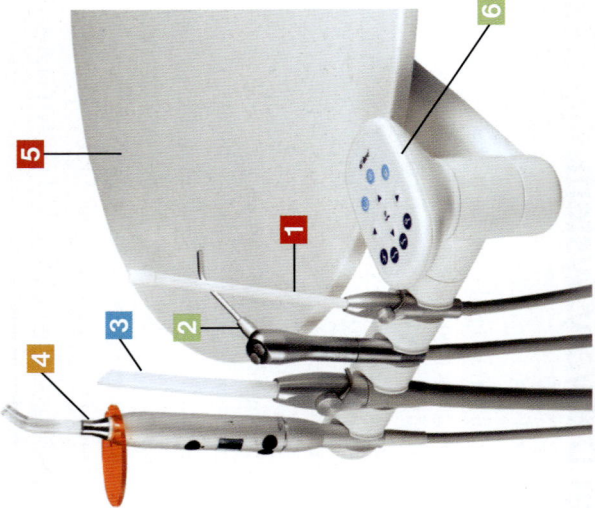

Dental Assistant Delivery System

Function ▶ To deliver dental care to patients as a chairside assistant

Characteristics ▶
1. Saliva ejector attached to the low-volume evacuation system tubing
2. Air/water syringe and tip attached to the tubing
3. High-volume evacuator tip attached to the tubing
4. Light curing device attached to the unit with protective shield
5. Bracket table for instrument setups
6. Chair adjustment device for height and reclining dental chair

Practice Notes ▶ Many different designs of dental delivery systems are available. Dental assistant delivery system is used to deliver dental care to patients.

Sterilization Notes ▶ Refer to manufacturing and CDC guidelines on purging dental lines, tubing, and disinfecting delivery system.

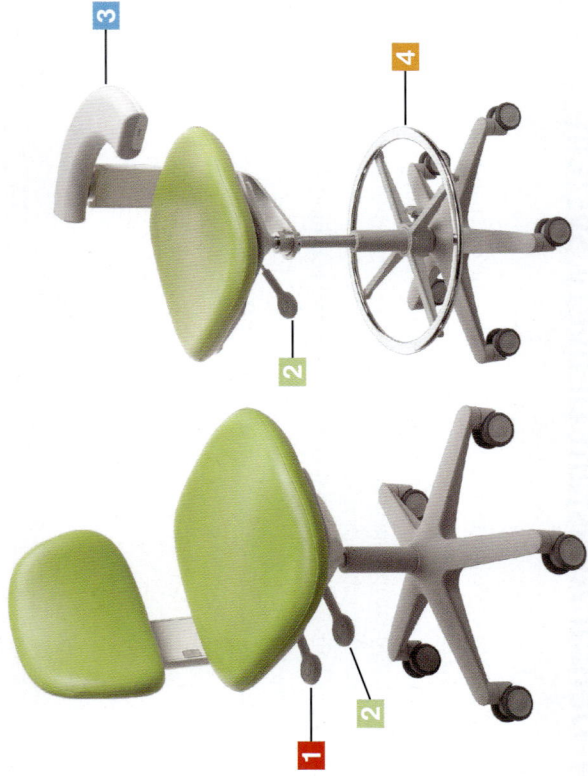

Dental Stools

Function ▶ To use providing treatment to a patient

Characteristics ▶
1. Operator chair—Adjustable back support is movable forward and backward
2. Operator and Assistant chair—Adjustable seat height
3. Adjustable torso support
4. Assistant chair—Adjustable foot ring under seat for feet support

Practice Notes ▶ Operator chair—Feet recommended to be placed flat on floor for ergonomically correct position

Assistant chair—Feet recommended to be placed on ring, bar underneath rib cage; while seated in the chair the assistant should be 4 to 6 inches above operator for ergonomically correct position.

Sterilization Notes ▶ Chairs must be disinfected (including the height adjustment lever) after each patient; refer to manufacturer's recommendation for disinfection of chairs.

Dental Handpieces

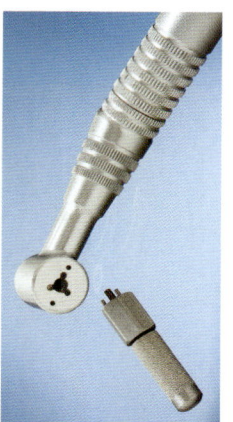
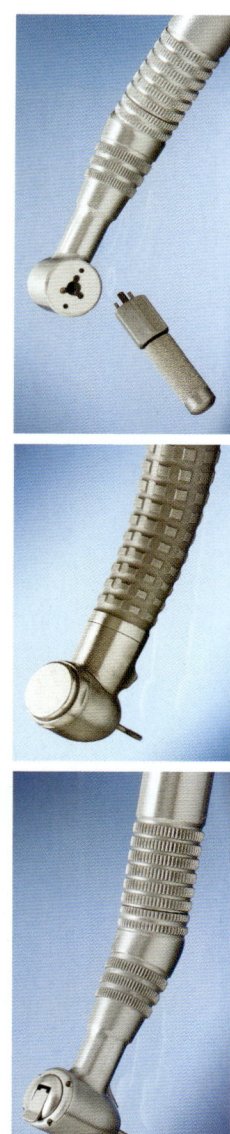

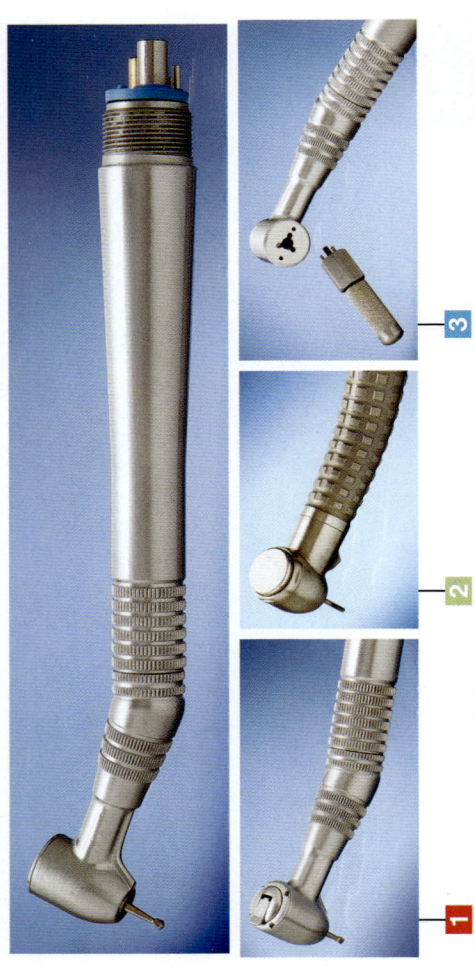

■ INSTRUMENT

High-Speed Handpiece

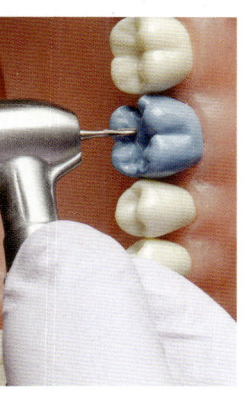

Functions ▶ To use with bur to cut tooth structure, to cut bone, to remove decay, and to modify or remove restorations

Example: Cavity preparation for restoration or crown

To use with bur for adjusting crowns and bridges for final fit

Characteristics ▶ Handpiece is run by air pressure at a maximum speed of 450,000 rotations per minute (rpm).

On high-speed handpiece, bur generates extreme amount of heat.

Handpiece sprays water/air or air on bur for cooling purposes to prevent damage to pulp.

Different styles of securing bur are available:

1 Power lever chuck **2** Push-button chuck

3 Conventional chuck—Need to secure bur and loosen bur in handpiece with wrench

Practice Notes ▶ Handpiece attaches to tubing on dental unit.

Sterilization Notes ▶ Most High-Speed Handpieces must be lubricated and precleaned according to the manufacturer's recommendation. Then, place in a sterilizing pouch with an internal process indicator, seal, then sterilize. OR, wrap with an internal process indicator inside and secure on the outside with process indicator tape, then sterilize. Verify appropriate color change has been achieved in external process indicator immediately after removal from sterilizer. Check internal process indicator before treatment. Refer to state regulations for any additional state requirements.

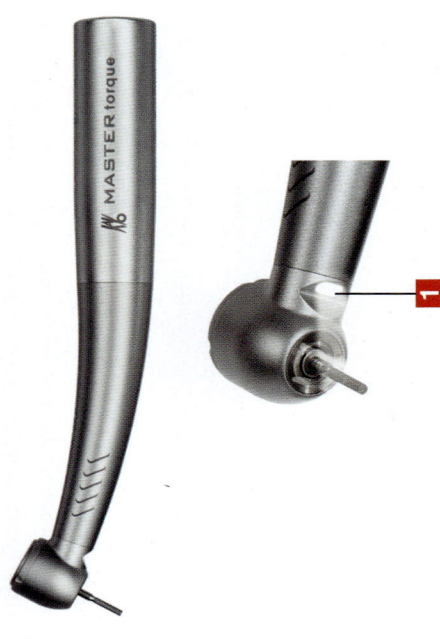

Fiberoptic High-Speed Handpiece

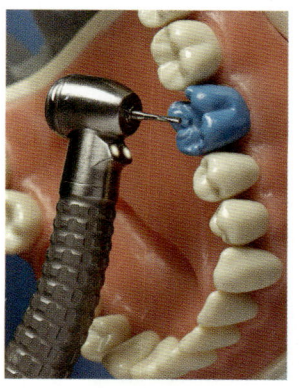

Functions ▶

To illuminate tooth during preparation for restoration
To provide light intraorally during use of handpiece
To use with bur to cut tooth structure, to cut bone, to remove decay, and to modify or remove restorations
Example: Cavity preparation for restoration or crown
To use with bur for adjusting crowns and bridges for final fit

Characteristics ▶

1 Light(s) at head of handpiece

Lights up working area while handpiece rotates
Same characteristics as high-speed handpiece

Practice Notes ▶

Handpiece attaches to tubing on dental unit.
Tubing has special adaptor for light availability.

Sterilization Notes ▶

Most fiberoptic High-Speed Handpieces must be lubricated and precleaned according to the manufacturer's recommendation. Then, place in a sterilizing pouch with an internal process indicator, seal, then sterilize. OR, wrap with an internal process indicator inside and secure on the outside with process indicator tape, then sterilize. Verify appropriate color change has been achieved in external process indicator immediately after removal from sterilizer. Check internal process indicator before treatment. Refer to state regulations for any additional state requirements.

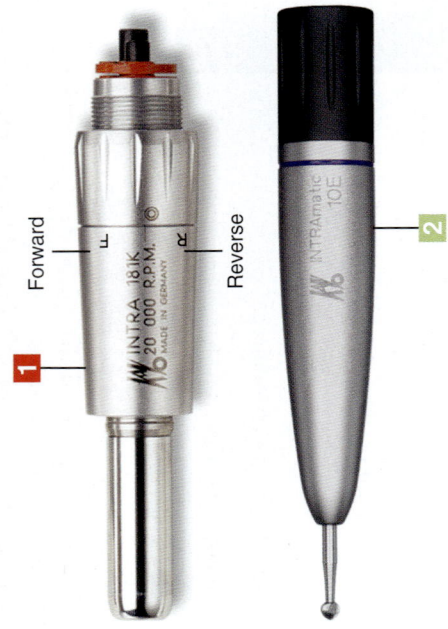

Forward

Reverse

■ INSTRUMENT

Slow-Speed Motor with Straight Handpiece Attachment

Functions ▸ To use with slow-speed attachments
To use straight attachment with long-shank straight bur

Characteristics ▸ 1 Slow-speed motor
2 Straight handpiece attachment (with bur attached)

Maximum speed of 30,000 rpm; used as adjunct to high-speed handpiece
Straight attachment—Used outside oral cavity, usually in a laboratory setting
Contra-angle or prophy angle attachments—Designed for intraoral use
Handpiece must be engaged in either forward or reverse.

Practice Notes ▸ Slow-Speed Motor attaches to tubing on dental unit.

Sterilization Notes ▸ Slow-Speed Motor with Straight Handpiece Attachment must be lubricated and precleaned according to the manufacturer's recommendation. Then, place in a sterilizing pouch with an internal process indicator, seal, then sterilize. OR, wrap with an internal process indicator inside and secure on the outside with process indicator tape, then sterilize. Verify appropriate color change has been achieved in external process indicator immediately after removal from sterilizer. Check internal process indicator before treatment. Refer to state regulations for any additional state requirements.

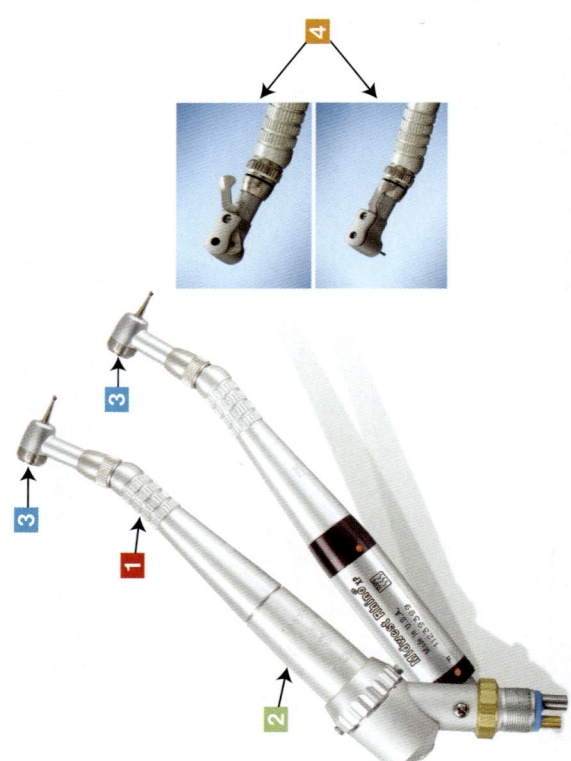

■ INSTRUMENT

Slow-Speed Motor with Contra-Angle Handpiece Attachment

Functions ▶ To use with burs for intraoral and extraoral procedures to remove decay, polish amalgam restorations, refine cavity preparation, adjust provisional and permanent crowns and bridges, adjust occlusal restorations, adjust partials and dentures, and to provide prophylaxis treatment

Characteristics ▶
1 Contra-angle attachment
2 Slow-speed motor
3 Push-button device to secure bur—Using friction grip bur

4 Latch-type attachment—Using latch-type bur
Top: latch open; *Bottom:* latch closed

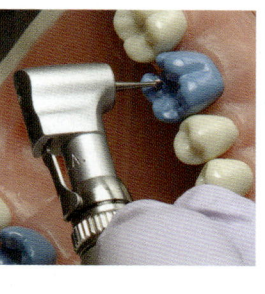

Contra-angle attaches to straight handpiece or to Slow-Speed Motor.
Types of Contra-Angle Attachments:
- Latch type—Latch-type bur, prophylaxis polishing cup or brush. Bur is secured by swivel of latch-type device in back of handpiece.
- Friction grip—Friction grip bur. Bur is secured by pushing back of handpiece.

Practice Notes ▶ Slow-Speed Motor attaches to tubing on dental unit.

Sterilization Notes ▶ Slow-Speed Motor with Contra-Angle Handpiece Attachment must be lubricated and precleaned according to the manufacturer's recommendation. Then, place in a sterilizing pouch with an internal process indicator, seal, then sterilize. OR, wrap with an internal process indicator inside and secure on the outside with process indicator tape, then sterilize. Verify appropriate color change has been achieved in external process indicator immediately after removal from sterilizer. Check internal process indicator before treatment. Refer to state regulations for any additional state requirements.

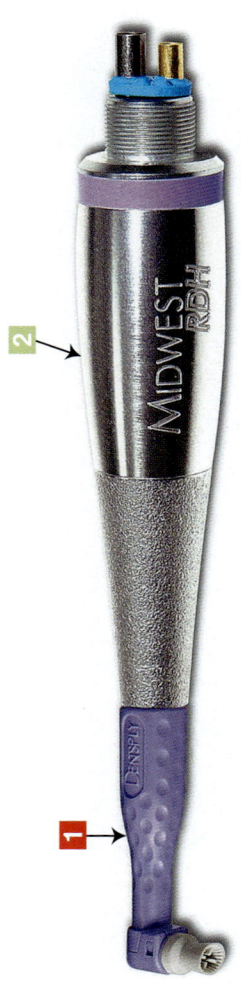

Prophy Slow-Speed Handpiece/Motor* with Disposable Prophy Angle Attachment

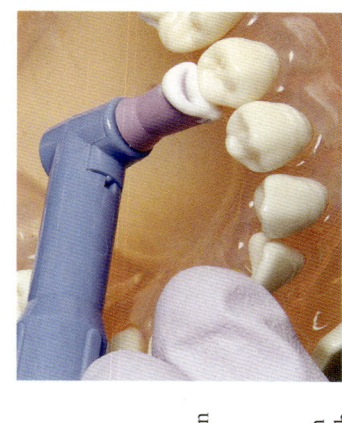

Function ▸ To polish teeth with prophylaxis/prophy cup or brush attachment

Characteristics ▸

1 Disposable prophy angle attachment (with rubber polishing cup)

2 Prophy Slow-Speed Handpiece/Motor

Prophy angle attaches to handpiece/motor.

Ergonomic shape for natural hand positioning

Lightweight design to reduce hand and wrist fatigue

Practice Notes ▸ Prophy Slow-Speed Handpiece/Motor attaches to tubing on dental unit.

Sterilization Notes ▸ Prophy Slow-Speed Handpiece/Motor must be lubricated and precleaned according to the manufacturer's recommendation. Then, place in a sterilizing pouch with an internal process indicator, seal, then sterilize. OR, wrap with an internal process indicator inside and secure on the outside with process indicator tape, then sterilize. Verify appropriate color change has been achieved in external process indicator immediately after removal from sterilizer. Check internal process indicator before treatment. Refer to state regulations for any additional state requirements. Disposable Prophy Angle Attachments (rubber polishing cup or brush) must be disposed of in garbage. Single use only.

* Referred to as RDH (Registered Dental Hygiene) Prophy Angle.

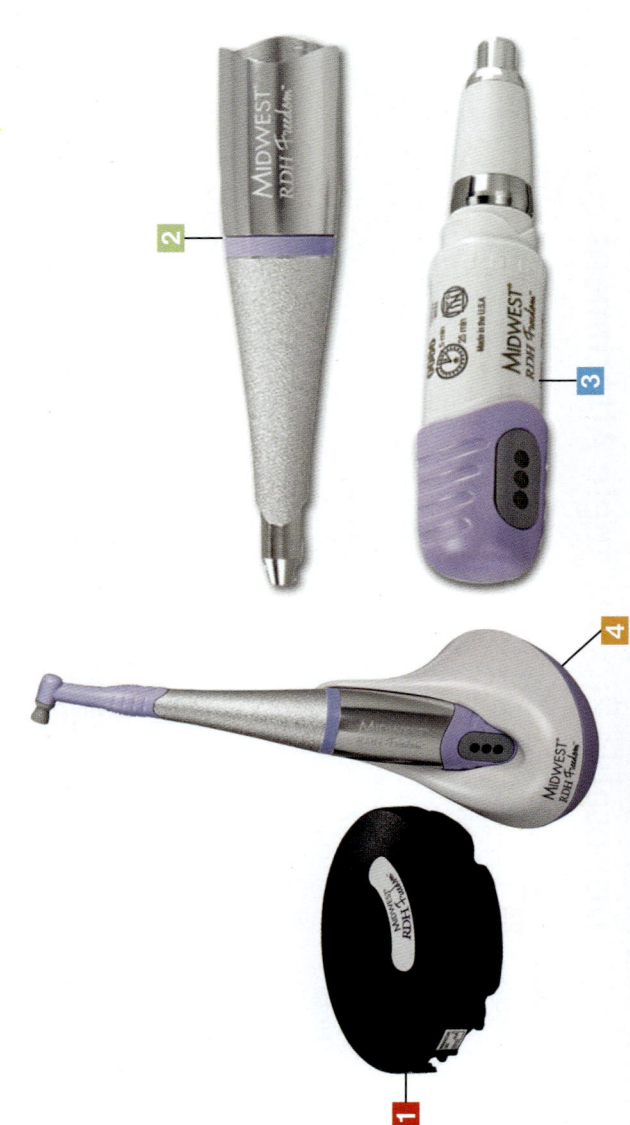

Rechargeable Prophy Slow-Speed Handpiece/Motor—RDH Freedom™

Function ▶ To polish teeth for prophylaxis with prophy cup and/or brush

Characteristics ▶ 1 Foot Pedal–Wireless–Cordless rechargeable
To operate Foot Pedal and control speed of handpiece
RDH Freedom™ Cordless Rechargable Prophy Handpiece
Parts:
2 Sheath—Handpiece Attachment
3 Motor
4 Cradle to hold the handpiece
Types of Prophy Angle Attachments:
- Disposable prophy cup—For polishing all surfaces of teeth. Refer to pages 96 & 97
- Disposable prophy brush—For polishing occlusal surfaces and deep grooves on lingual surfaces of anterior teeth. Refer to pages 96 & 97

Practice Notes ▶ Rechargeable handpiece is used mostly on prophylaxis and sealant tray setups.

Sterilization Notes ▶ RDH Motor should follow the manufacturer's recommendation for lubricating, precleaning. Then, place Sheath, Motor, and Attachments in a sterilizing pouch with an internal process indicator, seal, then sterilize. OR, wrap with an internal process indicator inside and secure on the outside with process indicator tape, then sterilize. Verify appropriate color change has been achieved in external process indicator immediately after removal from sterilizer. Check internal process indicator before treatment. Refer to state regulations for any additional state requirements. Disposable Prophy Angle Attachments (rubber polishing cup or brush) must be disposed of in garbage. Single use only. Cradle and Foot Pedal should have a barrier, otherwise disinfect according to manufacturer's recommendation.

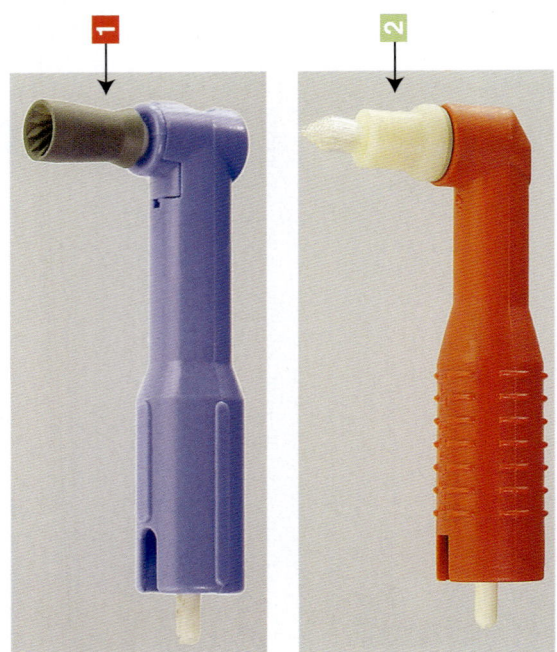

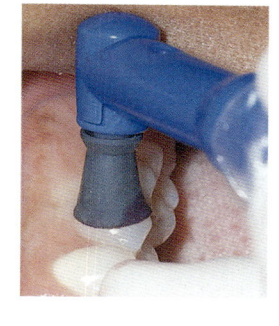

Disposable Prophy Angle Attachments for Slow-Speed Handpiece/Motor

■ INSTRUMENT

Function ▶ To polish teeth for prophylaxis

Characteristics ▶ Attaches to straight or prophy slow-speed handpiece/motor

Types:

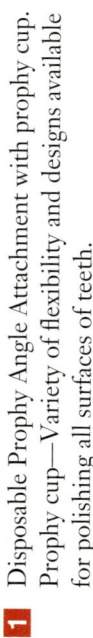

1 Disposable Prophy Angle Attachment with prophy cup. Prophy cup—Variety of flexibility and designs available for polishing all surfaces of teeth.

2 Disposable Prophy Angle Attachment with tapered brush—For polishing occlusal surfaces and deep grooves on lingual surfaces of anterior teeth.

Practice Note ▶ Disposable Prophy Angle Attachments are used mostly on prophylaxis and sealant tray setups.

Sterilization Notes ▶ Disposable Prophy Angle Attachments (rubber polishing cup or brush) must be disposed of in garbage. Single use only.

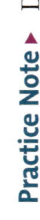

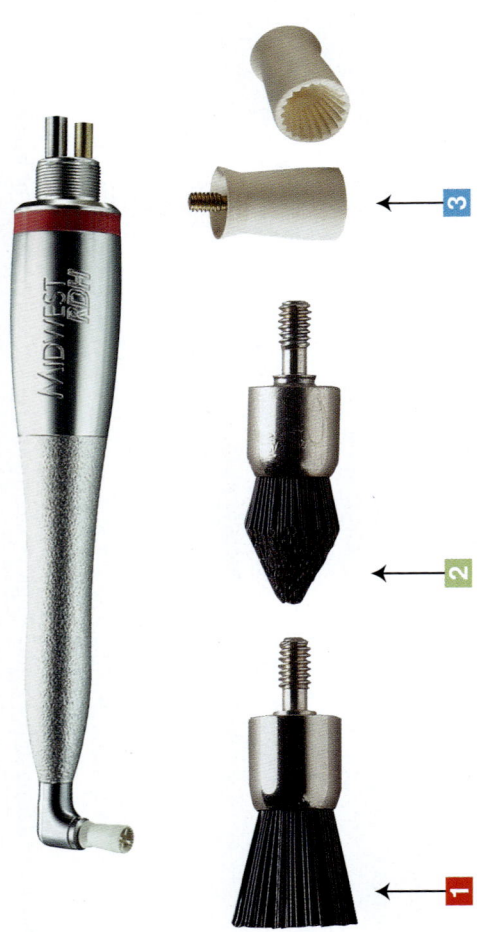

Prophy Angle Slow-Speed Handpiece/Motor*

Function ▶ To polish teeth for prophylaxis

Characteristics ▶ Prophy angle slow-speed handpiece/motor is one piece.
Disposable screw-type prophy cup or brush attaches to prophy angle slow-speed handpiece/motor.
Lightweight design to reduce hand and wrist fatigue
Ergonomic shape for natural hand positioning

Attachments:

1 Flat-end brush
2 Tapered-end brush
3 Prophy cup—Variety of flexibility and designs available

Practice Note ▶ Prophy Angle Slow-Speed Handpiece/Motor attaches to tubing on dental unit.

Sterilization Notes ▶ Prophy Angle Slow-Speed Handpiece/Motor must be lubricated and precleaned according to the manufacturer's recommendation. Then, place Motor and Attachments in a sterilizing pouch with an internal process indicator, seal, then sterilize. OR, wrap with an internal process indicator inside and secure on the outside with process indicator tape, then sterilize. Verify appropriate color change has been achieved in external process indicator immediately after removal from sterilizer. Check internal process indicator before treatment. Refer to state regulations for any additional state requirements. Disposable prophy polishing cup or brush must be disposed of in garbage. Single use only.

*Referred to as an RDH (Registered Dental Hygienist) prophy handpiece.

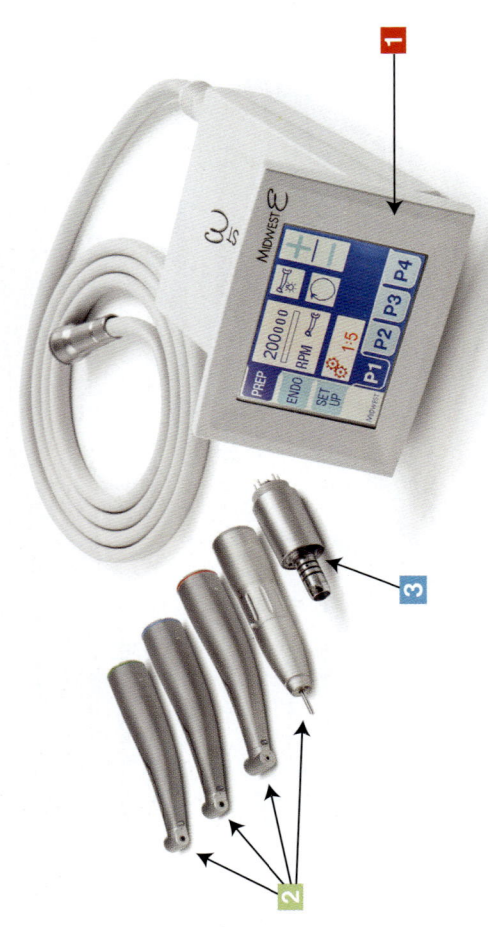

Electric Handpiece Unit and Handpiece Attachments

Functions ▶
To use with bur for intraoral cavity preparation
To use with bur with endodontic nickel-titanium rotary instruments
To use with bur for trimming of provisional crowns
To use with bur for adjusting permanent restorations, crowns, and bridges

Characteristics ▶
1 Electric Handpiece Unit
2 Electric Handpiece Attachments
3 Electric Handpiece Motor

Speed of handpiece can be set to specific rpms.

Practice Notes ▶
Handpiece attaches to tubing on electric handpiece unit.
Electric Handpiece is used with restorative, endodontic, and surgical tray setups.

Sterilization Notes ▶
Electric Handpiece Motor must be lubricated and precleaned according to the manufacturer's recommendation. Then, place Motor and Attachments in a sterilizing pouch with an internal process indicator, seal, then sterilize. OR, wrap with an internal process indicator inside and secure on the outside with process indicator tape, then sterilize. Verify appropriate color change has been achieved in external process indicator immediately after removal from sterilizer. Check internal process indicator before treatment. Refer to state regulations for any additional state requirements. Barriers should be used on the unit, or the manufacturer's recommendation should be followed for disinfecting the unit.

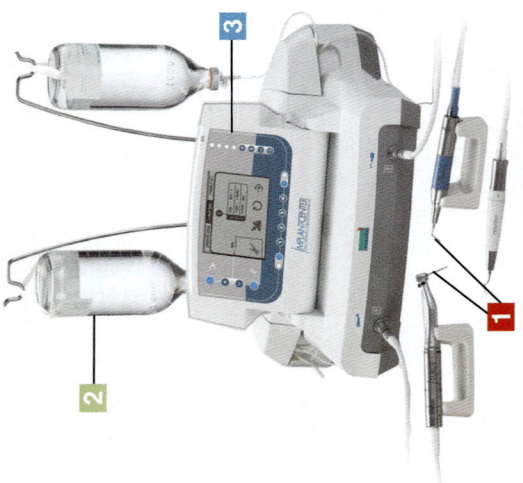

Surgical Electrical Handpiece Unit and Handpiece Attachments

Functions ▶

1. To use with depth drills for implants
2. To use with sterile water for cooling drilling system
3. Electric Handpiece Unit

Characteristics ▶

Straight and contra-angled (pictured) handpiece attachments available
Maximum speed of 40,000 rpm
Lower speed (e.g., 10–50 rpm) used for implant
Fiberoptic light available for these handpieces

Practice Note ▶

Surgical Electrical Handpiece Unit and Handpiece Attachments are used with surgical tray setups.

Sterilization Notes ▶

Surgical Electrical Handpiece Motor must be lubricated and precleaned according to the manufacturer's recommendation. Then, place Motor and Attachments in a sterilizing pouch with an internal process indicator, seal, then sterilize. OR, wrap with an internal process indicator inside and secure on the outside with process indicator tape, then sterilize. Verify appropriate color change has been achieved in external process indicator immediately after removal from sterilizer. Check internal process indicator before treatment. Refer to state regulations for any additional state requirements. Barriers should be used on the unit, or the manufacturer's recommendation should be followed for disinfecting the unit. Sterile water single use only.

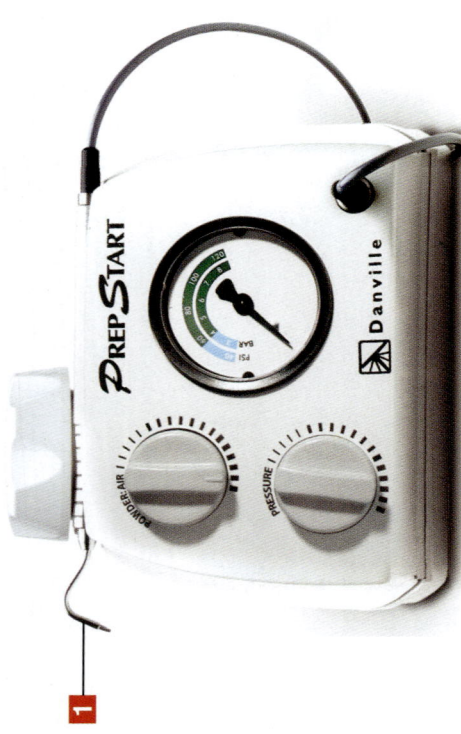

1

■ INSTRUMENT

Air Abrasion Unit and Handpiece Attachment

Functions ▶

To use for class I through class VI cavity preparation

To use for preparation of occlusal surface for sealants

Characteristics ▶

1 Handpiece attachment uses high pressure of alpha-alumina particles through small device that removes decay or prepares pit and fissures for sealants or restoration. Minimal use of anesthesia is required.

Practice Note ▶

Air Abrasion Unit and Handpiece Attachment are used with class I through class VI restorative tray setups and with sealant tray setups.

Sterilization Notes ▶

Air Abrasion Handpiece Attachments must be lubricated and precleaned according to the manufacturer's recommendation. Then, place Handpiece and Attachments in a sterilizing pouch with an internal process indicator, seal, then sterilize. OR, wrap with an internal process indicator inside and secure on the outside with process indicator tape, then sterilize. Verify appropriate color change has been achieved in external process indicator immediately after removal from sterilizer. Check internal process indicator before treatment. Refer to state regulations for any additional state requirements. Barriers should be used on the unit, or the manufacturer's recommendation should be followed for disinfecting the unit.

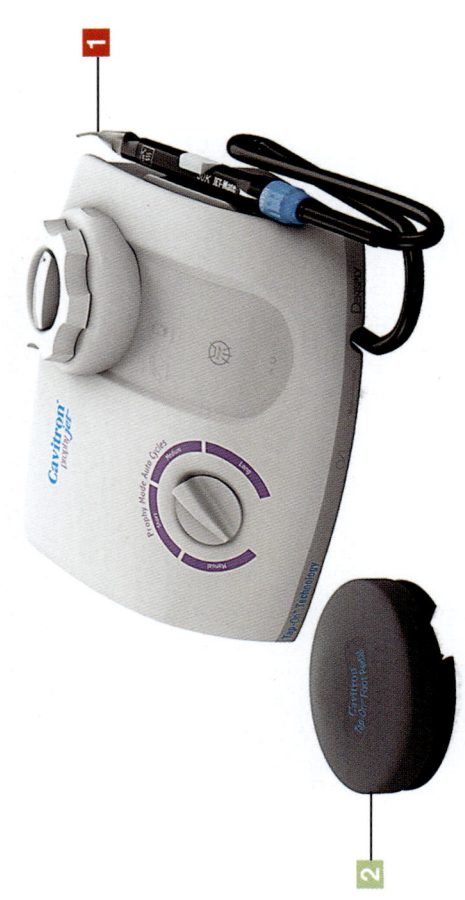

Air Polisher

Function ▶ To polish teeth by directing a high-pressure jet of pressurized air, water, and mild polishing agent of sodium bicarbonate

Characteristics ▶

1 Combination of slurry of water and powder cleans or debrides the tooth surface utilizing the Air Polisher Tip

2 Foot Pedal that controls the Air Polisher

Air Polisher has a self-contained water reservoir.

Air Polisher is connected to the dental unit water supply tubing.

Practice Note ▶ Air Polisher used in place of polishing teeth with prophy paste, prophy cup, and brush.

Sterilization Notes ▶ Air Polisher Unit Attachment tips must be precleaned. Then, place Attachments in a sterilizing pouch with an internal process indicator, seal, then sterilize. OR, wrap with an internal process indicator inside and secure on the outside with process indicator tape, then sterilize. Verify appropriate color change has been achieved in external process indicator immediately after removal from sterilizer. Check internal process indicator before treatment. Refer to state regulations for any additional state requirements. Barriers should be used on the Foot Pedal, Unit, and Attachments or the manufacturer's recommendation should be followed for disinfecting the unit and attachments.

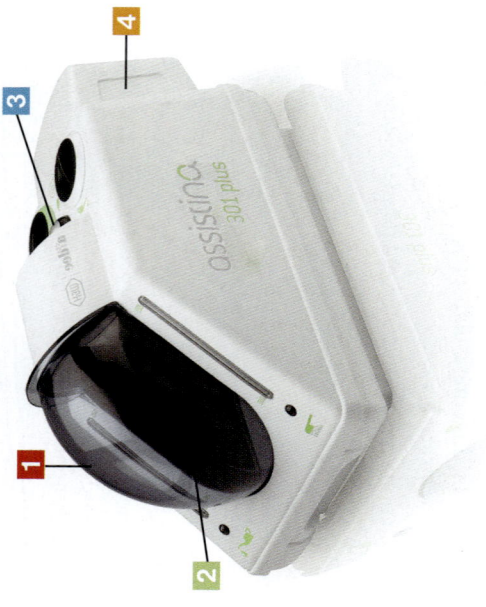

■ INSTRUMENT

Handpiece Maintenance System

Function ▶ To flush internal air/water coolant lines on high- and slow-speed handpieces

To remove debris within handpiece and prevent buildup

To lubricate handpiece

Characteristics ▶
1 Cover encloses system
2 Under cover connection for handpieces—Lift cover to access
3 Start button
4 Filter system

Universal adaptor for many styles of handpieces available
Handpiece Maintenance System
Cleans and lubricates before bagging to sterilized
Keeps aerosols contained and filters exhaust and air from unit

Practice Note ▶ To use, connect the instrument and close the cover and then push the start button for 2 seconds to begin automated delivery of service oil and cleaning liquid; cycle is complete in 35 seconds. Also refer to the instruction manual of the handpiece as different handpieces have to be lubricated different ways and at different times.

Sterilization Notes ▶ Refer to the manufacturer's recommendations for cleaning and disinfecting.

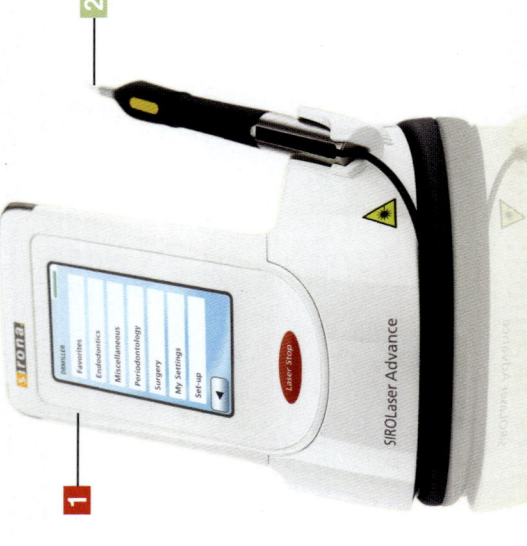

Laser Handpiece Unit and Laser Handpiece Attachment

Function ▶ To cut, vaporize, or cauterize soft tissue

Examples:

To remove lesions or tumors

To reduce excess tissue

To control bleeding

Characteristics ▶ Works by means of a highly concentrated light source
SIROLaser (pictured) operates at a wavelength of 980 nanometers and has a power output
varying from 0.5 to 7 watts.

Practice Notes ▶ 1 Laser Handpiece Unit

2 Laser Handpiece Attachment are used with specialty procedures.

Examples: Prosthodontics and Oral Surgery

Sterilization Notes ▶ Laser Handpiece must be lubricated and precleaned according to the manufacturer's recommendation. Then, place in a sterilizing pouch with an internal process indicator, seal, then sterilize. OR, wrap with an internal process indicator inside and secure on the outside with process indicator tape, then sterilize. Verify appropriate color change has been achieved in external process indicator immediately after removal from sterilizer. Check internal process indicator before treatment. Refer to state regulations for any additional state requirements. Barriers should be used on the unit, or the manufacturer's recommendation should be followed for disinfecting the unit.

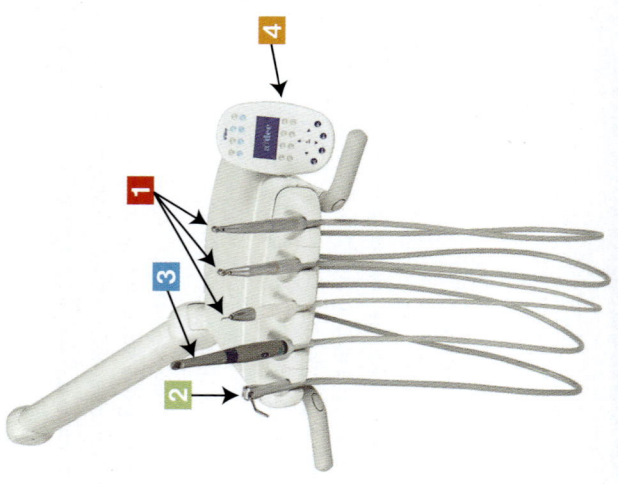

Dental Unit

Functions ▶

1. To provide a delivery system for handpieces and air/water syringe
2. To provide delivery system for air/water syringe
3. To provide intraoral camera
4. To provide a device for moving dental chair up, down, forward, and backward

Characteristics ▶ Delivery systems provide at least two tubings—one for high-speed handpieces and one for slow-speed handpiece. Above illustrates two tubing unit. Special mechanism required for fiberoptic handpiece

Practice Notes ▶ Different designs of dental delivery systems available in front, rear, or side delivery Air/water syringes available on one or both sides of operator or assistant's side

Barriers should be used on tubing, or the manufacturer's recommendation should be followed for disinfecting unit and tubing. Handpiece and Attachments must be lubricated and precleaned according to manufacturer's recommendation. Then place a sterilizing pouch with an internal process indicator, seal, then sterilize. OR, wrap with an internal process indicator inside and secure on the outside with process indicator tape, then sterilize. Verify appropriate color change has been achieved in external process indicator immediately after removal from sterilizer. Check internal process indicator before treatment. Refer to state regulations for any additional state requirements.

6

Burs and Rotary Attachments for Handpieces

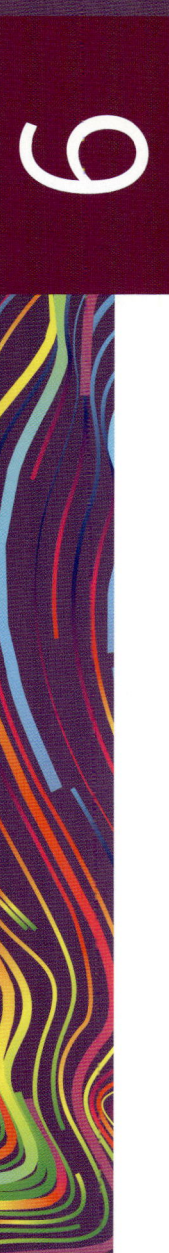

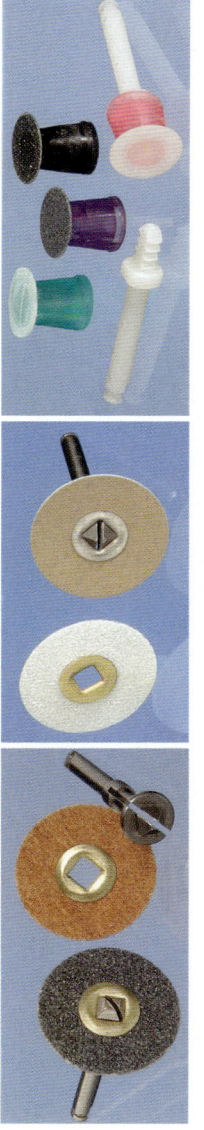

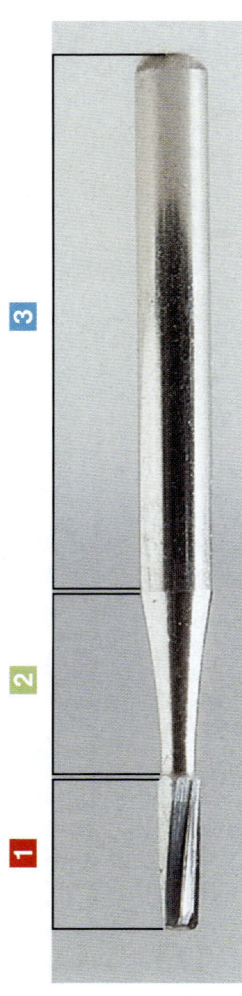

Bur

Function ▸ To be used in a high- or low-speed handpiece

Characteristics ▸ Parts:

1 Head: Part of bur that cuts, polishes, or finishes

- Available in a variety of shapes and sizes

2 Neck: Part of bur that tapers to connect shank to head

3 Shank: Part of bur that is inserted into the handpiece

- Length and style of shank vary depending on handpiece used.
- Bur with straight, long shank fits into straight slow-speed handpiece.
- Bur with latch-type shank fits into contra-angle slow-speed handpiece.
- Friction grip bur fits into high-speed handpiece (friction grip bur shown). Friction grip bur fits into high-speed handpiece; chuck, lever, or push button tightens bur into the handpiece.
- Bur with long shank used for surgical procedures

Sterilization Notes ▸ Bur must be precleaned. Then, place in a sterilizing pouch with an internal process indicator, seal, then sterilize. OR, wrap with an internal process indicator inside and secure on the outside with process indicator tape, then sterilize. Verify appropriate color change has been achieved in external process indicator immediately after removal from sterilizer. Check internal process indicator before treatment. Refer to state regulations for any additional state requirements. Or, the used bur must be disposed of in a sharps container.

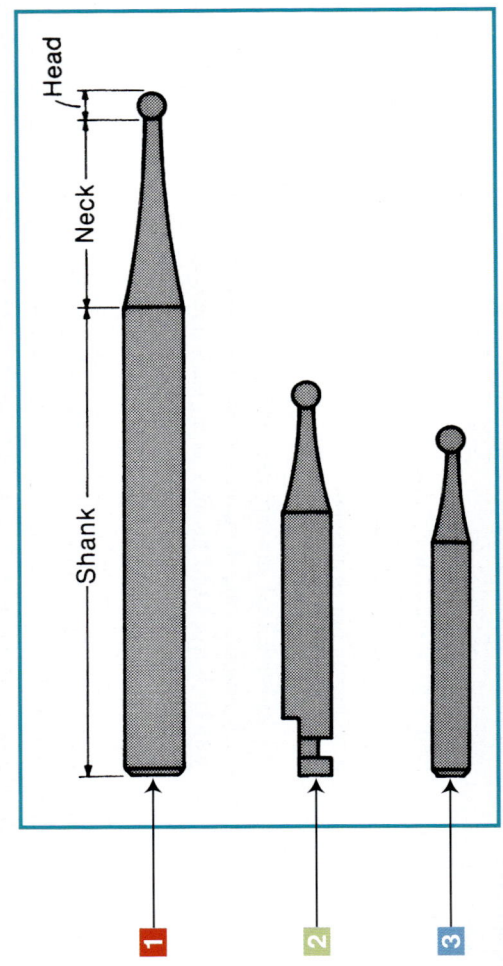

1
2
3

■ INSTRUMENT

Bur Shanks

Function ▸ To fit shank part of bur into handpiece

Characteristics ▸ Fit a variety of shanks into different styles of handpieces

Working or cutting end of the bur could be the same style or size, but shank could be different according to handpiece used

Examples:

1 No. 2 round bur in straight shank

2 No. 2 round bur in latch shank

3 No. 2 round bur in friction grip shank

Extra long shank used for surgical procedures

Sterilization Notes ▸ Burs must be precleaned. Then, place in a sterilizing pouch with an internal process indicator, seal, then sterilize. OR, wrap with an internal process indicator inside and secure on the outside with process indicator tape, then sterilize. Verify appropriate color change has been achieved in external process indicator immediately after removal from sterilizer. Check internal process indicator before treatment .Refer to state regulations for any additional state requirements. Or, the used bur must be disposed of in a sharps container.

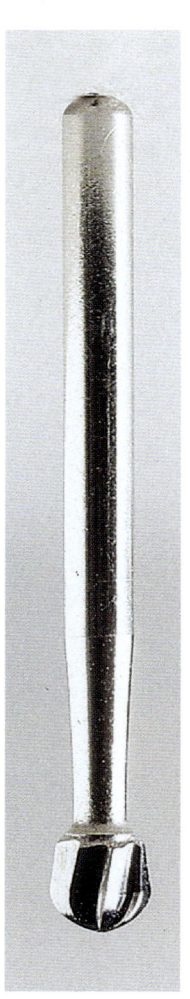

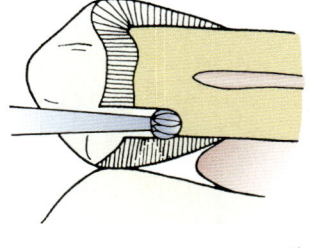

Round Bur

■ **INSTRUMENT**

Functions ▶

To remove caries from tooth structure

To open tooth for endodontic treatment

To create retention in cavity preparation

To use for many procedures on a tooth

Characteristics ▶

Range of sizes

Commonly used sizes: No. 1/4 to No. 10

Practice Notes ▶

Bur is inserted and secured in a handpiece.

Type of handpiece determines type of shank used.

Sterilization Notes ▶

A Round Bur must be precleaned. Then, place in a sterilizing pouch with an internal process indicator, seal, then sterilize. OR, wrap with an internal process indicator inside and secure on the outside with process indicator tape, then sterilize. Verify appropriate color change has been achieved in external process indicator immediately after removal from sterilizer. Check internal process indicator before treatment. Refer to state regulations for any additional state requirements. Or, the used bur must be disposed of in a sharps container.

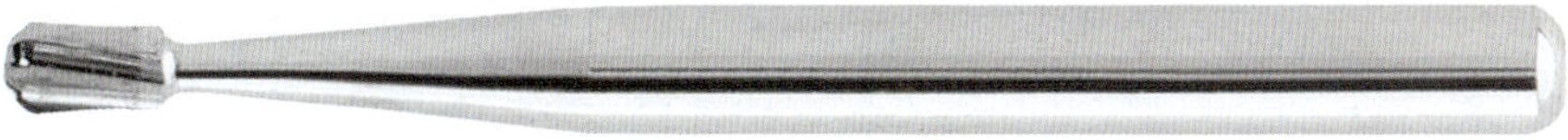

Pear-Shaped Bur

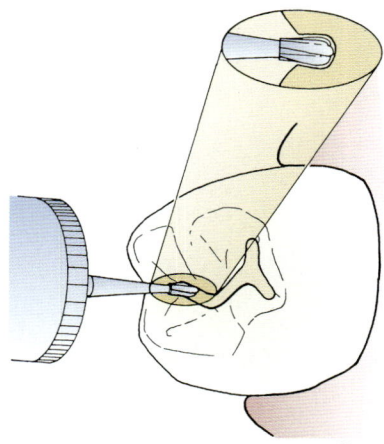

Functions ▸ To open tooth for a restoration

To remove caries

Characteristics ▸ Frequently used in preparation of composite restorations

Range of sizes

Commonly used sizes: No. 330 to No. 333

Bur head available in long

Example: No. 333L

Practice Notes ▸ Bur is inserted and secured in a handpiece.

Type of handpiece determines type of shank used.

Sterilization Notes ▸ Pear-Shaped Bur must be precleaned. Then, place in a sterilizing pouch with an internal process indicator, seal, then sterilize. OR, wrap with an internal process indicator inside and secure on the outside with process indicator tape, then sterilize. Verify appropriate color change has been achieved in external process indicator immediately after removal from sterilizer. Check internal process indicator before treatment. Refer to state regulations for any additional state requirements. Or, the used bur must be disposed of in a sharps container.

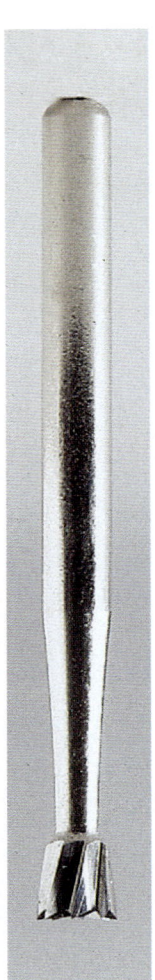

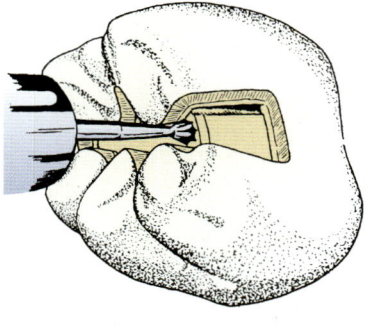

INSTRUMENT

Inverted Cone Bur

Functions ▶
To remove caries
To establish retention in tooth for cavity preparation

Characteristics ▶
Range of sizes
Commonly used sizes: No. 33½, No. 34, No. 37, No. 39

Practice Notes ▶
Bur is inserted and secured in a handpiece.
Type of handpiece determines type of shank used.

Sterilization Notes ▶
Inverted Cone Bur must be precleaned. Then, place in a sterilizing pouch with an internal process indicator, seal, then sterilize. OR, wrap with an internal process indicator inside and secure on the outside with process indicator tape, then sterilize. Verify appropriate color change has been achieved in external process indicator immediately after removal from sterilizer. Check internal process indicator before treatment. Refer to state regulations for any additional state requirements. Or, the used bur must be disposed of in a sharps container.

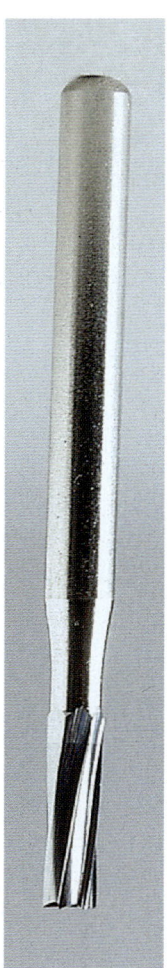

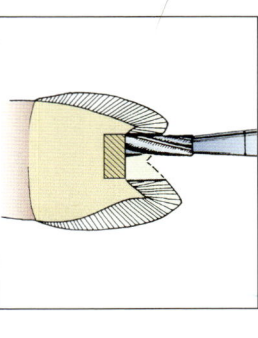

Straight Fissure Bur—Plain Cut

Functions ▶
To cut cavity preparation
To form inner walls of cavity preparation
To create retention grooves in walls of cavity preparation

Characteristics ▶
Cutting part of bur—Has parallel sides
Range of sizes—Commonly used: No. 56, No. 57, No. 58
May have short (S) or long (L) shank for adaptation to a variety of cavity preparations
Examples of short and long shank friction grip burs: No. 56S, No. 56L

Practice Notes ▶
Bur is inserted and secured in a handpiece.
Type of handpiece determines type of shank used.

Sterilization Notes ▶
Straight Fissure Bur—Plain Cut must be precleaned. Then, place in a sterilizing pouch with an internal process indicator, seal, then sterilize. OR, wrap with an internal process indicator inside and secure on the outside with process indicator tape, then sterilize. Verify appropriate color change has been achieved in external process indicator immediately after removal from sterilizer. Check internal process indicator before treatment. Refer to state regulations for any additional state requirements. Or, the used bur must be disposed of in a sharps container.

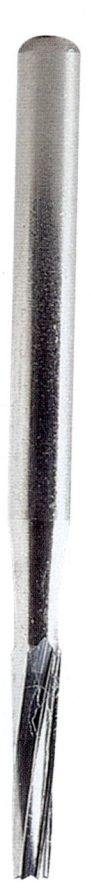

Tapered Fissure Bur—Plain Cut

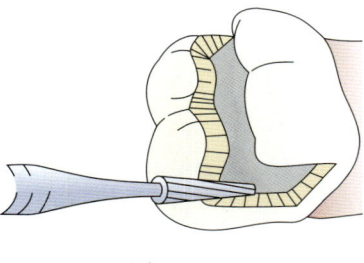

■ **INSTRUMENT**

Functions ▶
To cut cavity preparation
To form angles in walls of cavity preparation
To place retention grooves in walls of cavity preparation

Characteristics ▶
Cutting part of bur—Has tapered sides
Range of sizes—Commonly used: No. 168, No. 169, No. 170, No. 171
May have short (S) or long (L) shank for adaptation to a variety of cavity preparations
Examples of short and long shank friction grip burs: No. 168S, No. 171L

Practice Notes ▶
Bur is inserted and secured in a handpiece.
Type of handpiece determines type of shank used.

Sterilization Notes ▶
Tapered Fissure Bur—Plain Cut must be precleaned. Then, place in a sterilizing pouch with an internal process indicator, seal, then sterilize. OR, wrap with an internal process indicator inside and secure on the outside with process indicator tape, then sterilize. Verify appropriate color change has been achieved in external process indicator immediately after removal from sterilizer. Check internal process indicator before treatment. Refer to state regulations for any additional state requirements. Or, used bur must be disposed of in a sharps container.

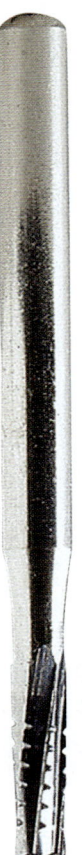

Straight Fissure Bur—Crosscut

Functions ▶
To cut cavity preparation
To form walls of cavity preparation
To create retention grooves in walls of cavity preparation

Characteristics ▶
Cutting part of bur—Has parallel sides with horizontal cutting edges
Range of sizes—Commonly used: No. 556, No. 557, No. 558
May have long (L) shank for adaptation to a variety of cavity preparations
Example of long shank friction grip bur: No. 556L

Practice Notes ▶
Bur is inserted and secured in a handpiece.
Type of handpiece determines type of shank used.

Sterilization Notes ▶
Straight Fissure Bur—Crosscut must be precleaned. Then, place in a sterilizing pouch with an internal process indicator, seal, then sterilize. OR, wrap with an internal process indicator inside and secure on the outside with process indicator tape, then sterilize. Verify appropriate color change has been achieved in external process indicator immediately after removal from sterilizer. Check internal process indicator before treatment. Refer to state regulations for any additional state requirements. Or, the used bur must be disposed of in a sharps container.

■ INSTRUMENT

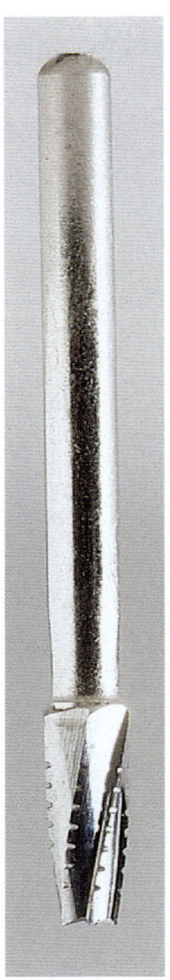

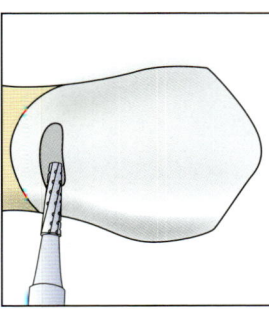

INSTRUMENT

Tapered Fissure Bur—Crosscut

Functions ▶

To cut cavity preparation

To form angles in walls of cavity preparation

To create retention grooves in walls of cavity preparation

Characteristics ▶

Cutting part of bur—Has tapered sides with horizontal cutting edges

Range of sizes—Commonly used: No. 699, No. 700, No. 701, No. 702, No. 703

May have long (L) shank for adaptation to a variety of cavity preparations

Example of long shank friction grip bur: No. 701L

Practice Notes ▶

Bur is inserted and secured in a handpiece.

Type of handpiece determines type of shank used.

Sterilization Notes ▶

Tapered Fissure Bur—Crosscut must be precleaned. Then, place in a sterilizing pouch with an internal process indicator, seal, then sterilize. OR, wrap with an internal process indicator inside and secure on the outside with process indicator tape, then sterilize. Verify appropriate color change has been achieved in external process indicator immediately after removal from sterilizer. Check internal process indicator before treatment. Refer to state regulations for any additional state requirements. Or, the used bur must be disposed of in a sharps container.

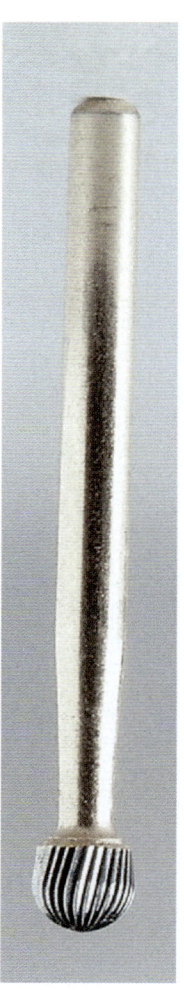

INSTRUMENT

Finishing Bur

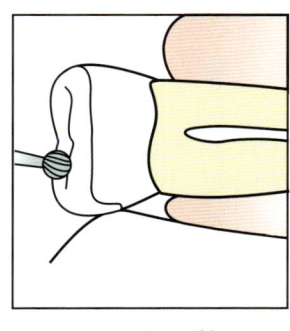

Functions ▸ To finish composite restoration

To finish restoration by restoring anatomy in tooth

To equilibrate or adjust occlusion

Characteristic ▸ Variety of shapes and sizes available

Finishing bur differs from the cutting burs as the working end or cutting end has an increased number of blades or flutes. An increased amount of blades will determine the greater amount of polishing capabilities.

Practice Notes ▸ Bur is inserted and secured in a handpiece.

Type of handpiece determines type of shank used.

Sterilization Notes ▸ Finishing Bur must be precleaned. Then, place in a sterilizing pouch with an internal process indicator, seal, then sterilize. OR, wrap with an internal process indicator inside and secure on the outside with process indicator tape, then sterilize. Verify appropriate color change has been achieved in external process indicator immediately after removal from sterilizer. Check internal process indicator before treatment. Refer to state regulations for any additional state requirements. Or, the used bur must be disposed of in a sharps container.

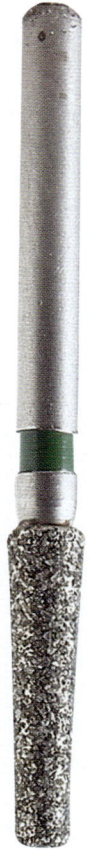

INSTRUMENT

Diamond Bur—Flat-End Taper

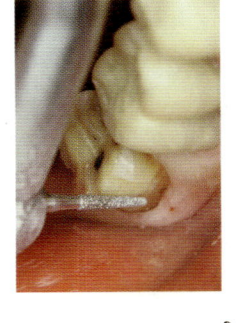

Function ▶ To reduce a tooth for crown preparation when a square shoulder is needed

Characteristics ▶ Range of grits—Superfine to coarse; grit designated by color band on shank of diamond bur or by letter after name of diamond bur

Superfine diamond burs—Used for finishing restorations

Variety of shapes and sizes

Practice Notes ▶ Bur is inserted and secured in a handpiece.

Type of handpiece determines type of shank used.

Sterilization Notes ▶ Diamond Bur—Flat-End Taper must be precleaned. Then, place in a sterilizing pouch with an internal process indicator, seal, then sterilize. OR, wrap with an internal process indicator inside and secure on the outside with process indicator tape, then sterilize. Verify appropriate color change has been achieved in external process indicator immediately after removal from sterilizer. Check internal process indicator before treatment. Refer to state regulations for any additional state requirements. Or, the used diamond bur must be disposed of in a sharps container.

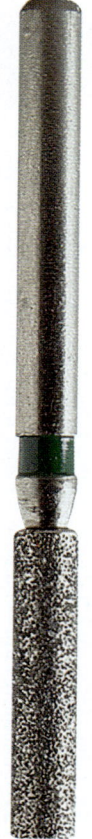

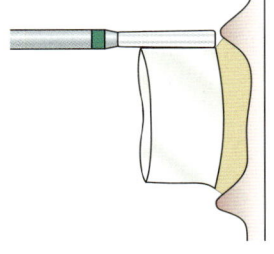

Diamond Bur—Flat-End Cylinder

Function ▶ To reduce a tooth for crown preparation when parallel walls and flat floors are needed

Characteristics ▶ Range of grits—Superfine to coarse; grit designated by color band on shank of diamond bur or by letter after name of diamond bur

Superfine diamond burs—Used for finishing restorations

Variety of shapes and sizes

Practice Notes ▶ Bur is inserted and secured in a handpiece.

Type of handpiece determines type of shank used.

Sterilization Notes ▶ Diamond Bur—Flat-End Cylinder must be precleaned. Then, place in a sterilizing pouch with an internal process indicator, seal, then sterilize. OR, wrap with an internal process indicator inside and secure on the outside with process indicator tape, then sterilize. Verify appropriate color change has been achieved in external process indicator immediately after removal from sterilizer. Check internal process indicator before treatment. Refer to state regulations for any additional state requirements. Or, the used bur must be disposed of in a sharps container.

■ INSTRUMENT

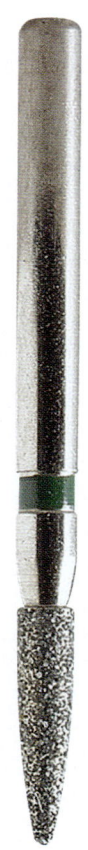

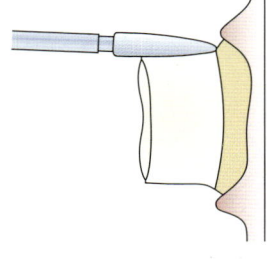

Diamond Bur—Flame

■ INSTRUMENT

Function ▲ To reduce a tooth for crown preparation for subgingival margins

Characteristics ▲ Range of grits—Superfine to coarse; grit designated by color band on shank of diamond bur or by letter after name of diamond bur
Superfine diamond burs—Used for finishing restorations
Variety of shapes and sizes

Practice Notes ▲ Bur is inserted and secured in a handpiece.
Type of handpiece determines type of shank used.

Sterilization Notes ▲ Diamond Bur—Flame must be precleaned. Then, place in a sterilizing pouch with an internal process indicator, seal, then sterilize. OR, wrap with an internal process indicator inside and secure on the outside with process indicator tape, then sterilize. Verify appropriate color change has been achieved in external process indicator immediately after removal from sterilizer. Check internal process indicator before treatment. Refer to state regulations for any additional state requirements. Or, the used bur must be disposed of in a sharps container.

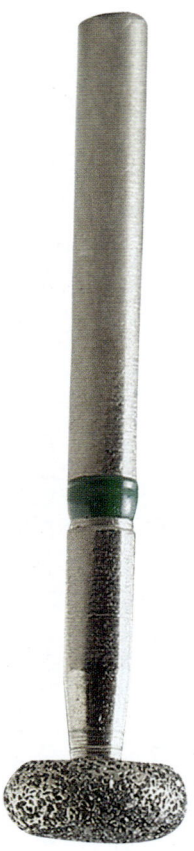

Diamond Bur—Wheel

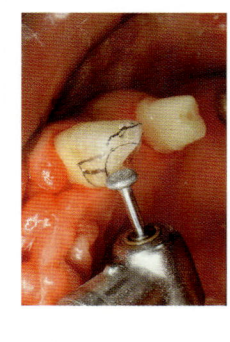

Function ▶ To reduce a tooth for crown preparation on lingual aspect of anterior teeth and to reduce bulk of incisal edges

Characteristics ▶ Range of grits—Superfine to coarse; grit designated by color band on shank of diamond bur or by letter after name of diamond bur

Superfine diamond burs—Used for finishing restorations
Variety of shapes and sizes

Practice Notes ▶ Bur is inserted and secured in a handpiece.
Type of handpiece determines type of shank used.

Sterilization Notes ▶ Diamond Bur—Wheel must be precleaned. Then, place in a sterilizing pouch with an internal process indicator, seal, then sterilize. OR, wrap with an internal process indicator inside and secure on the outside with process indicator tape, then sterilize. Verify appropriate color change has been achieved in external process indicator immediately after removal from sterilizer. Check internal process indicator before treatment. Refer to state regulations for any additional state requirements. Or, the used bur must be disposed of in a sharps container.

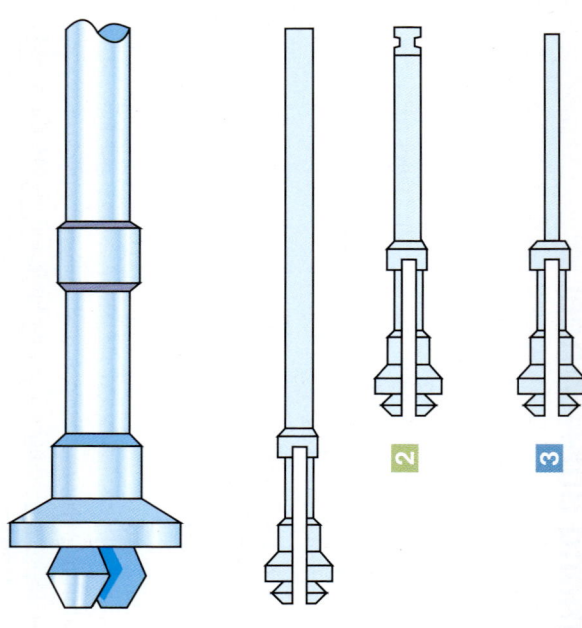

■ INSTRUMENT

Mandrel—Snap On

Function ▶ To attach discs to mandrel for finishing and polishing inside or outside oral cavity (mandrel is inserted into handpiece)

Characteristics ▶ Shank types:

1 Long shank—For straight slow-speed handpiece
2 Short latch-type shank—For contra-angle slow-speed handpiece
3 Friction grip shank—For high-speed handpiece

Plastic disposable Snap On Mandrels available

Practice Notes ▶ Mandrel is inserted and secured in a handpiece.
Type of handpiece determines type of shank used.

Sterilization Notes ▶ Mandrel—Snap On must be precleaned. Then, place in a sterilizing pouch with an internal process indicator, seal, then sterilize. OR, wrap with an internal process indicator inside and secure on the outside with process indicator tape, then sterilize. Verify appropriate color change has been achieved in external process indicator immediately after removal from sterilizer. Check internal process indicator before treatment. Refer to state regulations for any additional state requirements. Disposable snap-on mandrels should be disposed of in the garbage. Single use only.

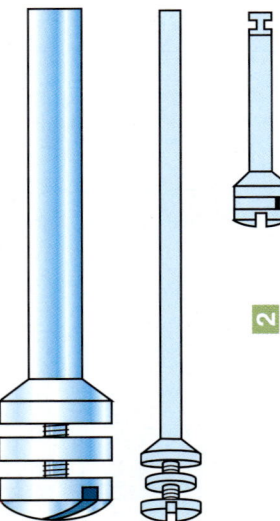

Mandrel—Screw On

Function ▶ To attach discs to mandrel for finishing and polishing inside or outside oral cavity (mandrel is inserted into handpiece)

Characteristics ▶ Shank types:

1 Long shank—For straight slow-speed handpiece

2 Short latch-type shank—For contra-angle or right-angle slow-speed handpiece

3 Friction grip shank—For high-speed handpiece

Practice Notes ▶ Mandrel is inserted and secured in a handpiece.
Type of handpiece determines type of shank used.

Sterilization Notes ▶ Mandrel—Screw On must be precleaned. Then, place in a sterilizing pouch with an internal process indicator, seal, then sterilize. OR, wrap with an internal process indicator inside and secure on the outside with process indicator tape, then sterilize. Verify appropriate color change has been achieved in external process indicator immediately after removal from sterilizer. Check internal process indicator before treatment. Refer to state regulations for any additional state requirements.

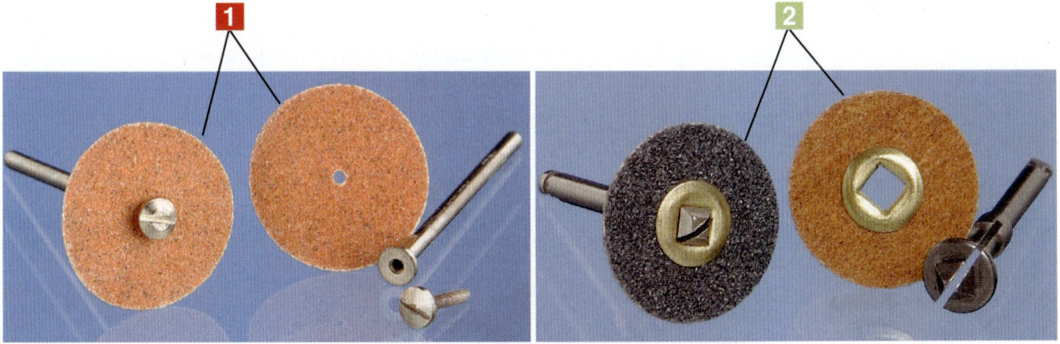

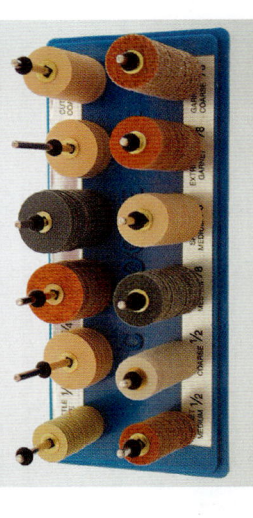

Sandpaper Disc with Screw-Type and Snap-On Mandrel

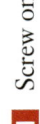

Functions ▶

To contour restorations

To polish restorative material use extra fine grit

Characteristics ▶

Range of grits—Coarse to extra fine

Darker color of disc denotes more abrasiveness

Two types:

1 Screw on

2 Snap on metal center

Sandpaper Disc organizer has a range of sizes and grits.

Sandpaper Disc is attached to either a snap-on mandrel or a screw-on mandrel, depending on the type of Sandpaper Disc being used.

Practice Notes ▶

Sterilization Notes ▶

Disposable Sandpaper Discs should be disposed of in the garbage Single use only. Mandrel must be precleaned. Then, place in a sterilizing pouch with an internal process indicator, seal, then sterilize. OR, wrap with an internal process indicator inside and secure on the outside with process indicator tape, then sterilize. Verify appropriate color change has been achieved in external process indicator immediately after removal from sterilizer. Check internal process indicator before treatment. Refer to state regulations for any additional state requirements.

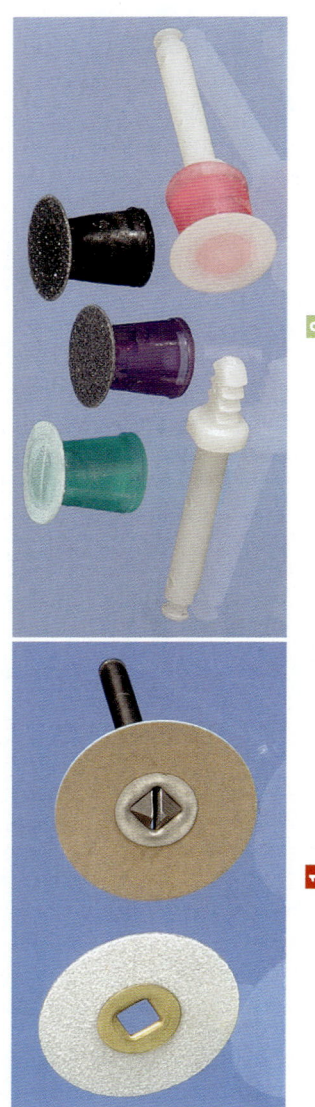

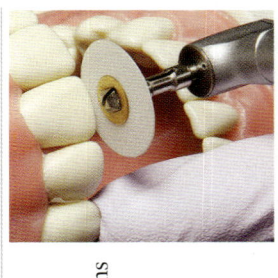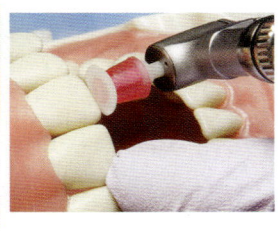

Composite Disc

Functions ▶

To contour restorations

To polish or smooth restorative material use extra fine grit

Characteristics ▶

Made from synthetic material to accommodate composite restorations

Range of grits—Coarse to extra fine

Darker color of disc denotes more abrasiveness

Variety of sizes

Two types available:

1 Snap on composite disc

2 Composite disc with disposable mandrel

Practice Notes ▶

Composite Disc is attached to either a snap-on mandrel or a screw-on mandrel, depending on the type of Composite Disc being used.

Sterilization Notes ▶

Disposable Composite Discs and disposable mandrel should be disposed of in the garbage. Single use only. Metal Mandrel must be precleaned. Then, place in a sterilizing pouch with an internal process indicator, seal, then sterilize. OR, wrap with an internal process indicator inside and secure on the outside with process indicator tape, then sterilize. Verify appropriate color change has been achieved in external process indicator immediately after removal from sterilizer. Check internal process indicator before treatment. Refer to state regulations for any additional state requirements.

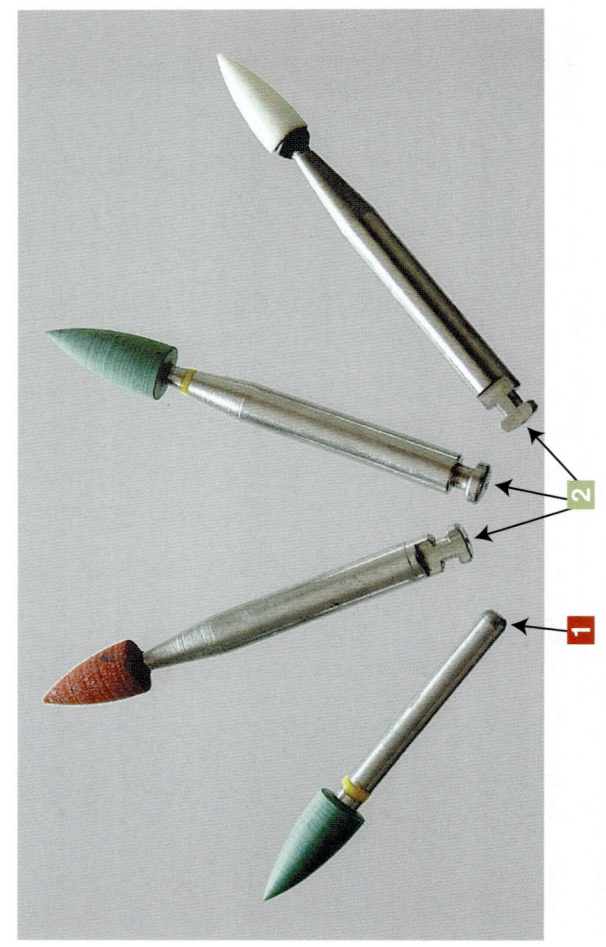

■ INSTRUMENT

Rubber Points

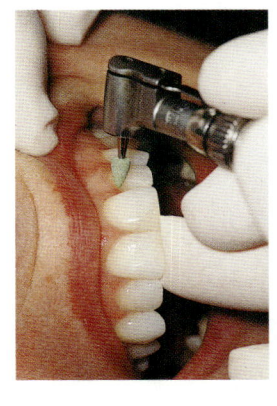

Function ▶ To polish restorations, amalgam, composite, and gold

Characteristics ▶ Types of polishing grits:
Brown points (brownies)—Abrasive
Green points (greenies)—Less abrasive than brownies
White points—Polishing point
Variety of shanks available for all types of rubber points:

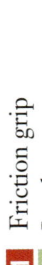

1 Friction grip
2 Latch type

Practice Notes ▶ Rubber Point is inserted and secured in a handpiece.
Type of handpiece determines type of shank used.

Sterilization Notes ▶ Rubber Point must be precleaned. Then, place in a sterilizing pouch with an internal process indicator, seal, then sterilize. OR, wrap with an internal process indicator inside and secure on the outside with process indicator tape, then sterilize. Verify appropriate color change has been achieved in external process indicator immediately after removal from sterilizer. Check internal process indicator before treatment. Refer to state regulations for any additional state requirements.

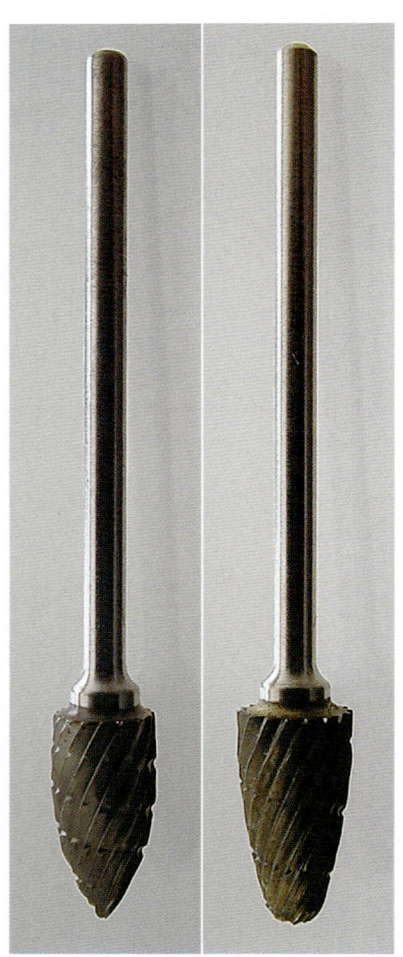

INSTRUMENT

Laboratory Bur—Acrylic Bur

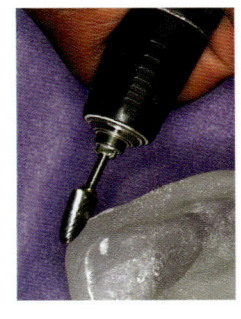

Function ▸ To cut models or trim acrylic in laboratory

Characteristics ▸ Long shank—For attachment to straight handpiece
Variety of sizes and shapes available

Practice Notes ▸ Laboratory Bur is inserted and secured in a slow-speed handpiece with a straight attachment.

Sterilization Notes ▸ Laboratory Bur—Acrylic Bur, when used on any patient's appliances, must be precleaned. Then, place in a sterilizing pouch with an internal process indicator, seal, then sterilize. OR, wrap with an internal process indicator inside and secure on the outside with process indicator tape, then sterilize. Verify appropriate color change has been achieved in external process indicator immediately after removal from sterilizer. Check internal process indicator before treatment. Refer to state regulations for any additional state requirements. Or, the used bur must be disposed of in a sharps container.

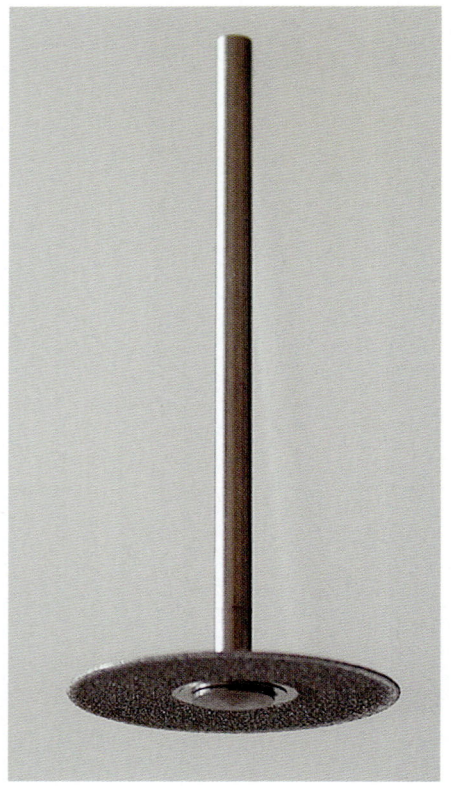

Laboratory Bur—Diamond Disc

INSTRUMENT

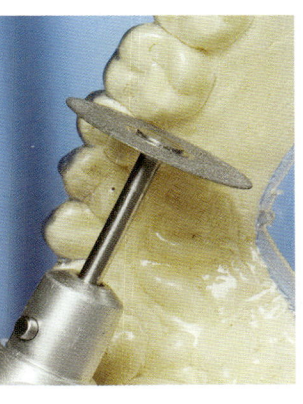

Function ▸ To contour or cut models in the laboratory

Characteristic ▸ Single- or double-sided cutting edge

Variety of sizes available

Practice Note ▸ Laboratory Bur—Diamond Disc is inserted and secured in a slow-speed handpiece with a straight attachment.

Sterilization Notes ▸ Laboratory Bur—Diamond Disc, when used on any patient's appliances, must be precleaned. Then, place in a sterilizing pouch with an internal process indicator, seal, then sterilize. OR, wrap with an internal process indicator inside and secure on the outside with process indicator tape, then sterilize. Verify appropriate color change has been achieved in external process indicator immediately after removal from sterilizer. Check internal process indicator before treatment. Refer to state regulations for any additional state requirements. Or, the used disc must be disposed of in a sharps container.

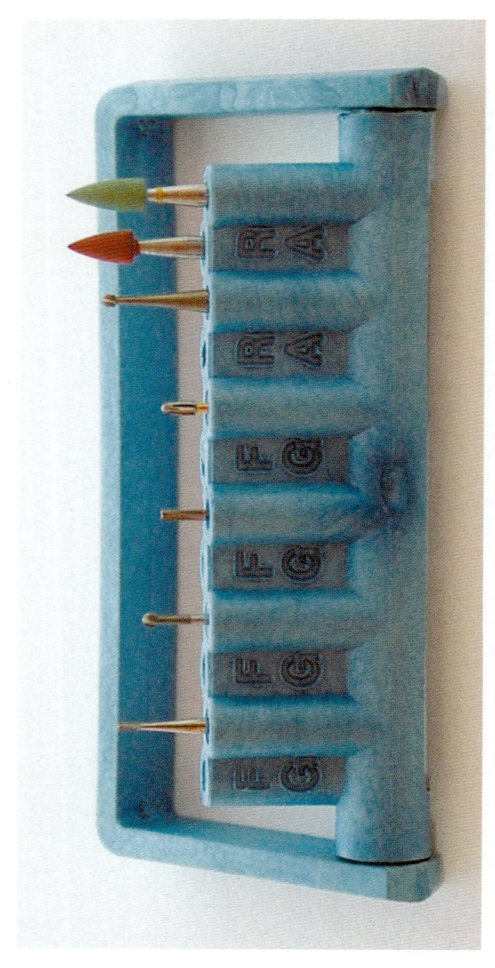

Magnetic Bur Block with Burs

■ INSTRUMENT

Function ▸ To be used on dental tray setups

Characteristics ▸ Magnetic to hold burs in place
Holds friction grip and latch-type burs
Variety of shapes and sizes available
Various colors available to coordinate with color of tray

Practice Note ▸ Magnetic Bur Blocks with Burs are used on most restorative tray setups.

Sterilization Notes ▸ Magnetic Bur Block with Burs must be precleaned. Then, place in a sterilizing pouch with an internal process indicator, seal, then sterilize. OR, wrap with an internal process indicator inside and secure on the outside with process indicator tape, then sterilize. Verify appropriate color change has been achieved in external process indicator immediately after removal from sterilizer. Check internal process indicator before treatment. Refer to state regulations for any additional state requirements. Or, the used bur must be disposed of in a sharps container.

7

Dental Dam Instruments

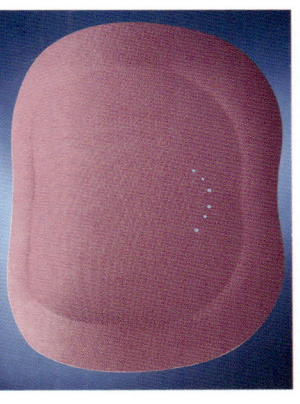

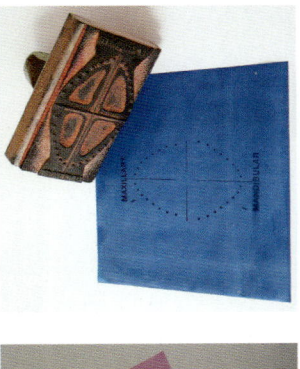

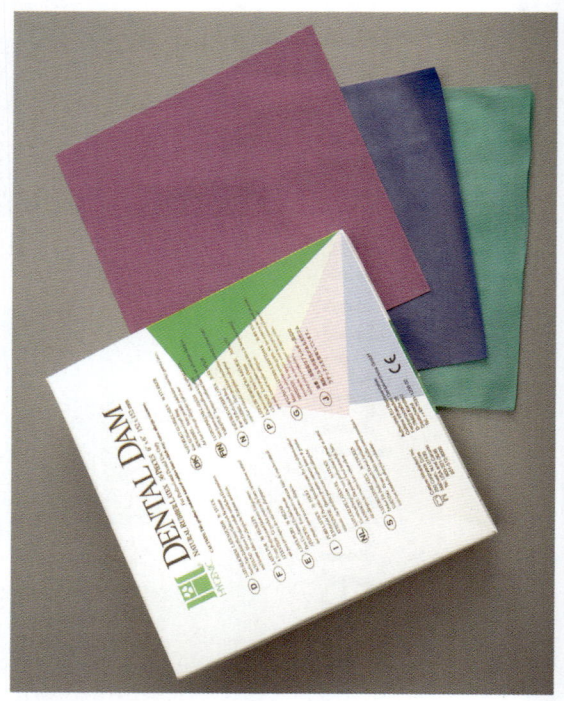

INSTRUMENT

Dental Dam

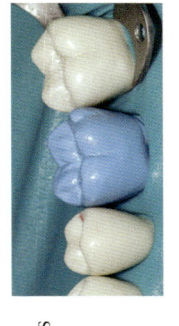

Function ▸ To isolate teeth for dental procedures

Characteristics ▸ Sizes—4 × 4, 5 × 5, 6 × 6, or continuous roll
Gauge or thickness—Thin, medium, heavy
Colors—Gray, green, blue, pastels
Latex free—Available in variety of gauge, thickness, and colors

Practice Notes ▸ Latex-free Dental Dam is used for patients who have latex allergies.

Sterilization Notes ▸ Dental Dam should be disposed of in garbage. Single use only.

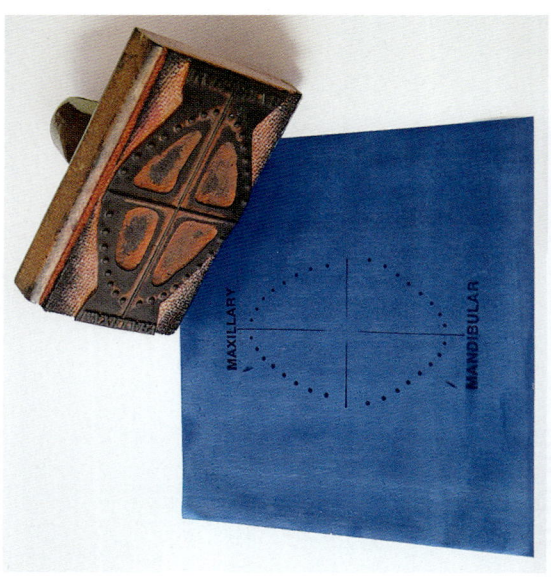

■ INSTRUMENT   Dental Dam Stamp

Function ▶ To mark holes on dental dam

Characteristics ▶ Has 32 dots that represent the adult dentition

Used as guide for punching holes in correct position

Practice Notes ▶ The oral cavity is examined before holes are marked and punched to adjust positioning to the patient's specific dentition.

Sterilization Notes ▶ Dental Dam Stamp should be disinfected according to the manufacturer's recommendation.

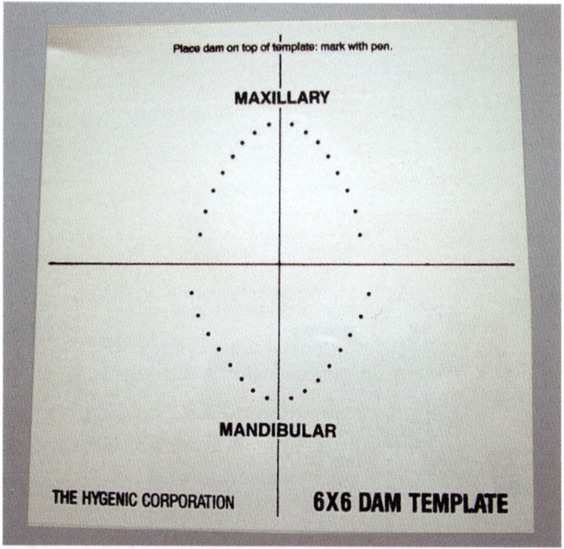

Place dam on top of template; mark with pen.

MAXILLARY

MANDIBULAR

6X6 DAM TEMPLATE

THE HYGENIC CORPORATION

Dental Dam Template

Function ▶ To use as a guide for marking and punching holes in correct position on dental dam

Characteristics ▶ Made of durable plastic

Has 32 dots that represent the adult dentition

Practice Notes ▶ The oral cavity is examined before holes are marked and punched to adjust positioning to the patient's specific dentition.

The dental dam is placed on the template, and the points where holes should be punched are marked with a pen.

Sterilization Notes ▶ Dental Dam Template should be disinfected according to the manufacturer's recommendation.

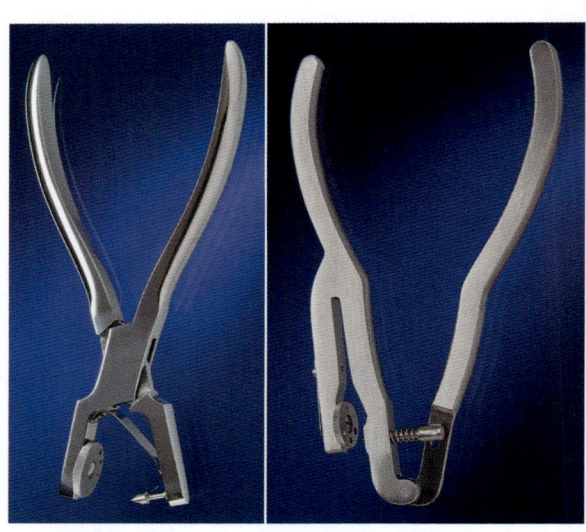

Dental Dam Punch

5 Largest hole
  (clamps)
4 Large hole
  (molars)
3 Medium hole
  (premolars)
2 Small hole
  (maxillary anteriors)
1 Smallest hole
  (mandibular anteriors)

Function ▶ To punch holes in dental dam for each individual tooth

Characteristics ▶ Designated hole size for each tooth for permanent dentition:

No. 5—Anchor tooth (largest)

No. 4—Molars

No. 3—Premolars

No. 2—Maxillary central and laterals, maxillary and mandibular cuspids

No. 1—Mandibular central and laterals (smallest)

Practice Notes ▶ The oral cavity is examined before holes are punched to accommodate the patient's specific dentition.

A space of 3 to 3.5 mm is maintained between holes.

Sterilization Notes ▶ Dental Dam Punch must be precleaned open and unlocked. Then, place in an open and unlocked position in a sterilizing pouch with an internal process indicator, seal, then sterilize. OR, wrap with an internal process indicator inside and secure on the outside with process indicator tape, then sterilize. Verify appropriate color change has been achieved in external process indicator immediately after removal from sterilizer. Check internal process indicator before treatment. Refer to state regulations for any additional state requirements.

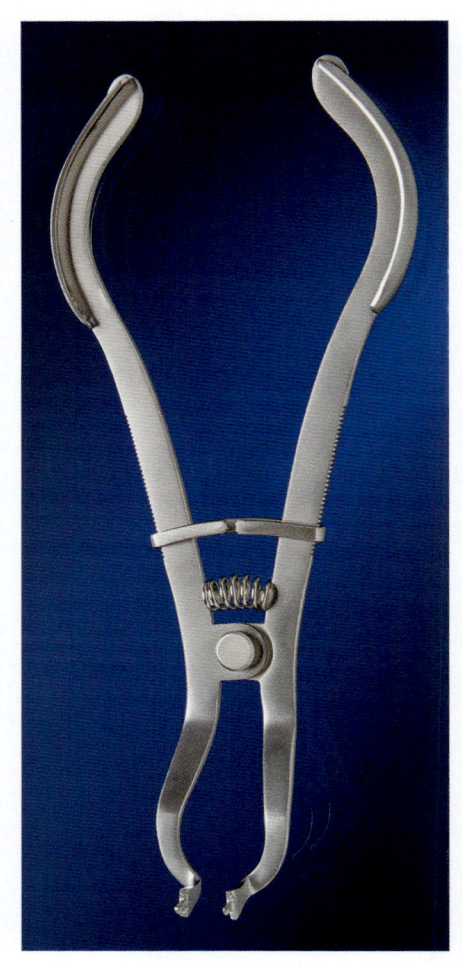

■ INSTRUMENT

Dental Dam Forceps

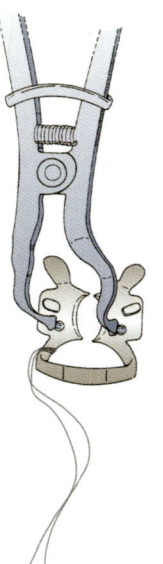

Function ▶ To place dental dam clamp on tooth and to remove clamp after procedure

Characteristics ▶ Beaks on forceps fit into dental dam clamp.

Forceps open with spring motion.

Bar between handle holds forceps in place while clamp is seated.

Practice Note ▶ Squeeze handles on Dental Dam Forceps to open working end.

Sterilization Notes ▶ Dental Dam Forceps must be precleaned open and unlocked. Then, place in an open and unlocked position in a sterilizing pouch with an internal process indicator, seal, then sterilize. OR, wrap with an internal process indicator inside and secure on the outside with process indicator tape, then sterilize. Verify appropriate color change has been achieved in external process indicator immediately after removal from sterilizer. Check internal process indicator before treatment. Refer to state regulations for any additional state requirements. For safety, dental floss (ligature tie) must be attached to each dental clamp before each use to allow for retrieval of clamp if dislodged and patient inhales or swallows.

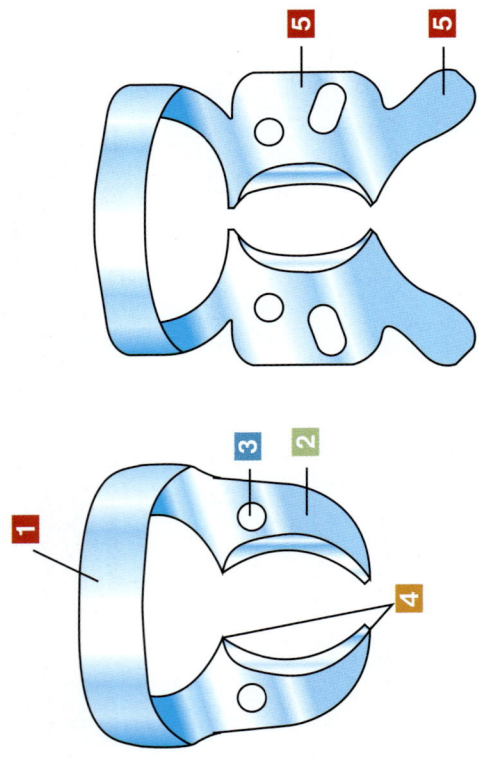

Dental Dam Clamp

Function ▶ To anchor and stabilize dental dam

Characteristics ▶ Parts:

1 Bow: Placed toward distal part of tooth

2 Jaws: Have four prongs that secure clamp on tooth

3 Holes: On jaws; designated for beaks on forceps to place clamp on tooth

4 Prongs: Designed to secure clamp on cervical part of tooth, beyond the height of contour

5 Winged clamps: Have extension of metal on jaws to hold dental dam away from tooth for better visibility. Wingless clamps do not have extra extension of metal.

For safety, dental floss, ligature tie, must be attached to each dental clamp before each use to allow for retrieval of clamp if dislodged and patient inhales or swallows.

Sterilization Notes ▶ Dental Dam Clamp must be precleaned. Then, place in a sterilizing pouch with an internal process indicator, seal, then sterilize. OR, wrap with an internal process indicator inside and secure on the outside with process indicator tape, then sterilize. Verify appropriate color change has been achieved in external process indicator immediately after removal from sterilizer. Check internal process indicator before treatment. Refer to state regulations for any additional state requirements.

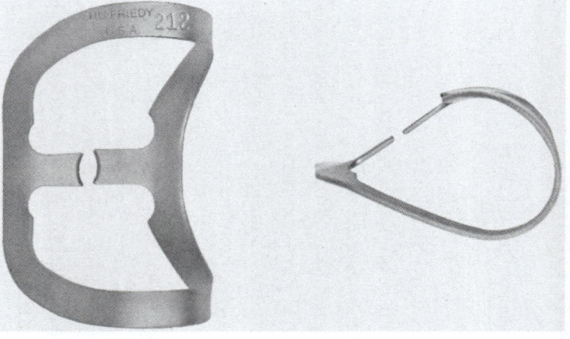

■ INSTRUMENT

Anterior Clamp

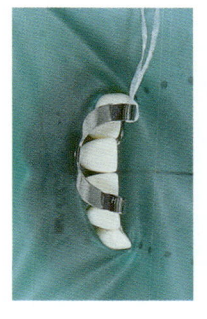

Function ▶ To anchor and stabilize dental dam

Characteristics ▶ Used only on anterior teeth
Example: Wingless clamp

Range of sizes available

Practice Notes ▶ Anterior Clamp is used on a dental dam setup for restorative and endodontic procedures.

For safety, dental floss (ligature tie) must be attached to each dental clamp before each use to allow for retrieval of clamp if dislodged and patient inhales or swallows.

Sterilization Notes ▶ Anterior Clamp must be precleaned. Then, place in a sterilizing pouch with an internal process indicator, seal, then sterilize. OR, wrap with an internal process indicator inside and secure on the outside with process indicator tape, then sterilize. Verify appropriate color change has been achieved in external process indicator immediately after removal from sterilizer. Check internal process indicator before treatment. Refer to state regulations for any additional state requirements.

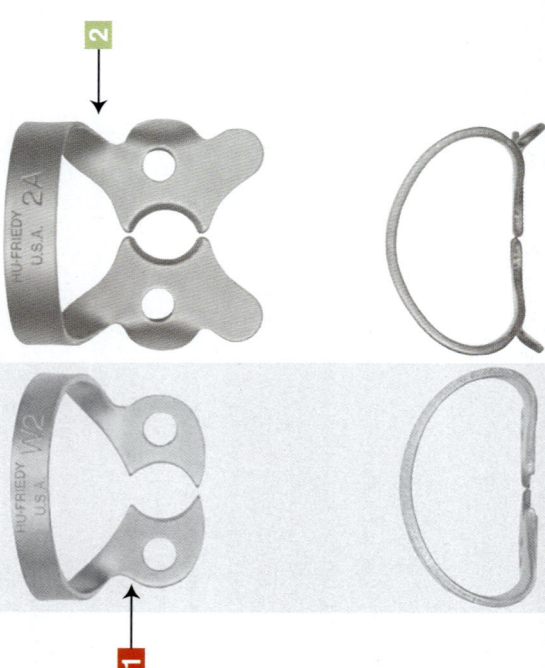

Premolar Clamp

Function ▶ To anchor and stabilize dental dam

Characteristics ▶ Clamp used is determined by tooth size.
Range of sizes available
Variety of styles
Examples:

1. Wingless clamp
2. Winged clamp

Practice Notes ▶ Premolar Clamp is used on a dental dam setup for restorative and endodontic procedures. For safety, dental floss (ligature tie) must be attached to each dental clamp before each use to allow for retrieval of clamp if dislodged and patient inhales or swallows.

Sterilization Notes ▶ Premolar Clamp must be precleaned. Then, place in a sterilizing pouch with an internal process indicator, seal, then sterilize. OR, wrap with an internal process indicator inside and secure on the outside with process indicator tape, then sterilize. Verify appropriate color change has been achieved in external process indicator immediately after removal from sterilizer. Check internal process indicator before treatment. Refer to state regulations for any additional state requirements.

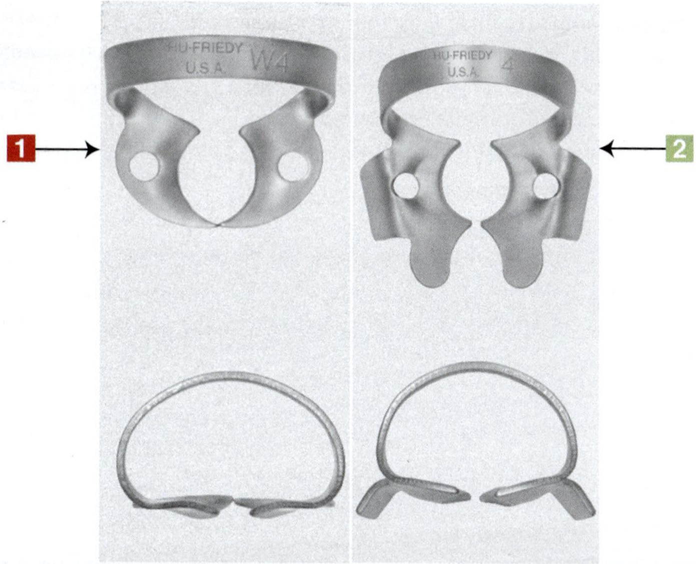
1
2
HU-FRIEDY
U.S.A.
W4
HU-FRIEDY
U.S.A.
4

Universal Clamp—Maxillary

Function ▸ To anchor and stabilize dental dam

Characteristics ▸ Used on right or left posterior molars
Range of sizes available
Variety of styles
Examples:

1 Wingless clamp
2 Winged clamp

Practice Notes ▸ Maxillary Clamp is used on a dental dam setup for restorative and endodontic procedures. For safety, dental floss (ligature tie) must be attached to each dental clamp before each use to allow for retrieval of clamp if dislodged and patient inhales or swallows.

Sterilization Notes ▸ Universal Maxillary Clamp must be precleaned. Then, place in a sterilizing pouch with an internal process indicator, seal, then sterilize. OR, wrap with an internal process indicator inside and secure on the outside with process indicator tape, then sterilize. Verify appropriate color change has been achieved in external process indicator immediately after removal from sterilizer. Check internal process indicator before treatment. Refer to state regulations for any additional state requirements.

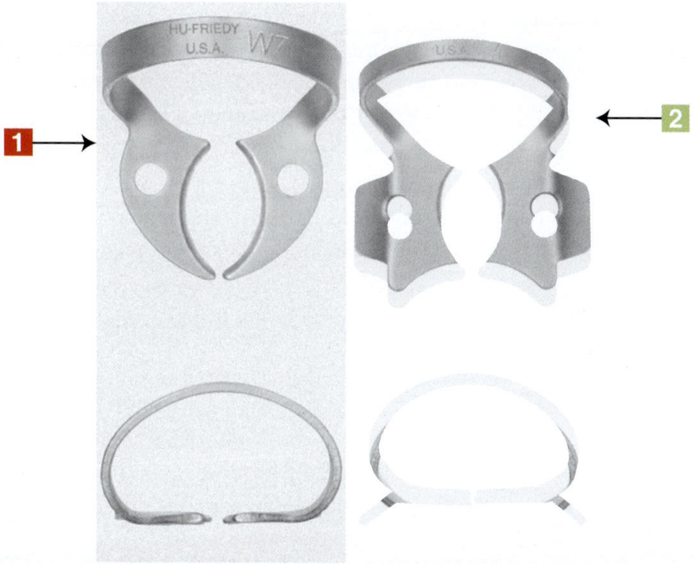
1
2
HU-FRIEDY
U.S.A.
W7
U.S.A.

Universal Clamp—Mandibular

Function ▶ To anchor and stabilize dental dam

Characteristics ▶ Used on right or left posterior molars

Range of sizes available

Variety of styles

Examples:

1 Wingless clamp

2 Winged clamp

Practice Notes ▶ Mandibular Clamp is used on a dental dam setup for restorative and endodontic procedures. For safety, dental floss (ligature tie) must be attached to each dental clamp before each use to allow for retrieval of clamp if dislodged and patient inhales or swallows.

Sterilization Notes ▶ Universal Mandibular Clamp must be precleaned. Then, place in a sterilizing pouch with an internal process indicator, seal, then sterilize. OR, wrap with an internal process indicator inside and secure on the outside with process indicator tape, then sterilize. Verify appropriate color change has been achieved in external process indicator immediately after removal from sterilizer. Check internal process indicator before treatment. Refer to state regulations for any additional state requirements.

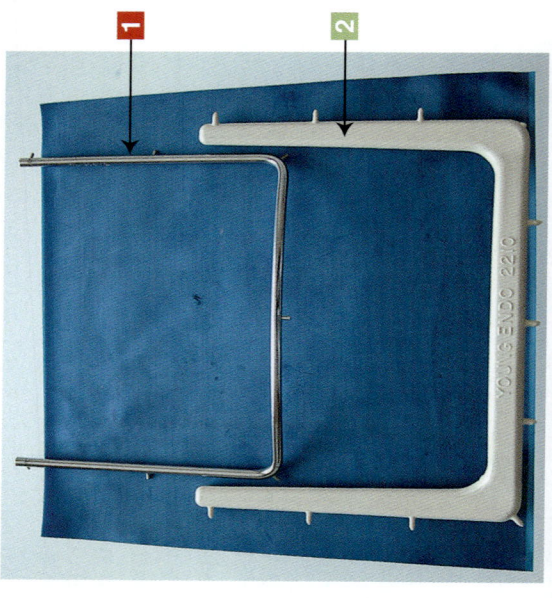

■ INSTRUMENT

Dental Dam Frame

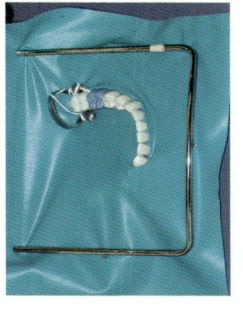

Function ▶ To hold dental dam away from teeth

Characteristics ▶
1 Metal frame
2 Plastic frame

Plastic frame—May be left on during radiographic exposures
Various styles of frames available

Practice Notes ▶ Dental Dam Frame is used on a dental dam setup for restorative and endodontic procedures.

Sterilization Notes ▶ Dental Dam Frame must be precleaned. Then, place in a sterilizing pouch with an internal process indicator, seal, then sterilize. OR, wrap with an internal process indicator inside and secure on the outside with process indicator tape, then sterilize. Verify appropriate color change has been achieved in external process indicator immediately after removal from sterilizer. Check internal process indicator before treatment. Refer to state regulations for any additional state requirements.

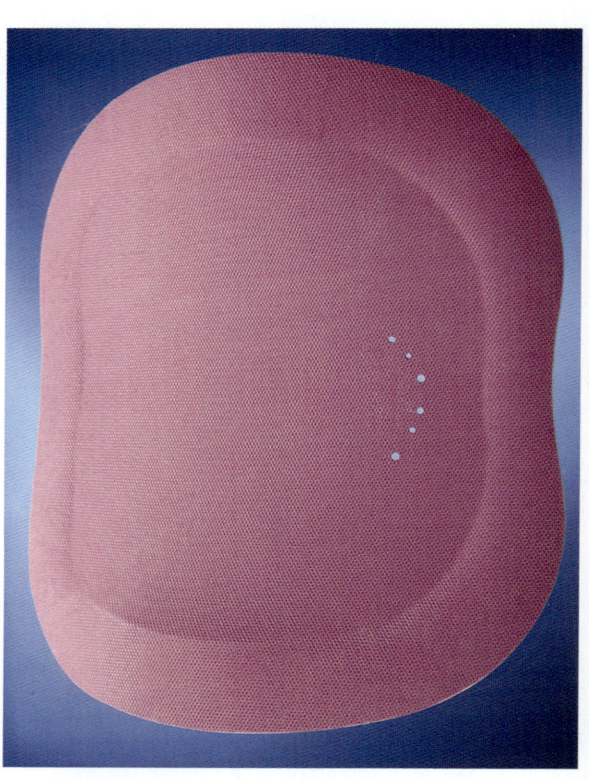

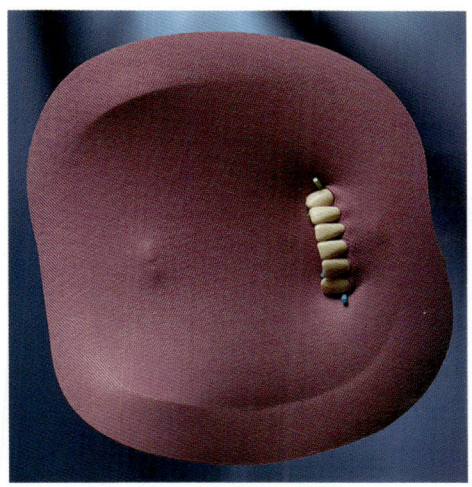

■ INSTRUMENT

Preframed Dental Dam

Function ▶ To isolate teeth for dental procedures

Characteristics ▶ Frame is attached to dental dam

Dental dams may come pre-punched—Additional holes can be punched

Practice Note ▶ Dental Dam is latex free. Shown in picture

Dam adjusts to the side for easy access for radiograph

Dam shown with secure ligatures to hold Dental Dam in place instead of Dental Dam clamp.

Sterilization Notes ▶ Dental Dam should be disposed of in garbage. Single use only.

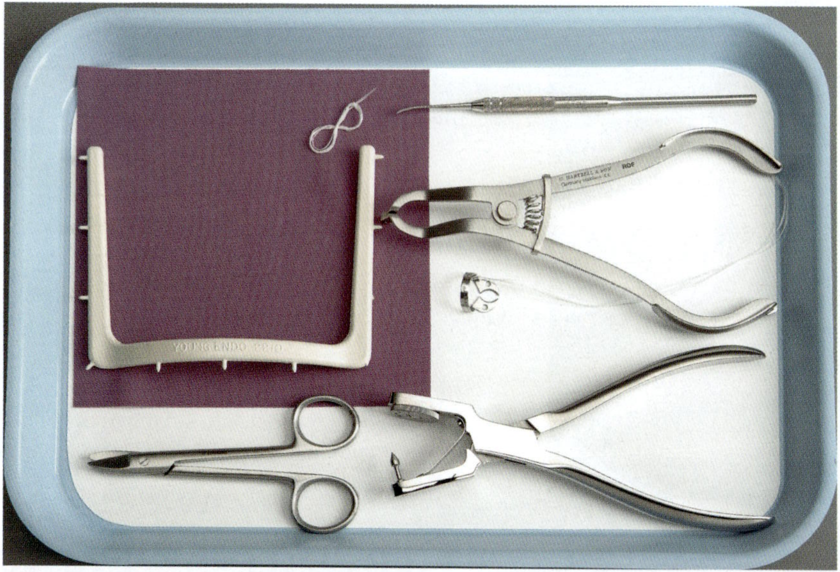

■ TRAY SETUP

Dental Dam

LEFT (TOP TO BOTTOM)

Dental Dam (latex free), dental floss, plastic Dental Dam Frame, crown and bridge scissors (see Chapter 10)

RIGHT (TOP TO BOTTOM)

Beavertail burnisher used to invert Dental Dam (see Chapter 8), Dental Dam Forceps, Dental Dam Clamp with stabilizing ligature tie (dental floss), Dental Dam Punch

Sterilization Notes ▶ Refer to each individual instrument for correct procedure for sterilization or disposal of material.

8

Amalgam Restorative Instruments

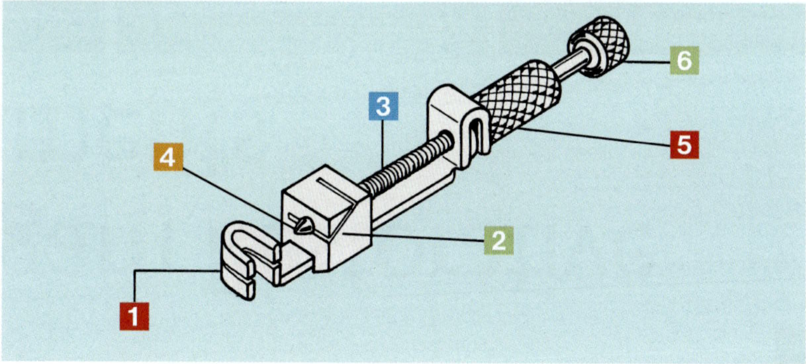
6
3
5
4
2
1

Tofflemire/Matrix Band Retainer

Function ▶ To hold and maintain stability of matrix band during condensation of restorative material for class II preparation

Characteristics ▶ Parts:

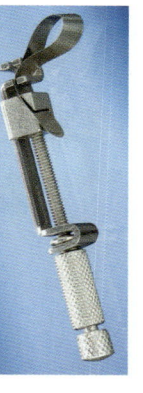

1 Guide slots: Straight slot; right and left slots for right or left quadrant

2 Diagonal slot: Slides up and down on spindle; matrix band is placed in slot, and spindle secures band in place; open slots are placed toward gingiva.

3 Spindle: Holds matrix band in retainer

4 Spindle pin: Stabilizes band in holder

5 Inner knob: Adjusts size of the loop of matrix band to fit around tooth and loosens band for removal

6 Outer knob: Positioned at end of spindle that tightens or loosens matrix band in retainer

Practice Notes ▶ Tofflemire Band Retainer is used on restorative tray setups.

The photo shown is for maxillary right quadrant and mandibular left quadrant.

Sterilization Notes ▶ Tofflemire Band Retainer must be precleaned with spindle disengaged. Then, place in an open position in a sterilizing pouch with an internal process indicator, seal, then sterilize. OR, wrap with an internal process indicator inside and secure on the outside with process indicator tape, then sterilize. Verify appropriate color change has been achieved in external process indicator immediately after removal from sterilizer. Check internal process indicator before treatment. Refer to state regulations for any additional state requirements.

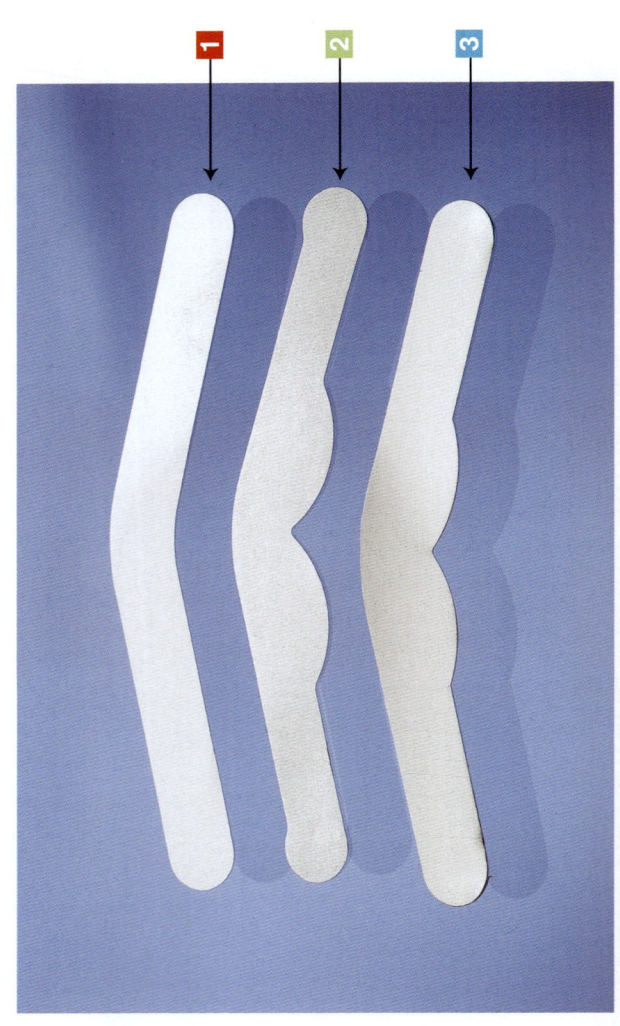

■ INSTRUMENT

Matrix Bands

Function ▸ To replace missing proximal wall or walls of cavity preparation for condensation of restorative material for class II preparations

Characteristics ▸ Variety of sizes, shapes, and thicknesses
Bands designed for specific types of restorations:

1. Universal band—For restorations on all posterior teeth except for teeth with deep cervical restorations—Example: MO, DO, MOD

2. Bands for teeth with deep cervical restorations—Example: Premolars that have a deep cervical restoration. Example: MO, DO, or MOD

3. Bands for larger teeth with deep cervical restorations—Example: Larger teeth such as molars that have a deep cervical restoration. Example: MO, DO, MOD

Variety of pediatric bands available for primary teeth

Practice Note ▸ Matrix Bands are used on amalgam, composite, buildup, and temporary filling tray setups.

Sterilization Notes ▸ Matrix Bands should be disposed of in a sharps container, and/or local and state regulations should be followed. Single use only.

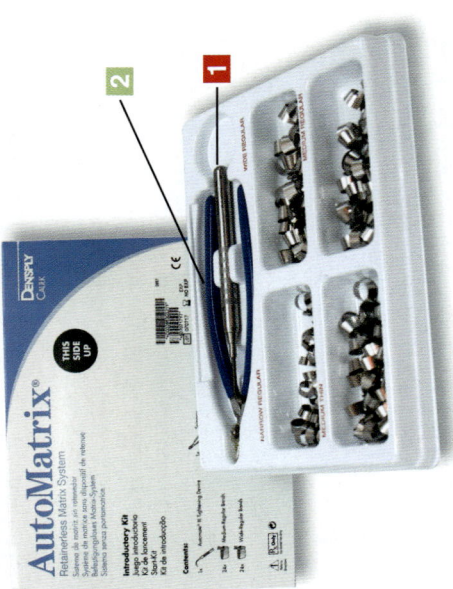

Matrix Band System

Function ▶ To replace missing proximal wall or walls of cavity preparation for condensation of restorative material for class II preparations

Characteristics ▶ Variety of matrix band systems: Pictured: AutoMatrix
Variety of sizes and shapes
Bands designed for specific teeth:

- Universal—Posterior teeth
- Molar—Larger molars
- Premolar—Medium size bands
- Pediatric—Primary teeth

Practice Notes ▶ 1 Tightening wrench is used to place, tighten, and loosen bands.

2 Removing pliers are used to remove bands.

Matrix Bands are used on amalgam, composite, buildup, and temporary filling tray setups.

Sterilization Notes ▶ Matrix Bands should be disposed of in sharps container, or local and state regulations should be followed. Single use only. Matrix Band Instruments must be precleaned open and unlocked. Then, place in an open and unlocked position in a sterilizing pouch with an internal process indicator, seal, then sterilize. OR, wrap with an internal process indicator inside and secure on the outside with process indicator tape, then sterilize. Verify appropriate color change has been achieved in external process indicator immediately after removal from sterilizer. Check internal process indicator before treatment. Refer to state regulations for any additional state requirements.

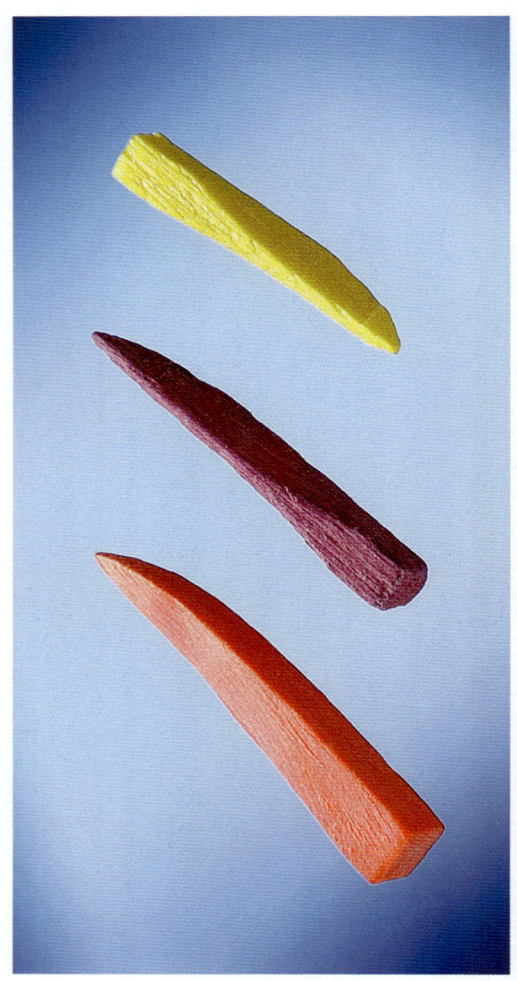

Wooden Wedges

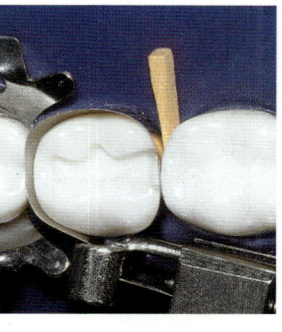

■ INSTRUMENT

Function ▶ To hold matrix band in place along gingival margin of class II, class III, or class IV preparation

Characteristics ▶ Wood or plastic
Triangular, round, or anatomical shapes (shown in picture)
Variety of sizes and shapes available to accommodate embrasure area

Practice Notes ▶ Wedges are placed in gingival embrasure area usually on the lingual.
Wedges are always set up with all types of matrix band systems for class II, class III, or class IV restorations.

Sterilization Notes ▶ Wooden Wedges should be disposed of in the garbage.
Single use only.

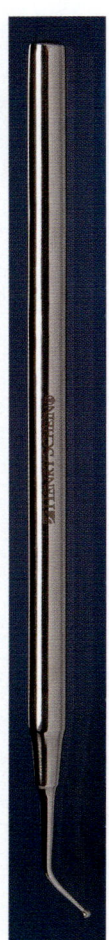

Liner Applicator

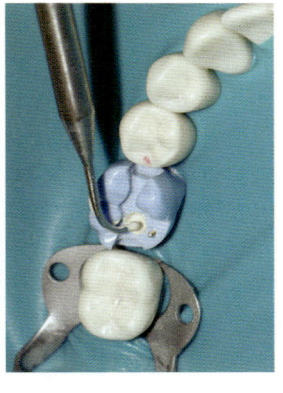

Function ▸ To place dental liner material (such as calcium hydroxide or glass ionomer) in cavity preparation

Characteristics ▸ Short or long handle
Single or double ended

Practice Notes ▸ Liner Applicator is used on amalgam, composite, crown and bridge, and temporary filling tray setups.
Also referred to as a Dycal instrument

Sterilization Notes ▸ Liner Applicator must be precleaned. Then, place in a sterilizing pouch with an internal process indicator, seal, then sterilize. OR, wrap with an internal process indicator inside and secure on the outside with process indicator tape, then sterilize. Verify appropriate color change has been achieved in external process indicator immediately after removal from sterilizer. Check internal process indicator before treatment. Refer to state regulations for any additional state requirements.

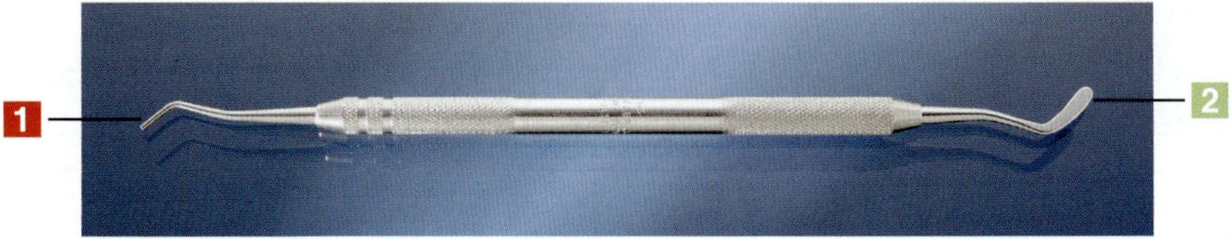
1
2

Woodson

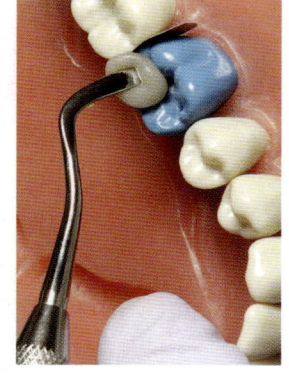

Functions ▶ To carry and place temporary restorative material for cavity preparation—Paddle end

To condense restorative material—Plugger end

To carry (paddle end) and condense a base (Plugger end)

Characteristics ▶ Double ended

Range of sizes available:

1 Plugger end available in variety of sizes

2 Paddle end available in different angles, sizes

Practice Notes ▶ Woodson is used on amalgam, composite, crown and bridge, temporary filling, and provisional crown tray setups.

Sterilization Notes ▶ Woodson must be precleaned. Then, place in a sterilizing pouch with an internal process indicator, seal, then sterilize. OR, wrap with an internal process indicator inside and secure on the outside with process indicator tape, then sterilize. Verify appropriate color change has been achieved in external process indicator immediately after removal from sterilizer. Check internal process indicator before treatment. Refer to state regulations for any additional state requirements.

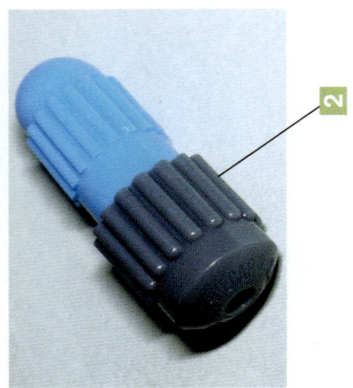

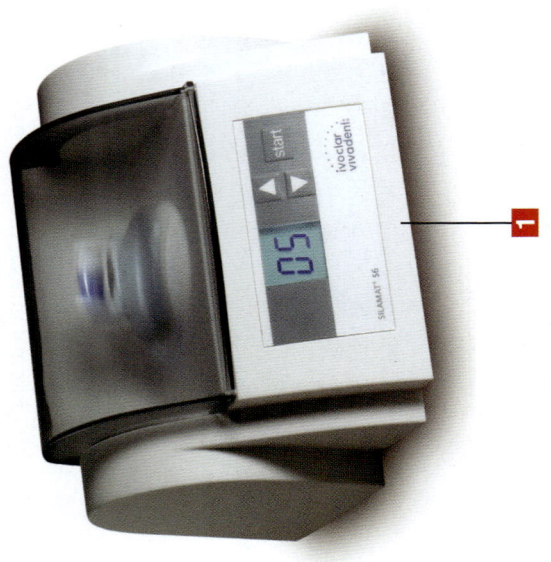

Amalgamator and Amalgam Capsule

Functions ▶

To mix alloy and mercury into amalgam in a capsule

To mix other types of restorative materials in a capsule

To mix precapsulated permanent and temporary cements

Characteristics ▶

1 Amalgamator

2 Preloaded amalgam capsules contain alloy, mercury, and pestle to aid mixing:

- Various types of capsules are available; they are activated manually by twisting or pushing or using a capsule activator.

Thin membrane separates materials until mixing occurs.

Practice Notes ▶

The process of mixing is called amalgamation or trituration.

The mixing time recommended by the manufacturer should be used.

Sterilization Notes ▶

Capsules must be disposed of in the garbage, or state regulations must be followed. Single use only. Excess amalgam must be disposed of as amalgam waste material. Refer to local and state regulations for disposal. Amalgamator should be handled with overgloves or precleaned and disinfected according to the manufacturer's recommendation.

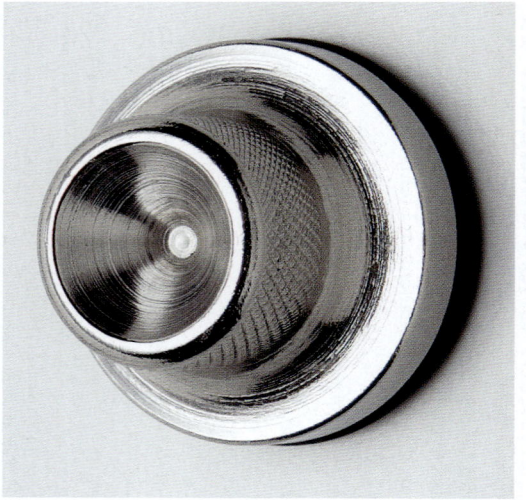

■ INSTRUMENT

Amalgam Well

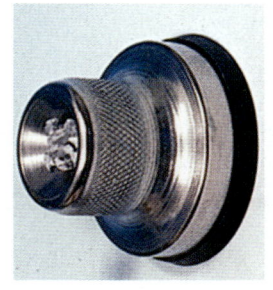

Functions ▶ To hold amalgam before it is placed in preparation
To hold amalgam while loading amalgam carrier

Characteristic ▶ Metal (shown in picture), plastic, or glass

Practice Notes ▶ Amalgam Well is used on the amalgam tray setup.

Sterilization Notes ▶ Amalgam Well must be precleaned. Then, place in a sterilizing pouch with an internal process indicator, seal, then sterilize. OR, wrap with an internal process indicator inside and secure on the outside with process indicator tape, then sterilize. Verify appropriate color change has been achieved in external process indicator immediately after removal from sterilizer. Check internal process indicator before treatment. Refer to state regulations for any additional state requirements. Excess amalgam must be disposed of as amalgam waste material. Refer to local and state regulations for disposal.

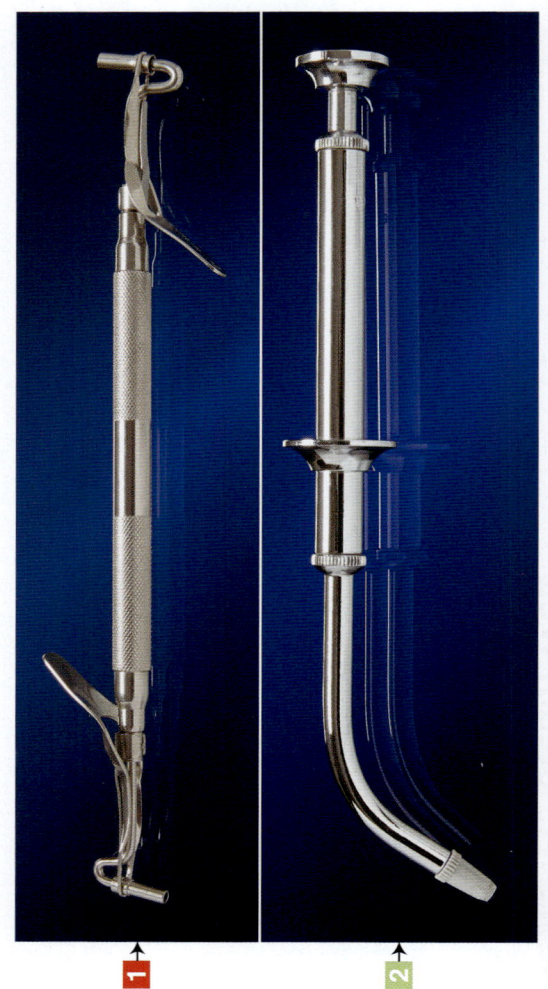

1

2

Amalgam Carrier

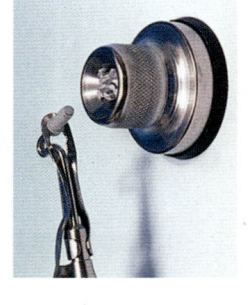

Function ▶ To carry and dispense amalgam into cavity preparation

Characteristics ▶ Single or double ended:

1 Double ended—One small end and one large end

2 Single ended—Plunger style

The inside of the hollow tubes is coated with metal or Teflon.

Practice Notes ▶ Amalgam is packed in hollow tubes and then transferred to the cavity preparation. Amalgam sticks in the carrier if it is not released immediately after the tubes are filled. Amalgam Carrier is used exclusively on amalgam tray setups.

Sterilization Notes ▶ Amalgam Carrier must be precleaned. Then, place in a sterilizing pouch with an internal process indicator, seal, then sterilize. OR, wrap with an internal process indicator inside and secure on the outside with process indicator tape, then sterilize. Verify appropriate color change has been achieved in external process indicator immediately after removal from sterilizer. Check internal process indicator before treatment. Refer to state regulations for any additional state requirements. Excess amalgam must be disposed of as amalgam waste material. Refer to local and state regulations for disposal.

1
2

Condenser (Plugger)—Smooth and Serrated

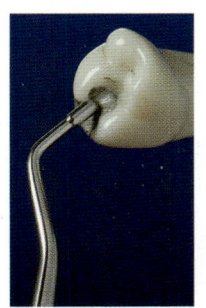

Functions ▶

To pack and condense amalgam into cavity preparation

To pack and condense other restorative materials

To pack and condense temporary filling material

Characteristics ▶

1 Smooth end small
2 Smooth end large

Round, flat, diamond shaped or serrated ends available

Single or double ended

• Double ended—One small end and one large end

Back action condenser available with right-angle working ends—
Accommodates difficult areas

Range of sizes available

Practice Notes ▶

Smooth and Serrated Condensers are used on amalgam, composite, and temporary filling tray setups.

Sterilization Notes ▶

Smooth and Serrated Condensers must be precleaned. Then, place in a sterilizing pouch with an internal process indicator, seal, then sterilize. OR, wrap with an internal process indicator inside and secure on the outside with process indicator tape, then sterilize. Verify appropriate color change has been achieved in external process indicator immediately after removal from sterilizer. Check internal process indicator before treatment. Refer to state regulations for any additional state requirements. Excess amalgam must be disposed of as amalgam waste material. Refer to local and state regulations for disposal.

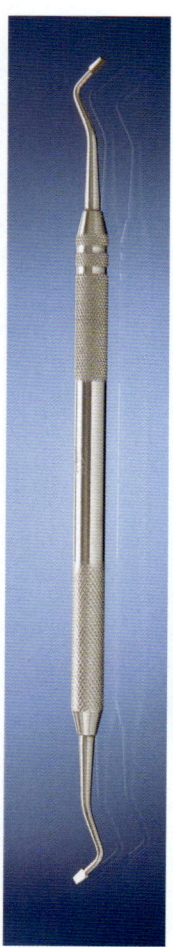

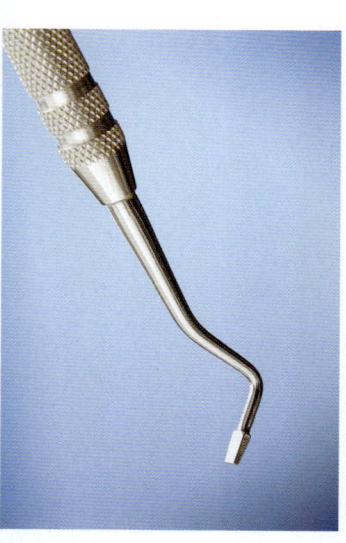

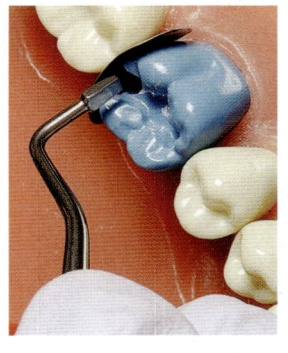

■ **INSTRUMENT**

Interproximal Condenser

Functions ▲ To pack and condense amalgam into interproximal areas of cavity preparation

To pack and condense other restorative materials

Characteristics ▲ Ends shaped to fit mesial or distal areas of cavity preparation

Smooth or serrated ends

Range of sizes available

Practice Note ▲ Interproximal Condenser is used on amalgam, composite, and temporary filling tray setups.

Sterilization Notes ▲ Interproximal Condenser must be precleaned. Then, place in a sterilizing pouch with an internal process indicator, seal, then sterilize. OR, wrap with an internal process indicator inside and secure on the outside with process indicator tape, then sterilize. Verify appropriate color change has been achieved in external process indicator immediately after removal from sterilizer. Check internal process indicator before treatment. Refer to state regulations for any additional state requirements. Excess amalgam must be disposed of as amalgam waste material. Refer to local and state regulations for disposal.

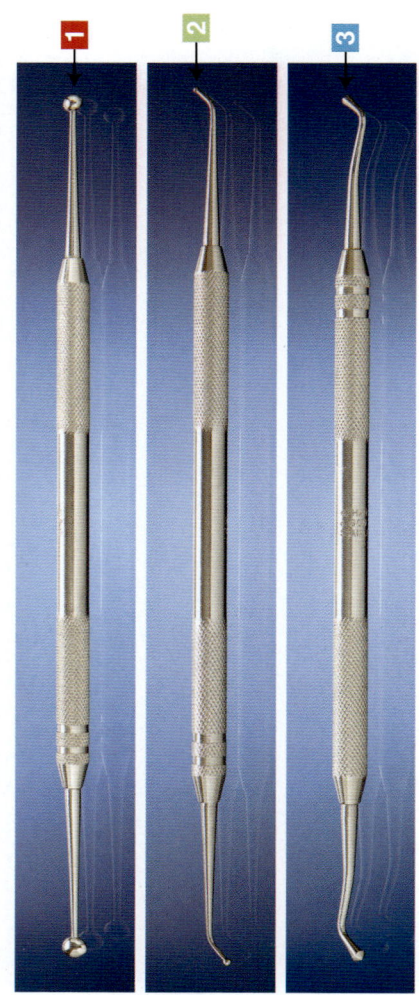

Burnishers—Football, Ball, and Acorn

Functions ▶

To smooth amalgam after condensing

To contour matrix band before placement

To perform initial shaping of amalgam

To burnish restorative material

To burnish temporary filling material

Characteristics ▶

1. Football burnisher
2. Ball burnisher
3. Acorn burnisher

Single or double ended—Some double ended burnishers may have two different types of burnishers

Practice Note ▶

Football, Ball, and Acorn Burnishers are used on amalgam, composite, and temporary filling tray setups.

Sterilization Notes ▶

Football, Ball, and Acorn Burnishers must be precleaned. Then, place in a sterilizing pouch with an internal process indicator, seal, then sterilize. OR, wrap with an internal process indicator inside and secure on the outside with process indicator tape, then sterilize. Verify appropriate color change has been achieved in external process indicator immediately after removal from sterilizer. Check internal process indicator before treatment. Refer to state regulations for any additional state requirements. Excess amalgam must be disposed of as amalgam waste material. Refer to local and state regulations for disposal.

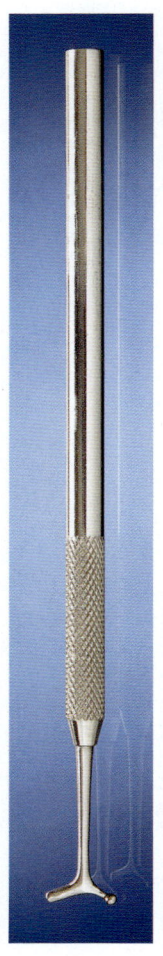

T-Ball Burnisher

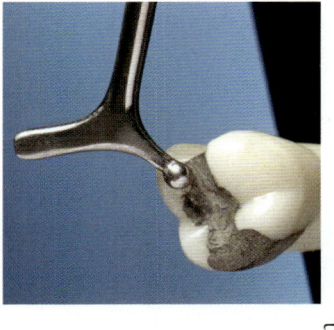

Functions ▸
To smooth amalgam after condensing
To contour matrix band before placement
To begin shaping of amalgam
To burnish restorative materials
To burnish temporary filling material

Characteristic ▸
Single ended

Practice Notes ▸
T-Ball Burnisher is used on amalgam, composite, and temporary filling tray setups.

Sterilization Notes ▸
T-Ball Burnisher must be precleaned. Then, place in a sterilizing pouch with an internal process indicator, seal, then sterilize. OR, wrap with an internal process indicator inside and secure on the outside with process indicator tape, then sterilize. Verify appropriate color change has been achieved in external process indicator immediately after removal from sterilizer. Check internal process indicator before treatment. Refer to state regulations for any additional state requirements. Excess amalgam must be disposed of as amalgam waste material. Refer to local and state regulations for disposal of amalgam.

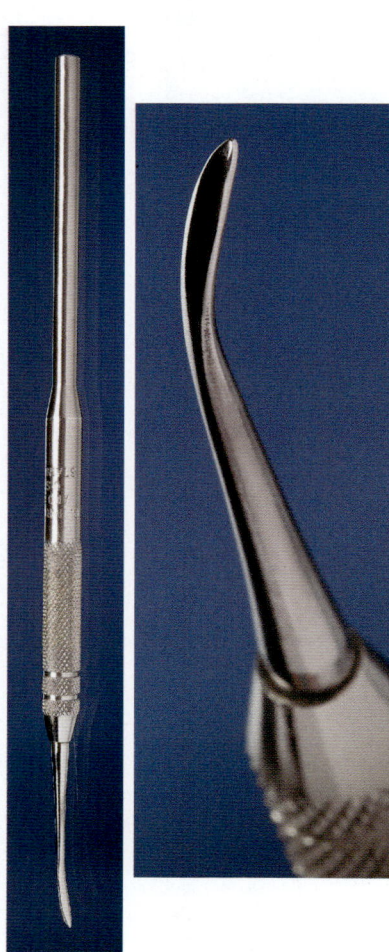

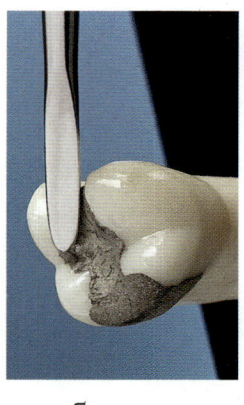

Beavertail Burnisher

Functions ▶

To smooth amalgam after condensing

To perform initial shaping and/or carving of amalgam

To invert dental dam (refer to dental dam tray setup in Chapter 7)

To burnish restorative materials

To burnish temporary filling material

Characteristic ▶

Single or double ended

Practice Note ▶

Beavertail Burnisher is used on amalgam, temporary filling, and dental dam tray setups.

Sterilization Notes ▶

Beavertail Burnisher must be precleaned. Then, place in a sterilizing pouch with an internal process indicator, seal, then sterilize. OR, wrap with an internal process indicator inside and secure on the outside with process indicator tape, then sterilize. Verify appropriate color change has been achieved in external process indicator immediately after removal from sterilizer. Check internal process indicator before treatment. Refer to state regulations for any additional state requirements. Excess amalgam must be disposed of as amalgam waste material. Refer to local and state regulations for disposal of amalgam.

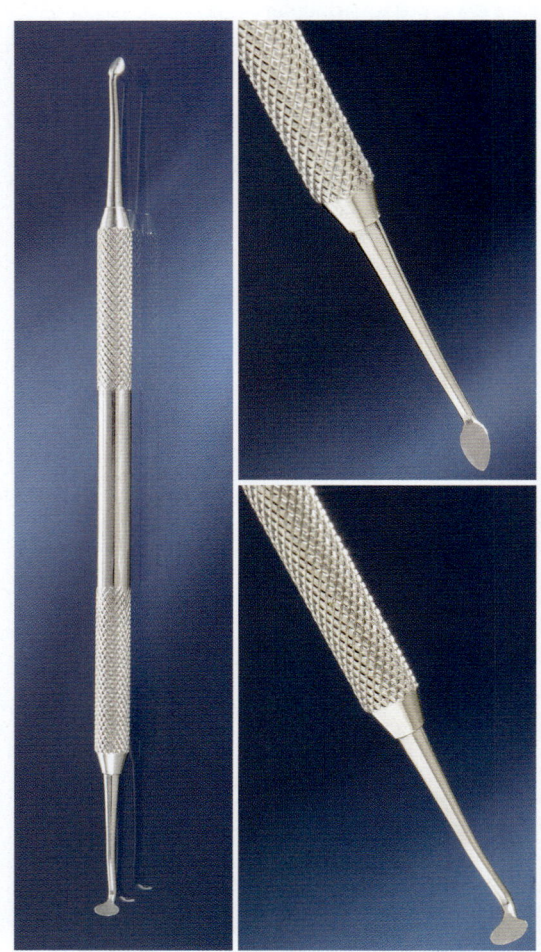

INSTRUMENT

Tanner Carver

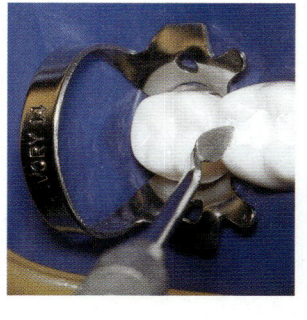

Functions ▶ To carve occlusal anatomy into amalgam restorations

To carve occlusal anatomy in other restorative and temporary filling materials

Characteristics ▶ Double ended—Two ends shaped differently

Ends shaped differently from those of discoid-cleoid carver

Practice Notes ▶ Tanner Carver is used on amalgam and temporary filling tray setups.

Sterilization Notes ▶ Tanner Carver must be precleaned. Then, place in a sterilizing pouch with an internal process indicator, seal, then sterilize. OR, wrap with an internal process indicator inside and secure on the outside with process indicator tape, then sterilize. Verify appropriate color change has been achieved in external process indicator immediately after removal from sterilizer. Check internal process indicator before treatment. Refer to state regulations for any additional state requirements. Excess amalgam must be disposed of as amalgam waste material. Refer to local and state regulations for disposal of amalgam.

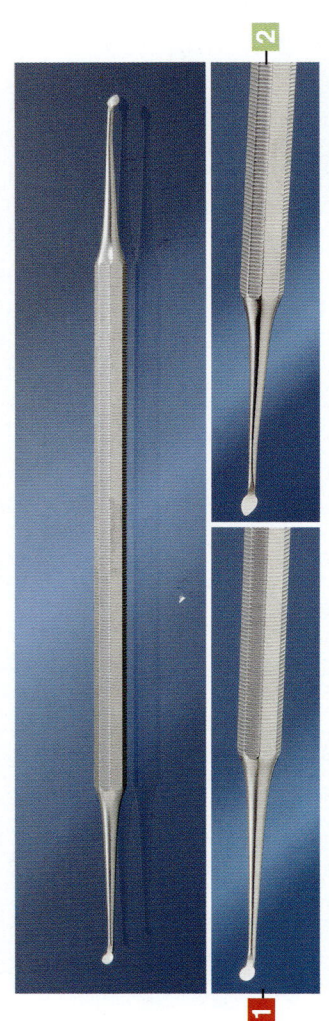

INSTRUMENT

Discoid-Cleoid Carver

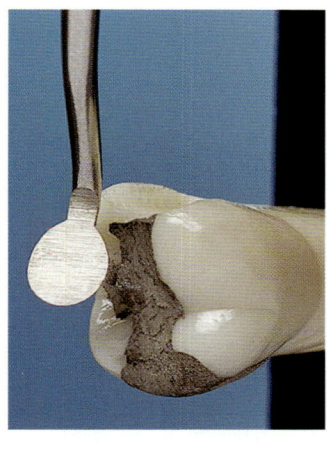

Functions ▶ To carve occlusal anatomy into amalgam restorations

To carve occlusal anatomy in other restorative and temporary filling materials

Characteristics ▶ Double ended—Two ends shaped differently:

1 Discoid end—Disc shaped

2 Cleoid end—Pointed

Ends shaped differently from those of Tanner carver

Practice Notes ▶ Discoid-Cleoid Carver is used on amalgam and temporary tray setups.

Sterilization Notes ▶ Discoid-Cleoid Carver must be precleaned. Then, place in a sterilizing pouch with an internal process indicator, seal, then sterilize. OR, wrap with an internal process indicator inside and secure on the outside with process indicator tape, then sterilize. Verify appropriate color change has been achieved in external process indicator immediately after removal from sterilizer. Check internal process indicator before treatment. Refer to state regulations for any additional state requirements. Excess amalgam must be disposed of as amalgam waste material. Refer to local and state regulations for disposal of amalgam.

1

2

Hollenback and Half-Hollenback Carvers

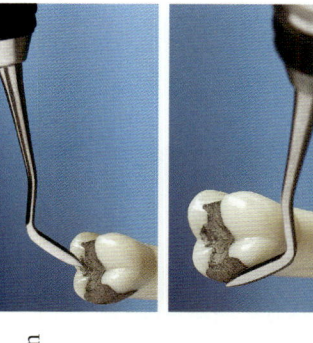

Functions ▶ To contour and carve occlusal and interproximal anatomy in amalgam restorations

To contour and carve occlusal and interproximal anatomy in other restorative and temporary filling materials

Characteristics ▶ 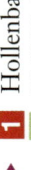 Hollenback

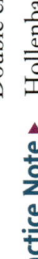 Half-Hollenback—Half the size of Hollenback carver

Double ended—Working ends protrude at different angles.

Practice Note ▶ Hollenback and Half-Hollenback Carvers are used on amalgam, composite, and temporary filling tray setups.

Sterilization Notes ▶ Hollenback and Half-Hollenback Carvers must be precleaned. Then, place in a sterilizing pouch with an internal process indicator, seal, then sterilize. OR, wrap with an internal process indicator inside and secure on the outside with process indicator tape, then sterilize. Verify appropriate color change has been achieved in external process indicator immediately after removal from sterilizer. Check internal process indicator before treatment. Refer to state regulations for any additional state requirements. Excess amalgam must be disposed of as amalgam waste material. Refer to local and state regulations for disposal of amalgam.

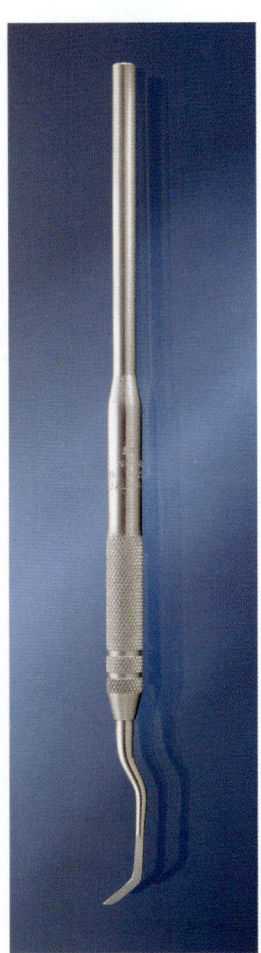

Gold Carving Knife

Functions ▸ To trim interproximal amalgam restoration, recreating contour of proximal wall(s)

To trim interproximal restorations with other restorative materials, recreating contour of proximal wall(s)

To remove flash composite material from interproximal areas

Characteristics ▸ Single or double ended

Variety of designs

Interproximal carving knife—Different styles available

Practice Notes ▸ Gold Carving Knife is used on amalgam and composite restorative tray setups.

Sterilization Notes ▸ Gold Carving Knife must be precleaned. Then, place in a sterilizing pouch with an internal process indicator, seal, then sterilize. OR, wrap with an internal process indicator inside and secure on the outside with process indicator tape, then sterilize. Verify appropriate color change has been achieved in external process indicator immediately after removal from sterilizer. Check internal process indicator before treatment. Refer to state regulations for any additional state requirements. Excess amalgam must be disposed of as amalgam waste material. Refer to local and state regulations for disposal of amalgam.

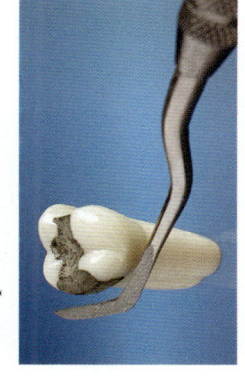

1

2

Articulating Paper Holder

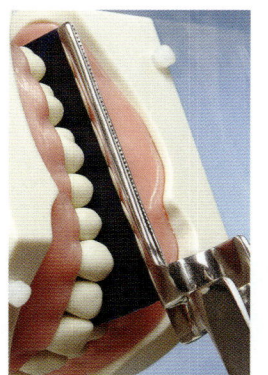

Functions ▶

To hold articulating paper in place

To check centric and lateral occlusion

Characteristics ▶

1 Metal articulating paper holder

2 Disposable articulating paper holder

Articulating paper—Blue (top) or red (bottom)

Paper variety—From thin to thick

Practice Notes ▶

Articulating Paper Holder and articulating paper are used on all restorative tray setups, including but not limited to amalgam, composite, fixed and removable prosthodontics, provisional crown, endodontics, orthodontic retainer delivery, and temporary filling tray setups.

Sterilization Notes ▶

Articulating Paper Holder (metal type) must be precleaned. Then, place in a sterilizing pouch with an internal process indicator, seal, then sterilize. OR, wrap with an internal process indicator inside and secure on the outside with process indicator tape, then sterilize. Verify appropriate color change has been achieved in external process indicator immediately after removal from sterilizer. Check internal process indicator before treatment. Refer to state regulations for any additional state requirements. Disposable Articulating Paper Holder and Articulating Paper should be disposed of in the garbage. Single use only. Excess amalgam must be disposed of as amalgam waste material. Refer to local and state regulations for disposal of amalgam.

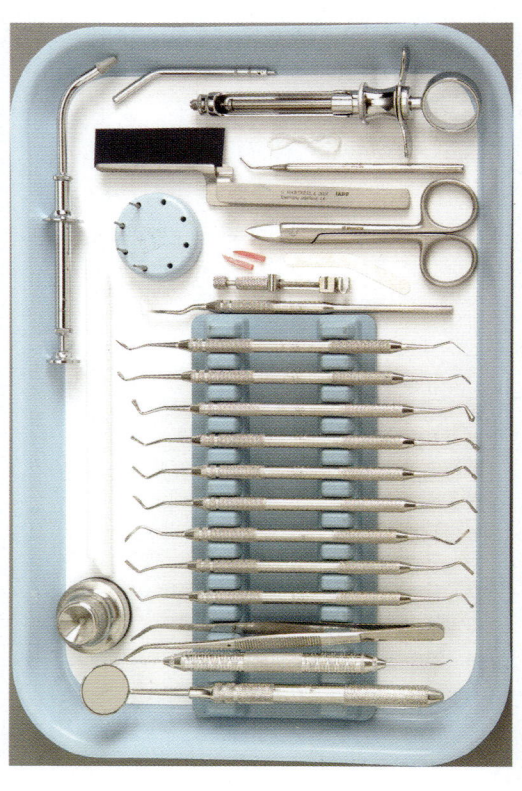

Amalgam

TOP ROW (LEFT TO RIGHT)

Amalgam well, HVE tip, burs in bur block, amalgam carrier-plunger style (very top of tray)

BOTTOM ROW (LEFT TO RIGHT)

Mouth mirror, explorer, cotton forceps (pliers), spoon excavator, enamel hatchet, mesial gingival margin trimmer, distal gingival margin trimmer, small condenser, large condenser, acorn burnisher, Tanner carver, half-Hollenback carver, gold carving knife, Tofflemire, wooden wedges, crown and bridge scissors, articulating paper holder and articulating paper, liner applicator, dental floss, anesthetic aspirating syringe, air/water syringe tip

Sterilization Notes ▶ Refer to each individual picture for correct procedure for instrument sterilization or disposal of instrument or material. Refer to other chapters for additional instruments on this tray setup that are not included in this chapter.

9

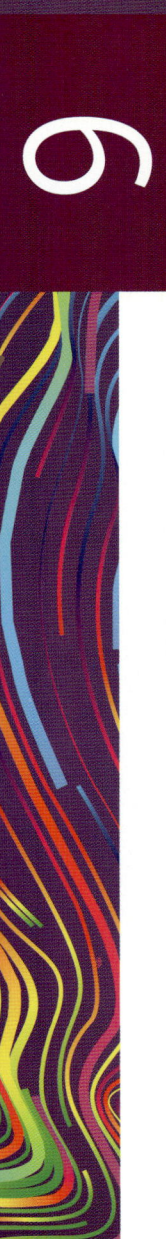

Composite Restorative Instruments

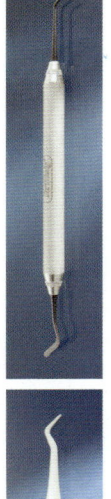

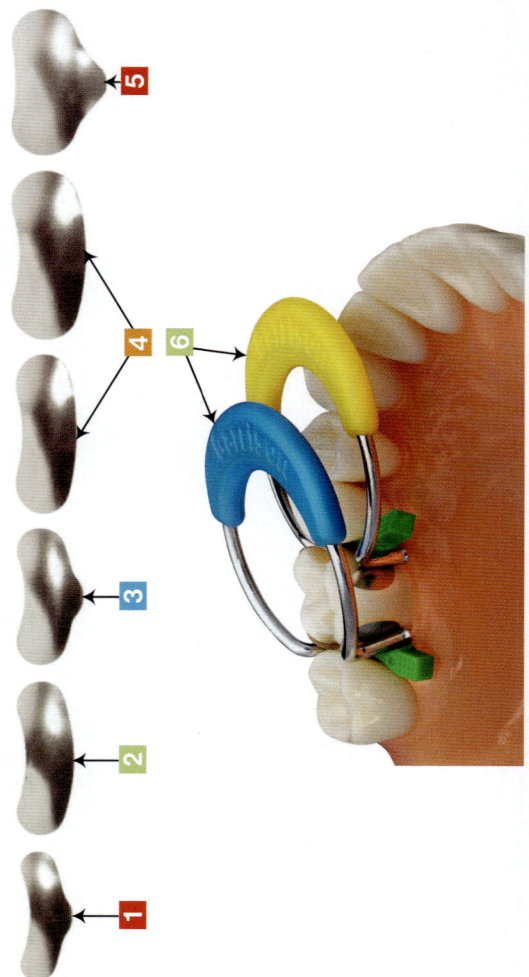

Sectional Matrix System

Function ▸ To replace missing proximal wall of cavity preparation for placement of composite material or other restorative materials for class II restorations

Characteristics ▸ Variety of sizes and shapes to accommodate restoration:

1. Pediatric band—Primary molar
2. Small band—Premolar, small molar
3. Extended small band—Premolar, molar, with deep cervical restoration
4. Standard band—Molar restoration
5. Large band—Deep cervical restoration
6. Tension rings—Different sizes to accommodate restoration

Placed to secure band on proximal wall

Placed on tooth with dental dam forceps (refer to page 170, Chapter 7)

Practice Notes ▸ Sectional Bands are used on amalgam, composite, buildup, and temporary filling tray setups. Classes III and IV composite restorations use a clear Mylar matrix strip.

Sterilization Notes ▸ Sectional Bands should be disposed of in sharps container, or state regulations should be followed. Single use only. Tension rings must be precleaned. Then, place in a sterilizing pouch with an internal process indicator, seal, then sterilize. OR, wrap with an internal process indicator inside and secure on the outside with process indicator tape, then sterilize. Verify appropriate color change has been achieved in external process indicator immediately after removal from sterilizer. Check internal process indicator before treatment. Refer to state regulations for any additional state requirements.

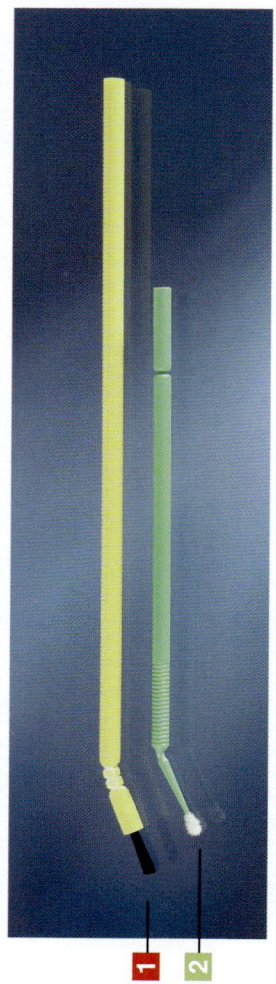

1
2

■ INSTRUMENT

Applicator

Functions ▸ To apply conditioning, primer, and bonding material to cavity preparation
To use with bonding procedures, sealants, and orthodontic band brackets

Characteristics ▸ Types:

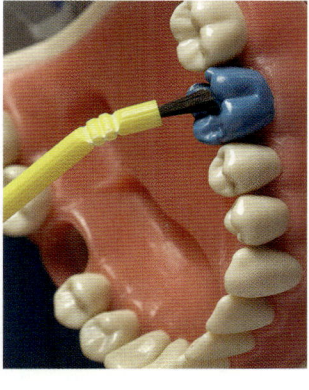

1 Disposable One-Piece Applicator—Several colors available for application of different materials; working end bends; various styles, sizes

2 Microbrush Applicator—Disposable, various styles, sizes

Practice Notes ▸ Applicators are used on composite, sealant tray setups and any procedure involving etching, primers, and bonding materials.

Sterilization Notes ▸ Disposable Applicator(s) should be disposed of in the garbage. Single use only.

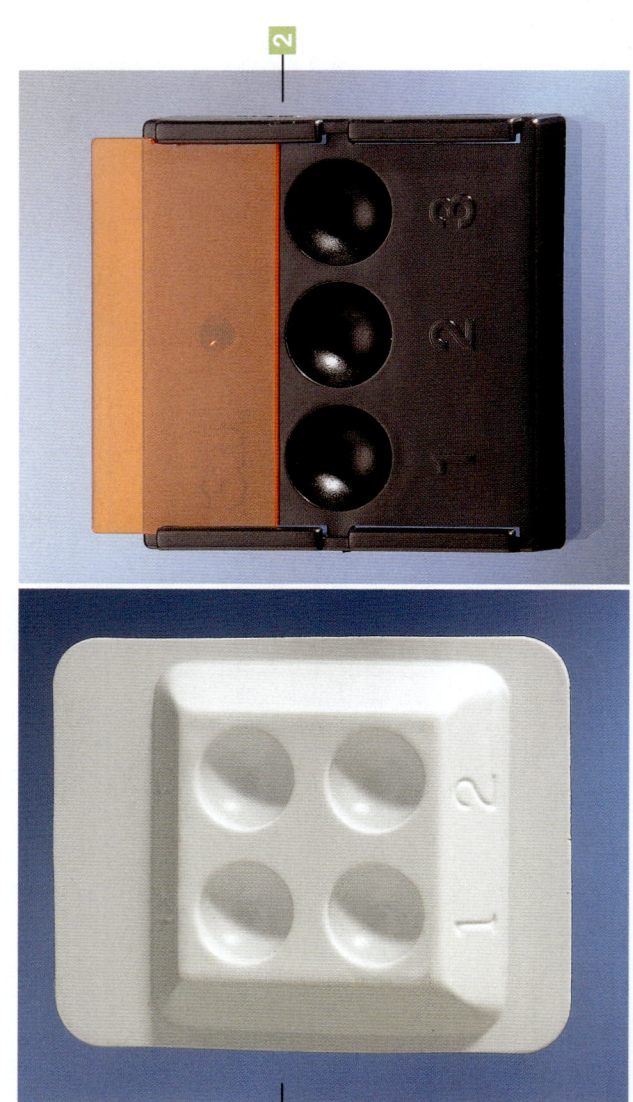

■ INSTRUMENT

Well for Composite Material

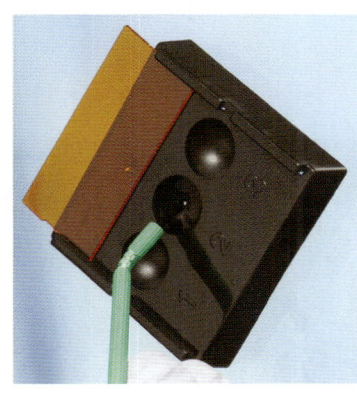

Function ▶ To hold material: etchant, primers, bonding, and composite

Characteristics ▶
1 Disposable (pictured) or autoclavable
2 Well with protective light cover

Labels on each well—Designate different materials
Variety of styles and colors available

Practice Notes ▶ Wells are also used on a sealant tray setup and any procedure involving etching, primers, and bonding.

Sterilization Notes ▶ Disposable Wells should be disposed of in the garbage. Reusable Well must be precleaned. Then, place in a sterilizing pouch with an internal process indicator, seal, then sterilize. OR, wrap with an internal process indicator inside and secure on the outside with process indicator tape, then sterilize. Verify appropriate color change has been achieved in external process indicator immediately after removal from sterilizer. Check internal process indicator before treatment. Refer to state regulations for any additional state requirements. Refer to manufacturer's recommendations.

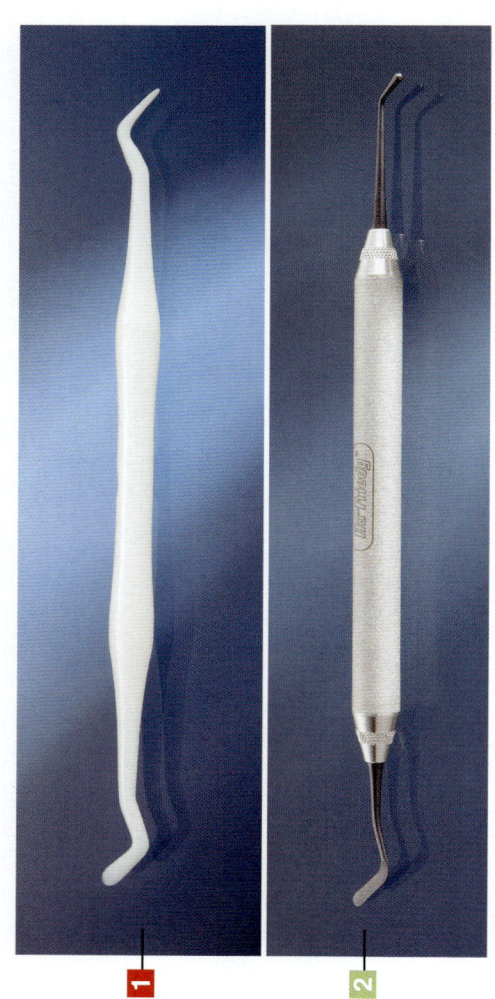

Composite Placement Instrument

Functions ▶
To carry composite material to the cavity preparation
To place, condense, and carve composite material in cavity preparation

Characteristics ▶
1 Plastic composite instrument—Plastic that can be sterilized
2 Metal composite instruments—Titanium nitride coating

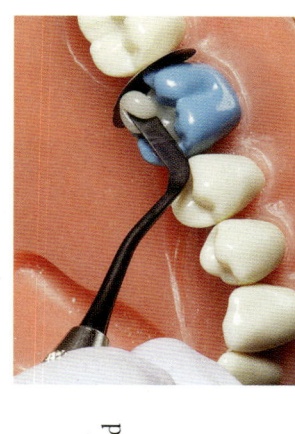

Double ended
Different angles on ends
Ends shaped differently, one to accommodate initial placement of material (paddle end) and the other end to condense, contour, and carve material
Variety of sizes, shapes, and angles available

Practice Notes ▶
Composite Placement Instrument is used on composite tray setups.

Sterilization Notes ▶
Composite Placement Instrument must be precleaned. Then, place in a sterilizing pouch with an internal process indicator, seal, then sterilize. OR, wrap with an internal process indicator inside and secure on the outside with process indicator tape, then sterilize. Verify appropriate color change has been achieved in external process indicator immediately after removal from sterilizer. Check internal process indicator before treatment. Refer to state regulations for any additional state requirements.

1

2

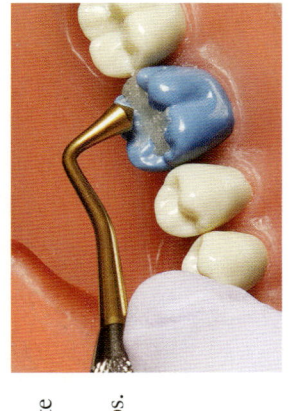

INSTRUMENT

Composite Burnisher

Functions ▸ To form occlusal anatomy in composite restorations

To achieve final contouring of anatomy, pits, fissures, and grooves

Characteristics ▸ Double ended—Different angle on either end

1 Composite Burnisher: Titanium nitride coating—Creates hard, smooth, nonstick surface that resists scratching, sticking, or discoloration of composite material

2 Acorn Burnisher (for composite restorations): Gold titanium nitride coating—Creates hard, smooth, nonstick surface that resists scratching, sticking, or discoloration of composite material

Practice Notes ▸ Composite Burnisher is used on composite tray setups.

Sterilization Notes ▸ Composite Burnisher must be precleaned. Then, place in a sterilizing pouch with an internal process indicator, seal, then sterilize. OR, wrap with an internal process indicator inside and secure on the outside with process indicator tape, then sterilize. Verify appropriate color change has been achieved in external process indicator immediately after removal from sterilizer. Check internal process indicator before treatment. Refer to state regulations for any additional state requirements.

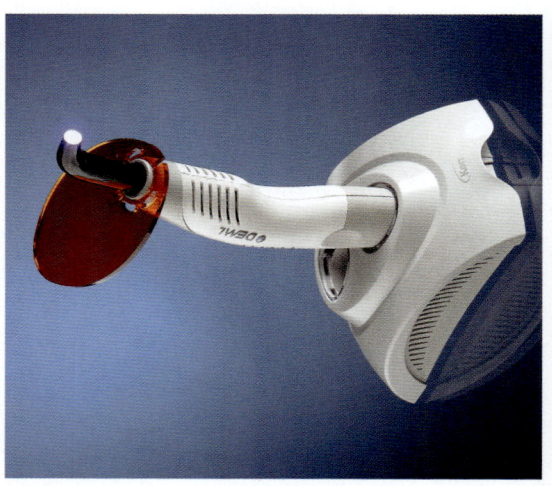

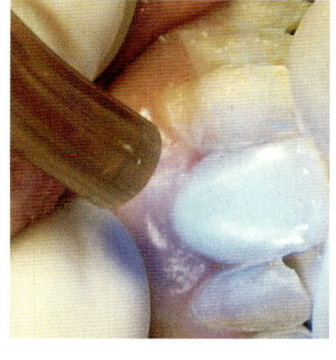

Curing Light—Battery Operated

Function ▸ To harden light-cured materials: Bonding agents, composite, sealants, buildup material

Characteristics ▸ Battery operated—Includes battery charger with extra battery

Practice Notes ▸ Material must be cured in increments of 2 mm or less to ensure complete setting.
Refer to manufacturer's recommendation for curing time.

Sterilization Notes ▸ A testing device should be used to check the accuracy of the Curing Light. Protective sleeves are available for the curing lights. Preclean and disinfect the wand and light using disinfectant solution according to the manufacturer's recommendation.

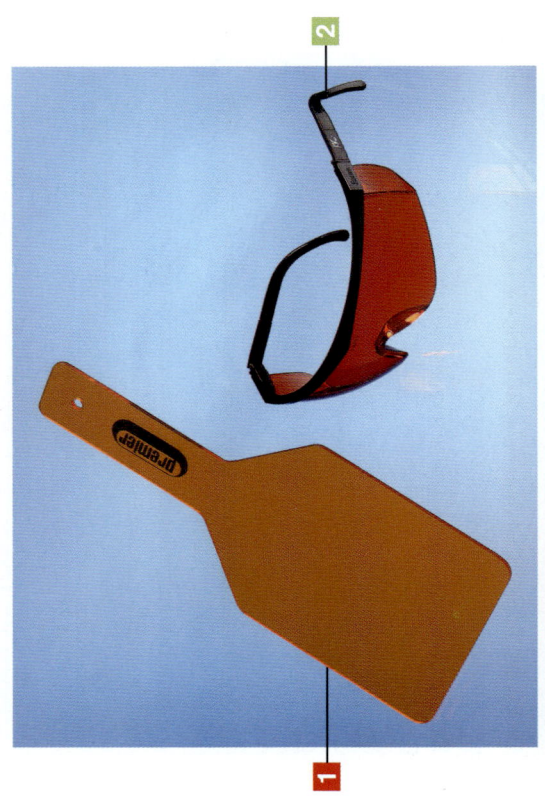

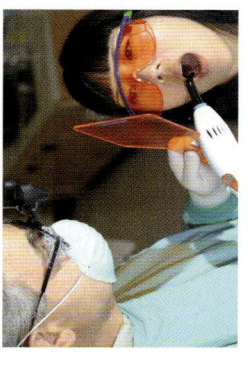

▪ INSTRUMENT

Protective Shield for Curing Light

Function ▸ To protect eyes during curing stage of light-cured material

Characteristics ▸ Orange color—Blocks harmful light to operator/assistant and patient's eyes
Protective shields also available on curing light (see Curing Light, page 242)

1 Paddle Shield style
2 Protective eyeglasses available for operator, assistant, and patient

Practice Notes ▸ Protective Shield must be used with all curing lights.

Sterilization Notes ▸ Protective Shield, paddle, glasses must be precleaned and disinfected according to the manufacturer's recommendation.

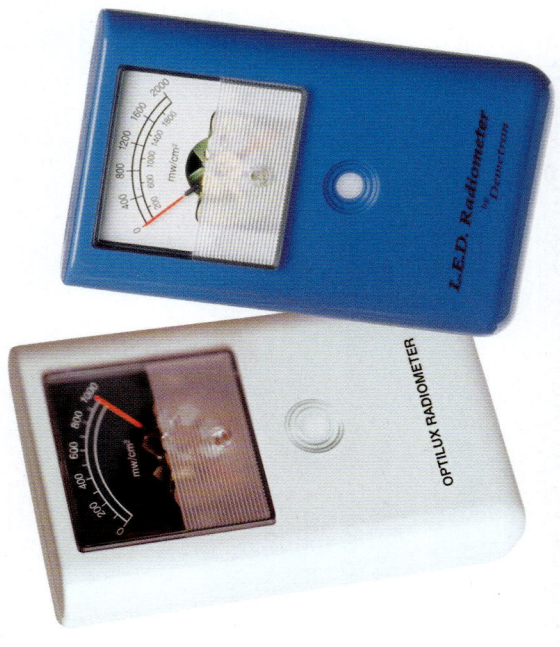

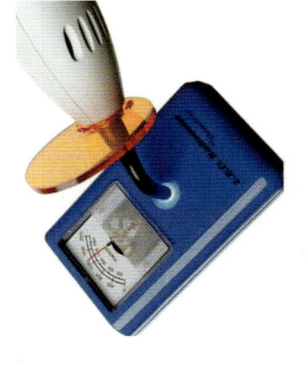

LED and Halogen Radiometers

Functions ▶ To accurately test the visible light output for the LED and halogen curing lights

To determine the accuracy of the LED and halogen lights that cure dental materials

Characteristics ▶ White—Halogen Radiometer

Blue—LED Radiometer

Practice Notes ▶ Loss of output of the curing lights will affect the amount of time needed to efficiently cure dental material.

Lights should be tested periodically to ensure lightbulb and battery are working efficiently.

Sterilization Notes ▶ Refer to manufacturer's recommendation for disinfecting Radiometers.

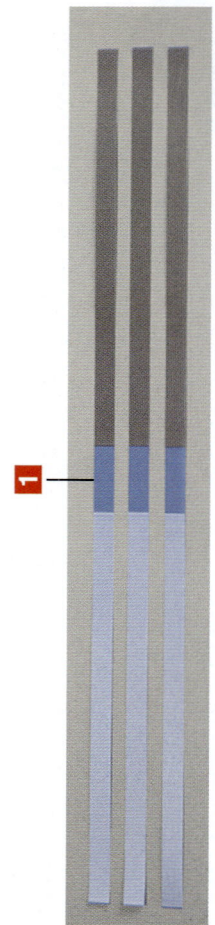

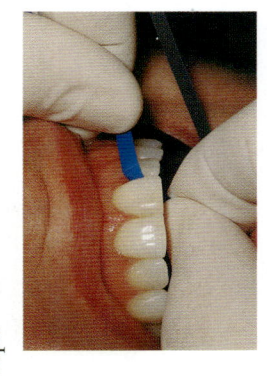

■ INSTRUMENT

Finishing Strip

Function ▶ To finish and smooth interproximal surface of restoration

Characteristics ▶ Abrasive textures available: Synthetic or sandpaper material

Different grit consistencies available

Different grit consistency is on either end of strip—See color difference.

Practice Notes ▶ Synthetic Finishing Strip

1 No abrasive material in center of strip; helps avoid removal of tooth structure while inserting the finishing strip interproximally.

Finishing Strip is used on composite and amalgam tray setups.

Sterilization Notes ▶ Finishing Strip should be disposed of in the garbage.

Single use only.

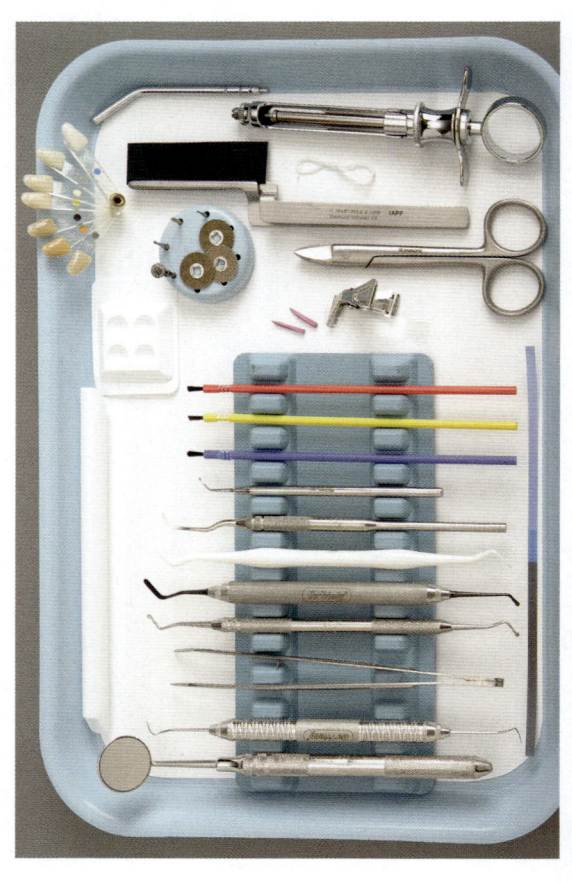

Composite Procedure—Class III and Class IV Composite Restorative

TOP ROW (FROM LEFT TO RIGHT)

High-volume evacuator (HVE) tip, well for composite material, burs and mandrel or discs in bur block, shade guide

BOTTOM ROW (FROM LEFT TO RIGHT)

Mouth mirror, explorer, cotton forceps (pliers), spoon excavator, composite placement instrument (titanium nitride coating), composite placement instrument (plastic), gold carving knife, liner applicator, three different colors of applicator brushes, wooden wedges, clear Mylar matrix strip and clamp to hold matrix, crown and bridge scissors, articulating paper holder and articulating paper, dental floss, anesthetic aspirating syringe, air/water syringe tip

Sterilization Notes ▶ Refer to each picture for correct procedure for instrument sterilization or disposal of material. Refer to other chapters for additional instruments on this tray setup that are not included in this chapter.

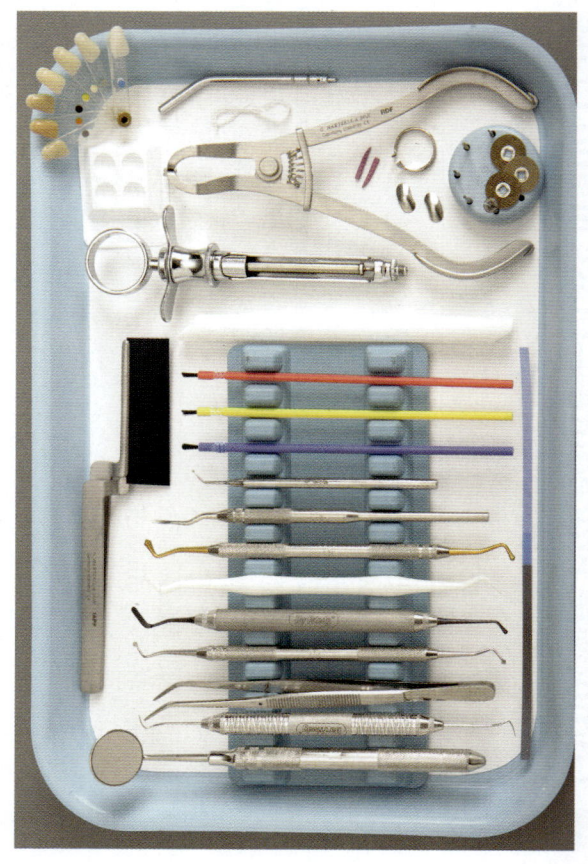

Composite Procedure—Class I, Class II, and Class V Composite Restorative

TOP ROW (LEFT TO RIGHT)

Articulating paper holder and articulating paper, well for composite material, shade guide

BOTTOM ROW (LEFT TO RIGHT)

Mouth mirror, explorer, cotton forceps (pliers), spoon excavator, composite placement instrument (titanium nitride coating), composite placement instrument (plastic), composite burnisher (gold–titanium nitride coating), gold carving knife, liner applicator, three different colors of applicator brushes, high-volume evacuator (HVE) tip, anesthetic syringe, dental dam forceps used for tension rings, (underneath forceps: matrix band, wooden wedges, tension rings, burs, mandrel/discs in bur block), dental floss, air/water syringe tip

BOTTOM OF TRAY

Finishing strip

Sterilization Notes ▶ Refer to each picture for correct procedure for instrument sterilization or disposal of material. Refer to other chapters for additional instruments on this tray setup that are not included in this chapter.

10

Fixed Prosthodontics Restorative Instruments

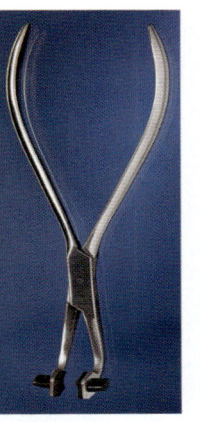

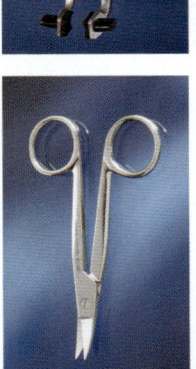

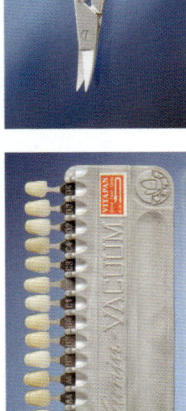

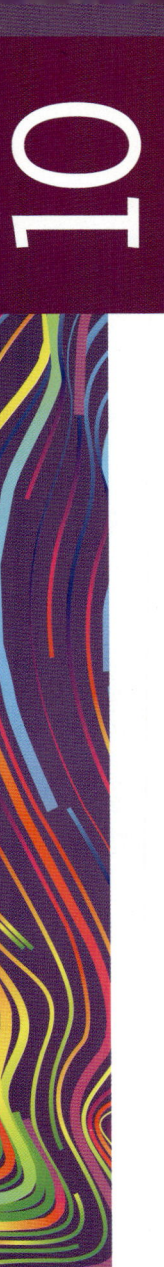

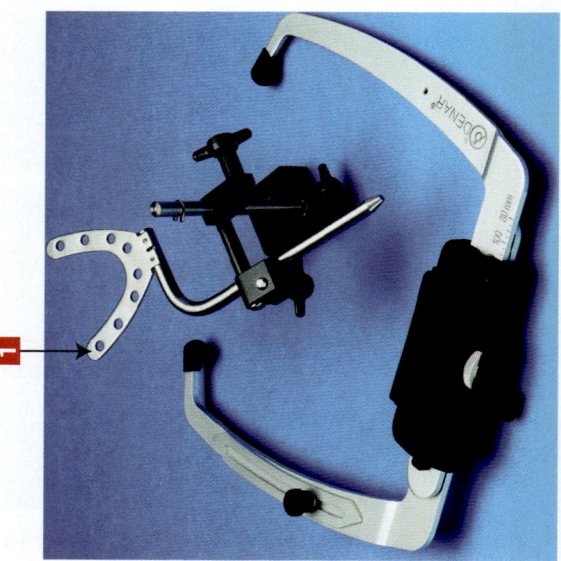

Facebow

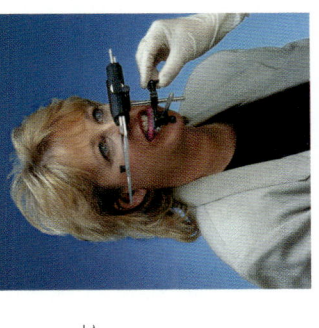

Functions ▶ To establish the centric relationship of the maxillary teeth to the mandibular teeth

To establish the position of the teeth when the temporal mandibular joint is aligned correctly

Characteristics ▶ Recording and establishing the centric occlusion assists in fabricating fixed prosthodontic restorations

1 Apply compound tabs or dental impression material on bite fork

Recording and establishing the centric occlusion assists in fabricating fixed and removable prosthodontic appliances

Example: Crowns, bridges, partials, and dentures.

Facebows are also used with orthodontic treatment assessment for mounting the impressions in correct occlusion

Practice Notes ▶ Facebow transfer applications are used in all phases of restorative dentistry.

Sterilization Notes ▶ Facebow outer appliances must be disinfected according to the manufacturer's recommendation. Bite Fork must be precleaned. Then, place in a sterilizing pouch with an internal process indicator, seal, then sterilize. OR, wrap with an internal process indicator inside and secure on the outside with process indicator tape, then sterilize. Verify appropriate color change has been achieved in external process indicator immediately after removal from sterilizer. Check internal process indicator before treatment. Refer to state regulations for any additional state requirements.

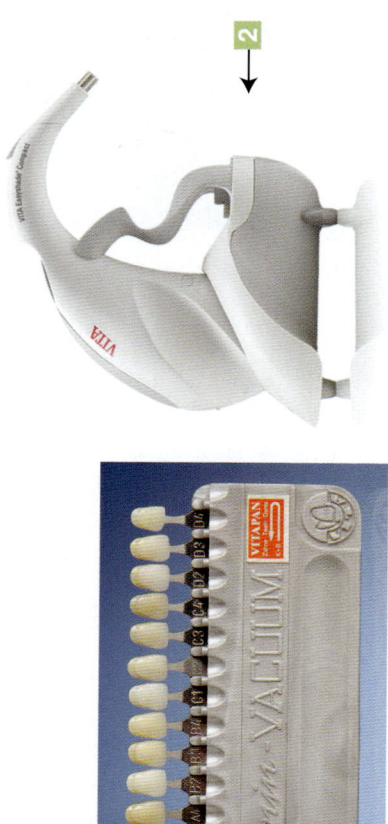

1

2

Shade Guides/Digital Color Imaging

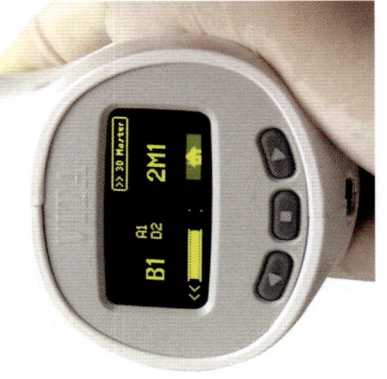

■ INSTRUMENT

Functions ▶ To select a shade for permanent fixed restorations
Example: Crowns, veneers, bridges

To select a shade for removable appliances
Example: Partials, dentures

Characteristics ▶
1. Many different shade guides are available.
2. Many different digital or computerized shade guides are available.

Practice Notes ▶ Each tooth may have different shades: one for the gingival third, one for the body or middle third, and one for the incisal edge (usually needed for anteriors).

Sterilization Notes ▶ Shade Guides must be disinfected according to the manufacturer's recommendation.

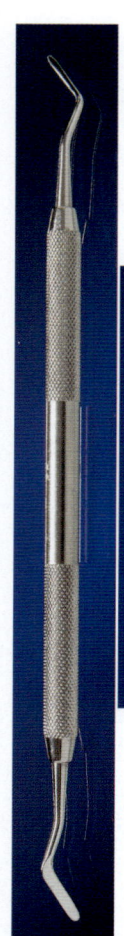

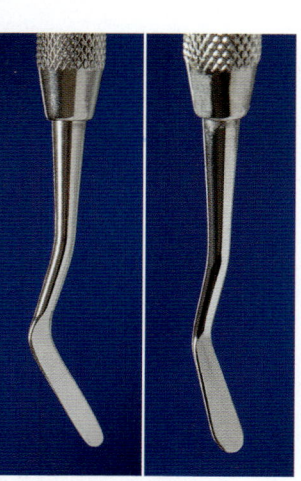

■ INSTRUMENT

Gingival Retraction Cord Instrument

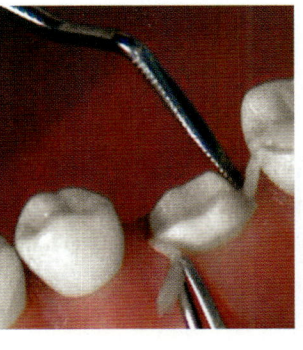

Function ▶ To place gingival retraction cord in sulcus area after tooth is prepared for a crown and before final impressions are taken

Characteristics ▶ Smooth or serrated edges
Double ended—Different angle on each end
Variety of styles

Practice Notes ▶ Gingival Retraction Cord instrument is mainly used on crown and bridge tray setup unless gingiva needs to be retracted for a restorative procedure.

Sterilization Notes ▶ Gingival Retraction Cord Instrument must be precleaned. Then, place in a sterilizing pouch with an internal process indicator, seal, then sterilize. OR, wrap with an internal process indicator inside and secure on the outside with process indicator tape, then sterilize. Verify appropriate color change has been achieved in external process indicator immediately after removal from sterilizer. Check internal process indicator before treatment. Refer to state regulations for any additional state requirements. Gingival retraction cord instrument should be disposed of in the garbage.

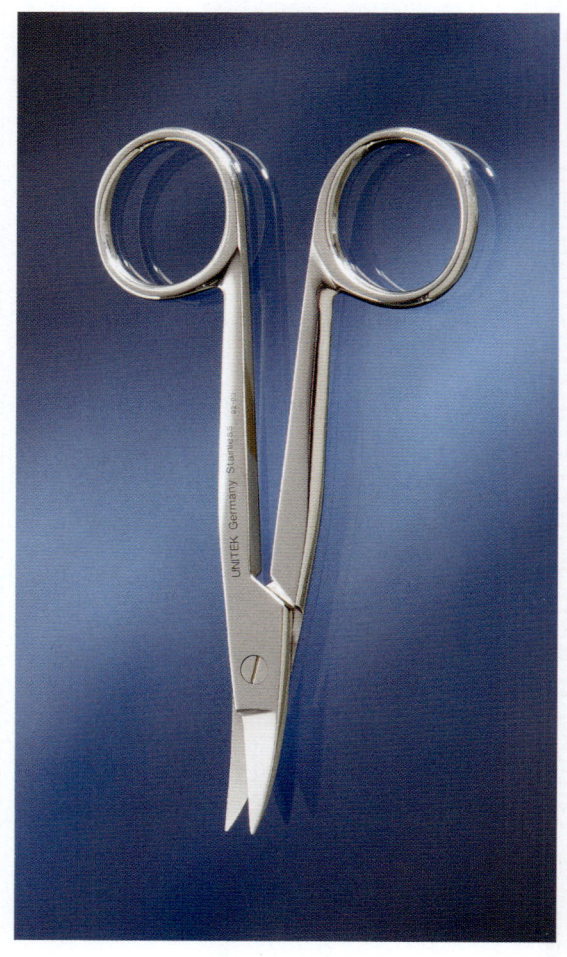

Crown and Bridge Scissors

Functions ▶
To trim aluminum temporary crowns on gingival side
To trim custom temporary crowns
To cut gingival retraction cord
To trim matrix bands
To cut dental dam septum

Characteristics ▶
Short cutting edges—Can be straight or curved, narrow or wide
Variety of sizes

Practice Notes ▶
Crown and Bridge Scissors are used on other restorative tray setups.

Sterilization Notes ▶
Crown and Bridge Scissors must be precleaned, open, and unlocked. Then, place in an open and unlocked position in a sterilizing pouch with an internal process indicator, seal, then sterilize. OR, wrap with an internal process indicator inside and secure on the outside with process indicator tape, then sterilize. Verify appropriate color change has been achieved in external process indicator immediately after removal from sterilizer. Check internal process indicator before treatment. Refer to state regulations for any additional state requirements.

■ **INSTRUMENT**

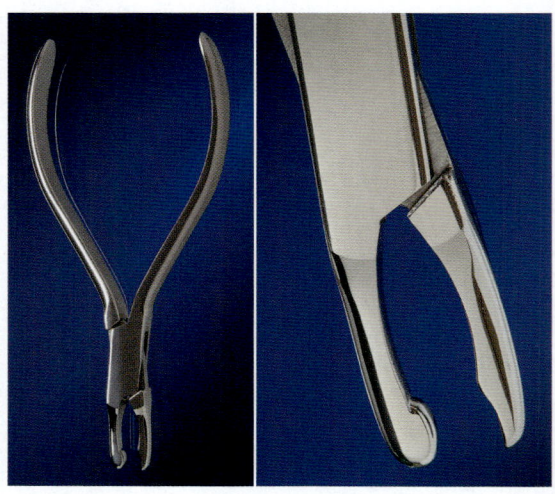

Contouring Pliers

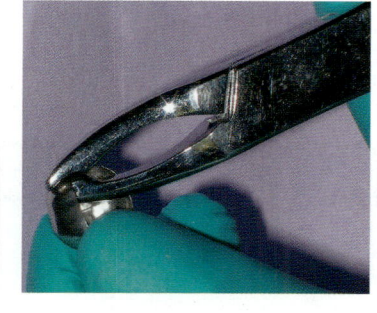

■ INSTRUMENT

Function ▶ To crimp and contour marginal edge of temporary crown or stainless steel crown

Characteristics ▶ Commonly used type: Johnson
Range of sizes available

Practice Notes ▶ Contouring Pliers are mainly used on crown and bridge tray setup.

Sterilization Notes ▶ Contouring Pliers must be precleaned, open, and unlocked. Then, place in an open and unlocked position in a sterilizing pouch with an internal process indicator, seal, then sterilize. OR, wrap with an internal process indicator inside and secure on the outside with process indicator tape, then sterilize. Verify appropriate color change has been achieved in external process indicator immediately after removal from sterilizer. Check internal process indicator before treatment. Refer to state regulations for any additional state requirements.

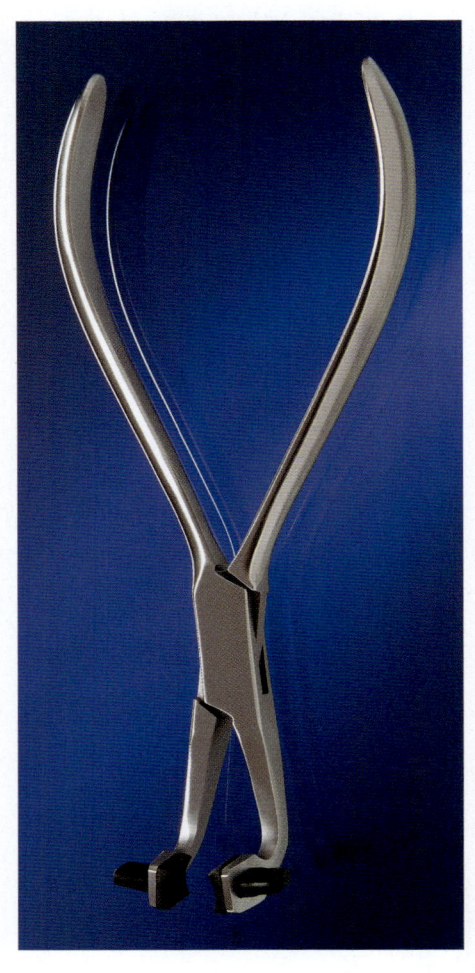

Provisional Crown–Removing Forceps

INSTRUMENT

Function ▸ To remove provisional crown from tooth

Characteristic ▸ Range of sizes available

Practice Notes ▸ Provisional Crown–Removing Forceps are mainly used on crown and bridge tray setup.

Sterilization Notes ▸ Provisional Crown–Removing Forceps must be precleaned, open, and unlocked. Then, place in an open and unlocked position in a sterilizing pouch with an internal process indicator, seal, then sterilize. OR, wrap with an internal process indicator inside and secure on the outside with process indicator tape, then sterilize. Verify appropriate color change has been achieved in external process indicator immediately after removal from sterilizer. Check internal process indicator before treatment. Refer to state regulations for any additional state requirements.

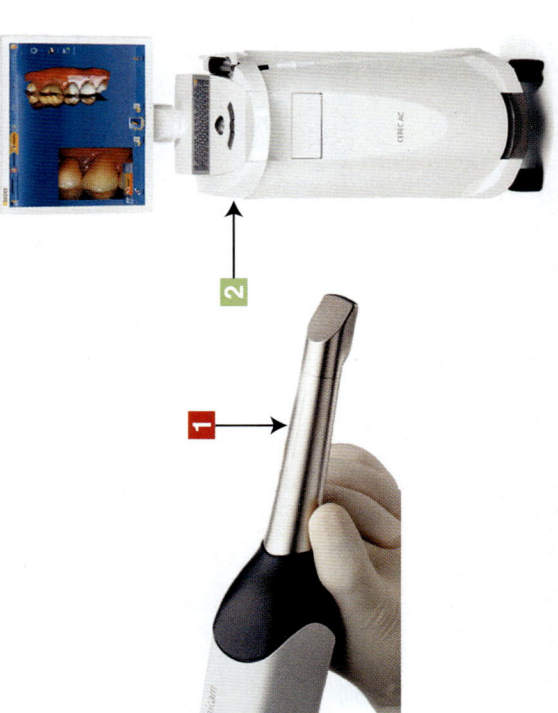

CAD/CAM Machine

Functions ▶ To take a computer image of a tooth with an intraoral scanner that connects to a computer

To construct the anatomy, gingival margins, occlusal and mesial/distal contacts of the crown on the computer

To create 3D digital models for diagnostic purposes

To send the information from the unit to the milling machine. Refer to Milling Machine.

Characteristics ▶ **1** Intraoral scanner

2 CAD/CAM in-office system with attached scanner and computer screen

Crown is made of porcelain or other type materials.

Practice Notes ▶ CAD/CAM allows the patient to have one appointment for a crown. Scanning the crown preparation, then milling the crown for seating/cementing.

CAD/CAM scans intraoral digital images creating virtual models.

Sterilization Notes ▶ Barriers should be used for the intraoral scanner. Barriers or overgloves should be used for manipulating the computer on the CAD/CAM-CEREC Machine. Otherwise, refer to the manufacturer's recommendation for disinfecting.

269

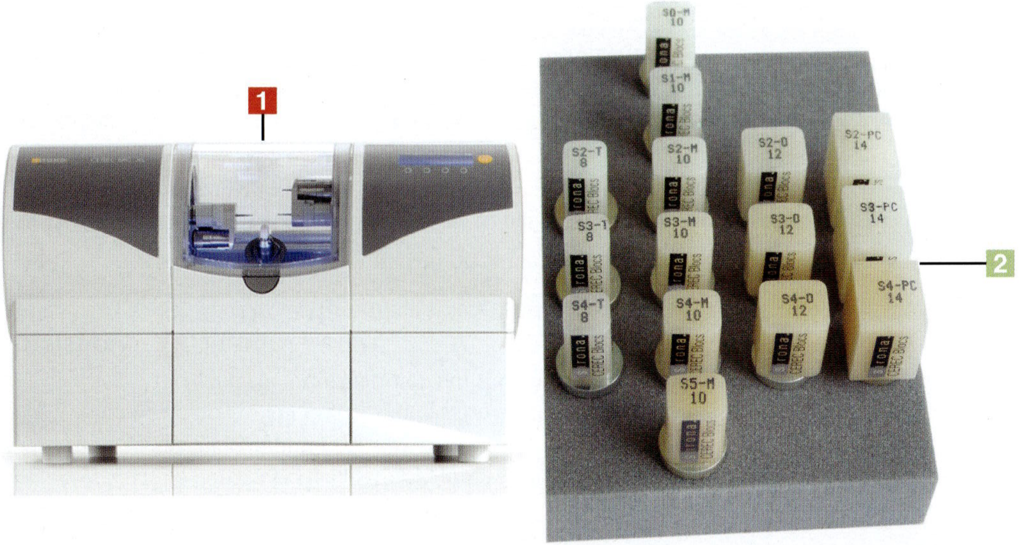
1
2
S0-M 10
S1-M 10
S2-M 10
S3-M 10
S4-M 10
S5-M 10
S2-T 8
S4-T 8
S2-O 12
S3-O 12
S4-O 12
S2-PC 14
S3-PC 14
S4-PC 14

CAD/CA Milling Machine

Functions ▶ To mill the crown with the image taken from the camera that connects to the CAD/CAM

Characteristics ▶
1. Milling machine
2. Ceramic blocks that are placed in the milling machine to fabricate the crown

As shown different shades are available.

Practice Notes ▶ CAD/CAM machine allows the patient to have one appointment for preparing and seating a crown.

Sterilization Notes ▶ Refer to manufacturer's recommendation for disinfecting.

Courtesy of TEMREX Corporation

Bite Stick

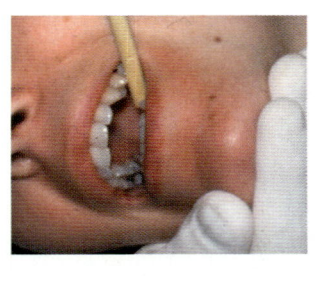

INSTRUMENT

Function ▶ To seat permanent crown while patient bites in centric occlusion

Characteristics ▶ One end square and the other end round for specific uses
Range of sizes available

Practice Notes ▶ Bite Stick is primarily used on crown and bridge tray setup.
Other styles of biting devices to seat a crown are mostly available in disposable devices

Sterilization Notes ▶ Bite Stick and other disposable seating devices should be disposed of in the garbage. One time use only.

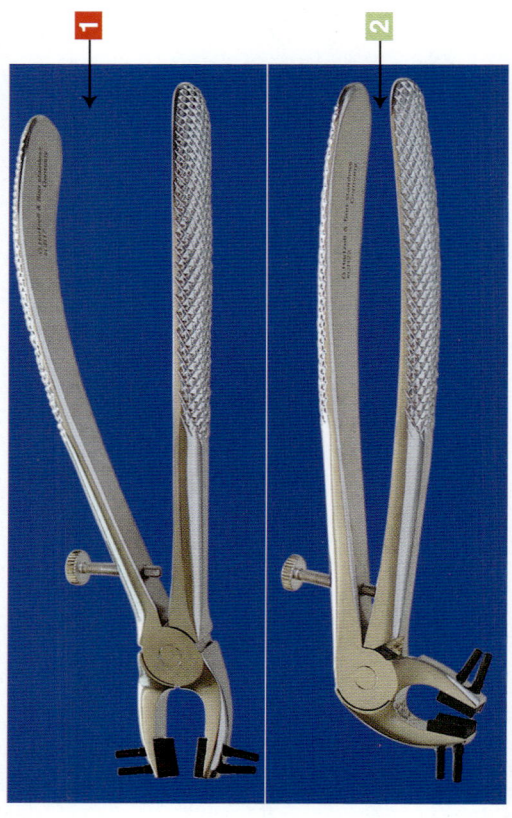

■ INSTRUMENT

Trial Crown Remover

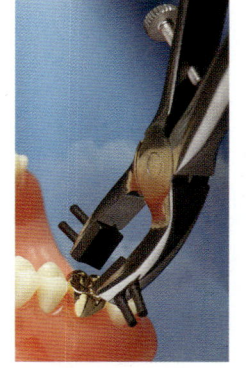

Functions ▶

To remove permanent crown from tooth during try-in phase
To remove provisional crown

Characteristics ▶

Types:

1 Maxillary trial crown remover
2 Mandibular trial crown remover

Replaceable pads—Provide nonslipping, tight grip

Practice Notes ▶

Trial Crown Remover is mainly used on crown and bridge tray setup.

Sterilization Notes ▶

Trial Crown Remover must be precleaned, open, and unlocked. Then, place in an open and unlocked position in a sterilizing pouch with an internal process indicator, seal, then sterilize. OR, wrap with an internal process indicator inside and secure on the outside with process indicator tape, then sterilize. Verify appropriate color change has been achieved in external process indicator immediately after removal from sterilizer. Check internal process indicator before treatment. Refer to state regulations for any additional state requirements.

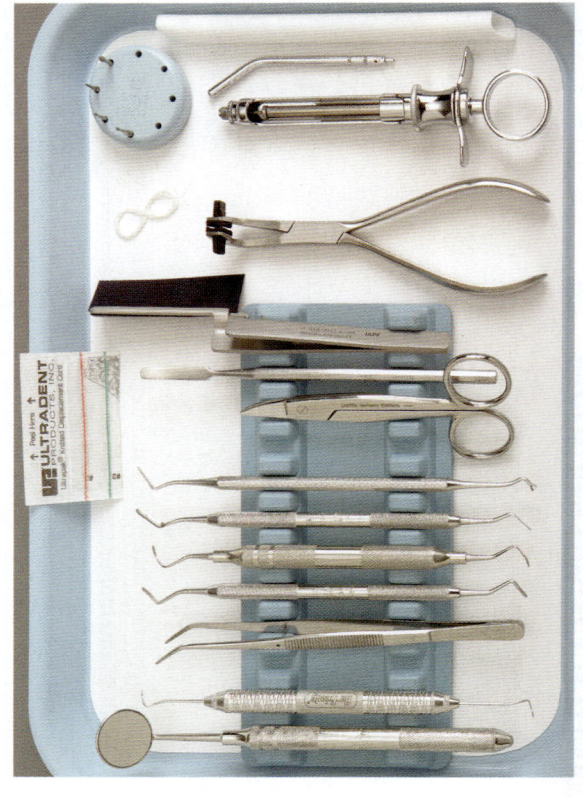

Crown and Bridge Preparation

TOP ROW (LEFT TO RIGHT)

Gingival retraction cord, dental floss, burs in bur block

BOTTOM ROW (LEFT TO RIGHT)

Mouth mirror, explorer, cotton forceps (pliers), spoon excavator, curette, gingival retraction cord instrument, Woodson, crown and bridge scissors, flexible cement mixing spatula, articulating paper holder and articulating paper, provisional crown–removing forceps, anesthetic aspirating syringe, air/water syringe tip, high-volume evacuation (HVE) tip

Sterilization Notes ▶ Refer to each picture for correct procedure for instrument sterilization or disposal of material. Refer to other chapters for additional instruments on this tray setup that are not included in this chapter.

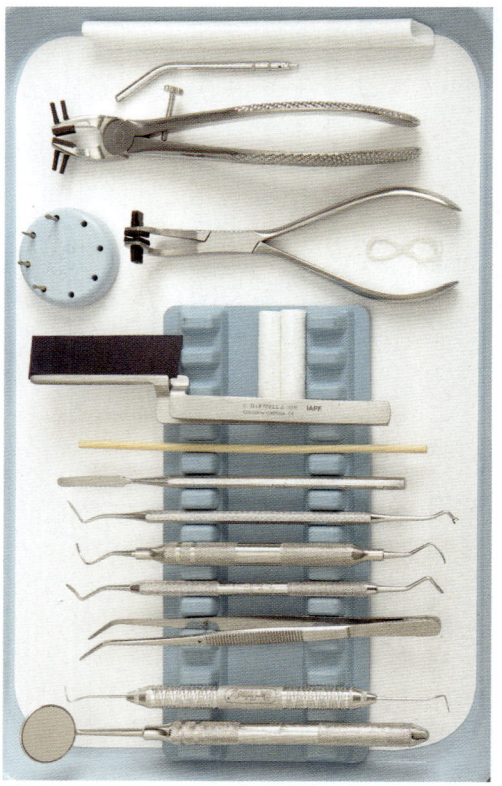

Crown and Bridge Cementation

TOP ROW (LEFT TO RIGHT)
Burs in bur block

BOTTOM ROW (LEFT TO RIGHT)
Mouth mirror, explorer, cotton forceps (pliers), spoon excavator, curette, Woodson, flexible cement mixing spatula, wooden bite stick, articulating paper holder and articulating paper, cotton rolls, provisional crown–removing forceps, dental floss (under provisional crown–removing forceps), trial crown remover (maxillary), air/water syringe tip, high-volume evacuation (HVE) tip

Sterilization Notes ▶ Refer to each picture for correct procedure for instrument sterilization or disposal of material. Refer to other chapters for additional instruments on this tray setup that are not included in this chapter.

Endodontic Instruments

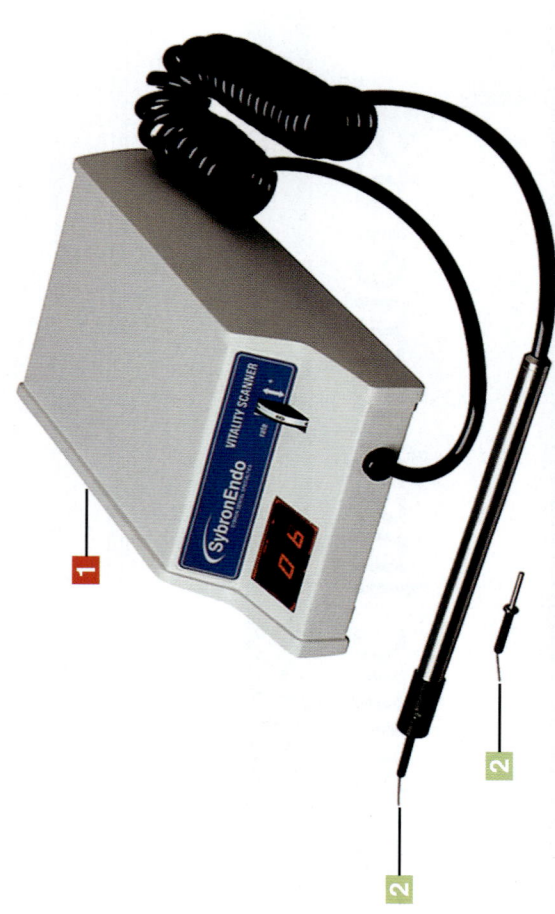

Vitalometer/Pulp Tester

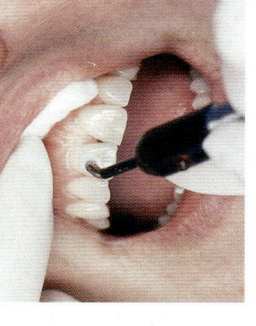

Function ▶ To test vitality of pulp in teeth

Characteristics ▶ Two types—Electronic and Digital with digital readout
Electric or battery operated

Practice Notes ▶ **1** The Pulp Tester sends an impulse of electric current to the pulp, causing a reaction. The current is increased by small increments until the patient indicates feeling a sensation. Toothpaste is applied to the tip of the electrode to conduct electricity.
2 The tip is placed on the surface of a natural tooth, facial and/or lingual. Each root and pulp on the tooth is tested.
Vitalometer is used exclusively with endodontic tray setups.

Sterilization Notes ▶ Vitalometer tip must be precleaned. Then, place in a sterilizing pouch with an internal process indicator, seal, then sterilize. OR, wrap with an internal process indicator inside and secure on the outside with process indicator tape, then sterilize. Verify appropriate color change has been achieved in external process indicator immediately after removal from sterilizer. Check internal process indicator before treatment. Refer to state regulations for any additional state requirements. Barriers should be used on the unit or the manufacturer's recommendation for disinfection of unit should be followed.

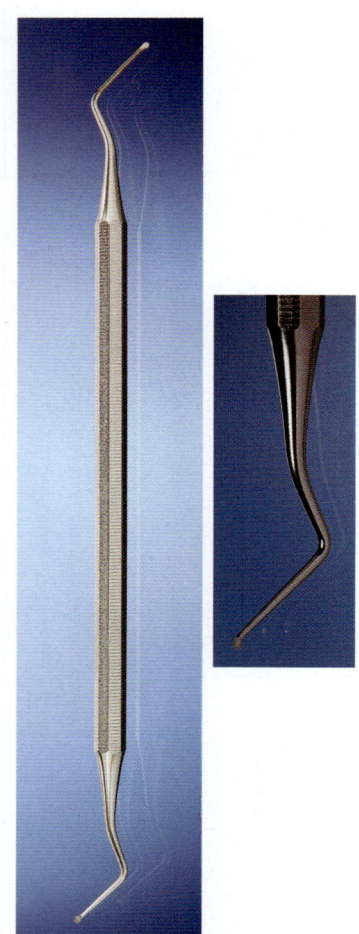

■ INSTRUMENT

Endodontic Long-Shank Spoon Excavator

Function ▶ To reach deep into the canal to remove coronal pulp tissue, decay, and temporary cements

Characteristics ▶ Long shank to reach deep into cavity preparation

Double ended

Range of sizes available

Practice Notes ▶ Endodontic Long-Shank Spoon is used exclusively on endodontic tray setups.

Sterilization Notes ▶ Endodontic Long-Shank Spoon Excavator must be precleaned. Then, place in a sterilizing pouch with an internal process indicator, seal, then sterilize. OR, wrap with an internal process indicator inside and secure on the outside with process indicator tape, then sterilize. Verify appropriate color change has been achieved in external process indicator immediately after removal from sterilizer. Check internal process indicator before treatment. Refer to state regulations for any additional state requirements.

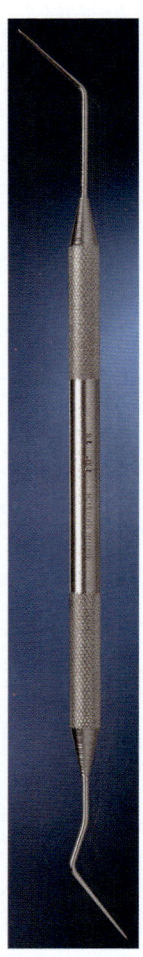

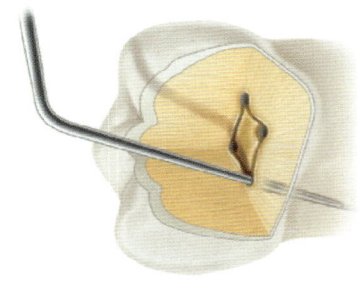

■ INSTRUMENT

Endodontic Explorer

Function ▶ To locate opening of small canal orifices for endodontic procedure

Characteristics ▶ Double ended

Working end—Longer than regular explorer to reach opening of canals

Practice Note ▶ Endodontic Explorer is used exclusively on endodontic tray setups.

Sterilization Notes ▶ Endodontic Explorer must be precleaned. Then, place in a sterilizing pouch with an internal process indicator, seal, then sterilize. OR, wrap with an internal process indicator inside and secure on the outside with process indicator tape, then sterilize. Verify appropriate color change has been achieved in external process indicator immediately after removal from sterilizer. Check internal process indicator before treatment. Refer to state regulations for any additional state requirements.

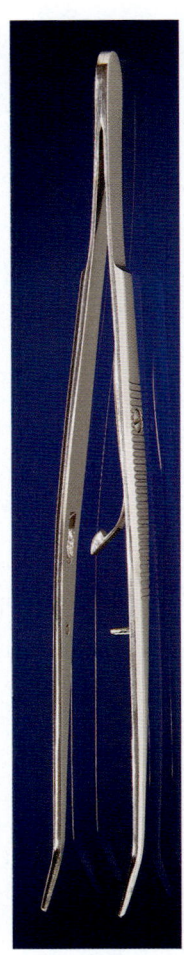

Endodontic Locking Forceps (Pliers)

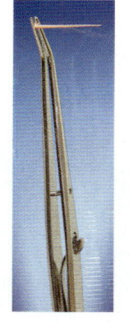

Function ▶ To grasp and lock material for transfer into and out of oral cavity

Characteristic ▶ Similar to regular cotton forceps except for locking mechanism to secure material on the working end of the forceps (pliers)

Practice Note ▶ Endodontic Locking Forceps are used on endodontic tray setup and could also be used on restorative tray setups.

Sterilization Notes ▶ Endodontic Locking Forceps must be precleaned open and unlocked. Then, place in an open and unlocked position in a sterilizing pouch with an internal process indicator, seal, then sterilize. OR, wrap with an internal process indicator inside and secure on the outside with process indicator tape, then sterilize. Verify appropriate color change has been achieved in external process indicator immediately after removal from sterilizer. Check internal process indicator before treatment. Refer to state regulations for any additional state requirements.

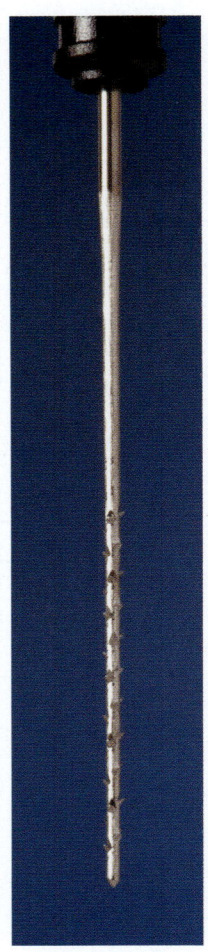

■ INSTRUMENT

Broach

Function ▶ To remove pulp tissue from canal(s)

Characteristics ▶ Working end—Barbed wire protrusions on shaft grab and remove vital or nonvital pulp fibers

Handles—Color coded according to size

Range of sizes—Diameter increases with size.

Practice Notes ▶ Endodontic Broach is used exclusively on endodontic tray setups.

Sterilization Notes ▶ Endodontic Broach must be disposed of in a sharps container. For single use only.

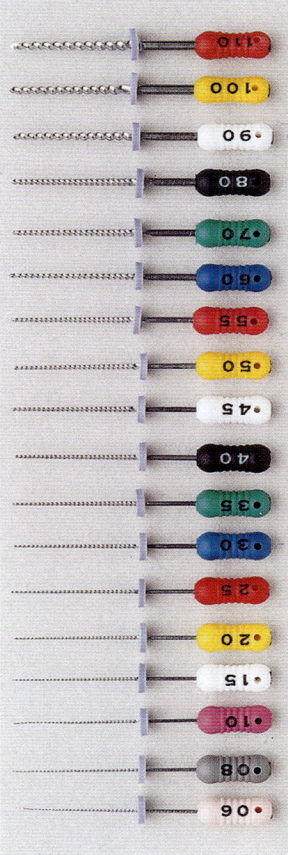

■ INSTRUMENT

Endodontic File—K Type

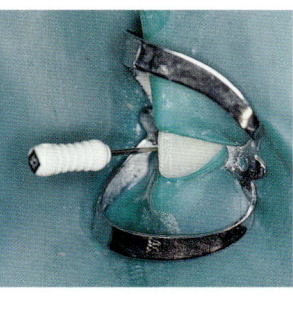

Functions ▶
To clean inside walls of canal
To contour inner walls of canal

Characteristics ▶
Twisted design—More twists per millimeter than reamer
Used with push–pull motion
Handles—Color coded according to size
Range of sizes—To accommodate width of canal, diameter increases with size.
Available in different lengths
Examples: 21 mm, 25 mm, 31 mm

Practice Note ▶
Endodontic File—K Type is used exclusively on endodontic tray setups.

Sterilization Notes ▶
Endodontic File—K Type must be precleaned. Then, place in a sterilizing pouch with an internal process indicator, seal, then sterilize. OR, wrap with an internal process indicator inside and secure on the outside with process indicator tape, then sterilize. Verify appropriate color change has been achieved in external process indicator immediately after removal from sterilizer. Check internal process indicator before treatment. Refer to state regulations for any additional state requirements. OR, used File must be disposed of in a sharps container. Rubber stopper on the file should be disposed of in the garbage.

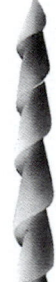

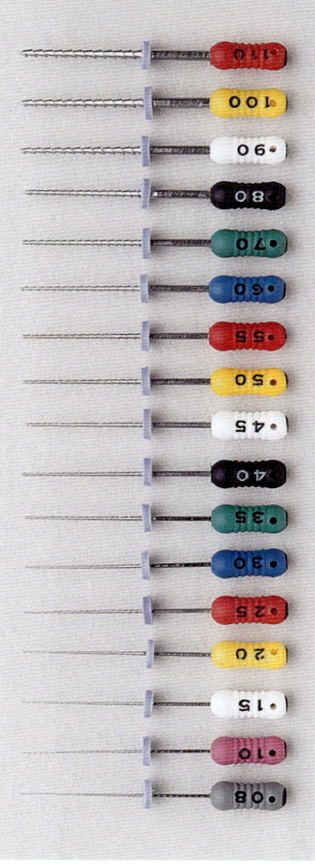

■ INSTRUMENT

Endodontic File—Hedstrom

Functions ▸ To clean inside walls of canal
To enlarge and smooth inner walls of canal

Characteristics ▸ Triangular cutting edge
Handles—Color coded according to size
Range of sizes—To accommodate width of canal, diameter increases with size.
Available in different lengths
Examples: 21 mm, 25 mm, 31 mm

Practice Note ▸ Endodontic File—Hedstrom is used exclusively on endodontic tray setups.

Sterilization Notes ▸ Endodontic File—Hedstrom must be precleaned. Then, place in a sterilizing pouch with an internal process indicator, seal, then sterilize. OR, wrap with an internal process indicator inside and secure on the outside with process indicator tape, then sterilize. Verify appropriate color change has been achieved in external process indicator immediately after removal from sterilizer. Check internal process indicator before treatment. Refer to state regulations for any additional state requirements. OR, used File must be disposed of in a sharps container. Rubber stopper on the file should be disposed of in the garbage.

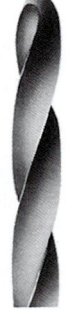

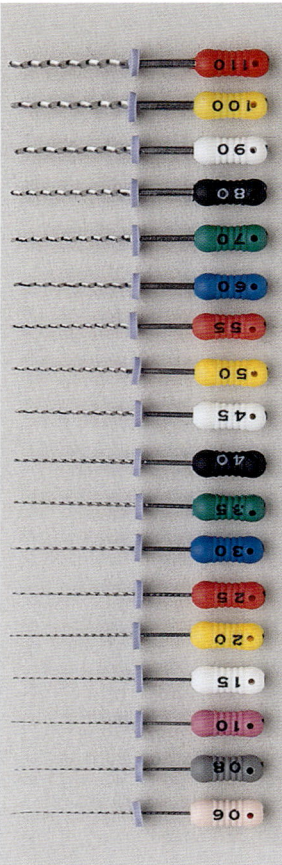

Reamer

Functions ▲

To cut and smooth dentinal walls of canal

To enlarge inner walls of canal

Characteristics ▲

Twisted triangular cutting edge Reamer is similar to K-type file, but cutting edge is farther apart and has fewer twists per millimeter

Used with twisting motion

Handles—Color coded according to size

Range of sizes—To accommodate width of canal, diameter increases with size.

Available in different lengths

Examples: 21 mm, 25 mm, 31 mm

Practice Note ▲

Reamer is used exclusively on endodontic tray setups.

Sterilization Notes ▲

Reamer must be precleaned. Then, place in a sterilizing pouch with an internal process indicator, sealed then sterilized. OR, wrapped with an internal process indicator inside and secured on the outside with process indicator tape, then sterilize. Verify appropriate color change has been achieved in external process indicator immediately after removal from sterilizer. Check internal process indicator before treatment. Refer to state regulations for any additional state requirements. Or used Reamer must be disposed of in a sharps container. Rubber stopper on the file should be disposed of in the garbage.

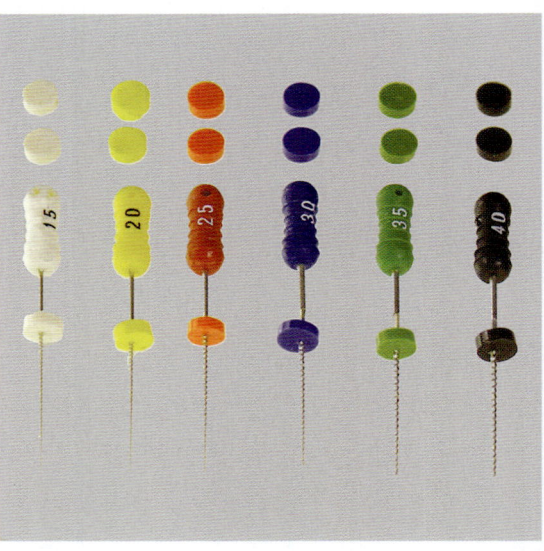

Endodontic Stoppers

Function ▶ To place onto an intracanal instrument such as a file or reamer to help determine length of canal

Characteristics ▶ Files or reamers are measured from stopper to apex of root to determine length of canal. Radiographs also help determine length. Stoppers are made from rubber, silicone, or plastic.

Practice Notes ▶ Endodontic Stoppers are color coded to correspond to a particular file or reamer, or a single color of stopper is used for all files or reamers. Endodontic Stoppers are used exclusively on endodontic tray setups.

Sterilization Notes ▶ Endodontic Stoppers should be disposed of in the garbage. Single use only.

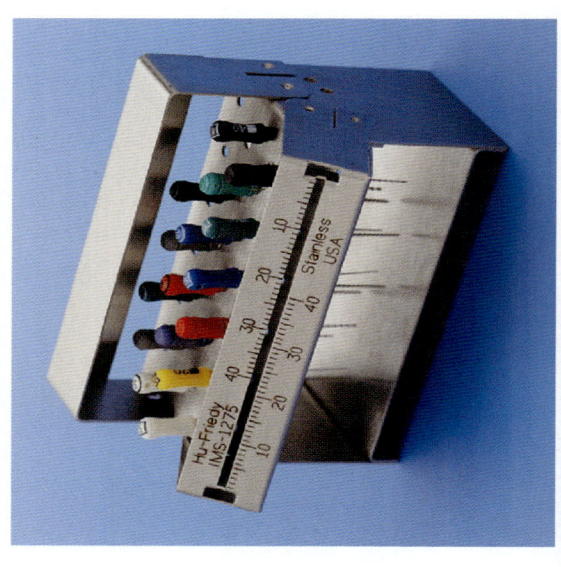

■ INSTRUMENT

Endodontic Stand

Functions ▸ To hold endodontic files and reamers
To measure endodontic files and reamers with millimeter ruler etched in container; may be measured from right or left side of stand

Characteristic ▸ Container closes with endodontic files and reamers for sterilization processes.

Practice Note ▸ Endodontic Stand is used exclusively with endodontic tray setups.

Sterilization Notes ▸ File or Reamer in Endodontic Stand and Endodontic Stand must be precleaned. Then, place in a sterilizing pouch with an internal process indicator, seal, then sterilize. OR, wrap with an internal process indicator inside and secure on the outside with process indicator tape, then sterilize. Verify appropriate color change has been achieved in external process indicator immediately after removal from sterilizer. Check internal process indicator before treatment. Refer to state regulations for any additional state requirements. Or used file or reamer must be disposed of in a sharps container. Rubber stopper on the file should be disposed of in the garbage. Single use only.

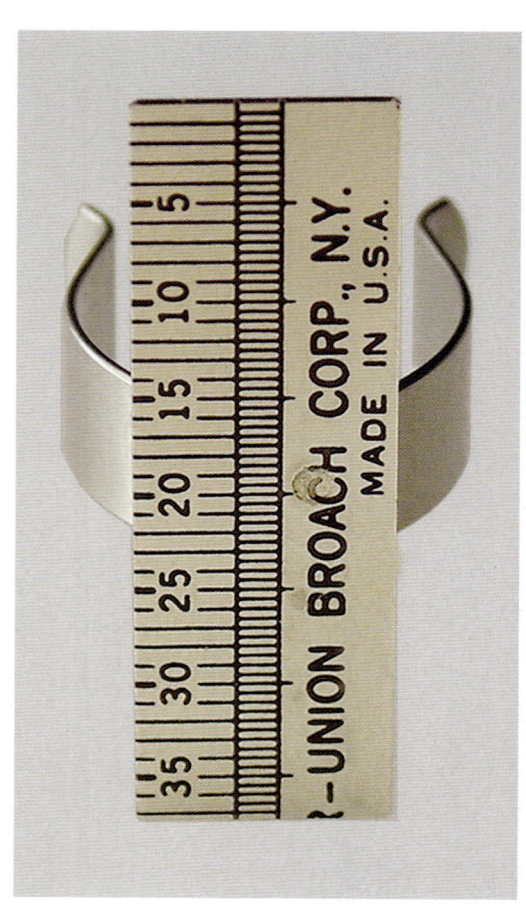

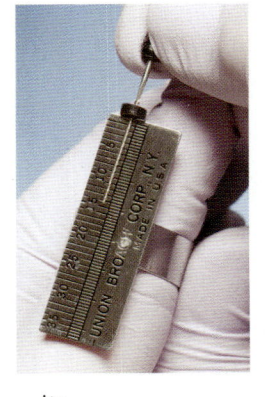

Endodontic Millimeter Ruler

■ INSTRUMENT

Function ▶ To measure files, reamers, other instruments, and materials in millimeter increments

Characteristic ▶ Variety of designs

Practice Notes ▶ Endodontic Millimeter Ruler could be used in areas of dentistry other than on endodontic tray setups.

Sterilization Notes ▶ Endodontic Millimeter Ruler must be precleaned. Then, place in a sterilizing pouch with an internal process indicator, seal, then sterilize. OR, wrap with an internal process indicator inside and secure on the outside with process indicator tape, then sterilize. Verify appropriate color change has been achieved in external process indicator immediately after removal from sterilizer. Check internal process indicator before treatment. Refer to state regulations for any additional state requirements.

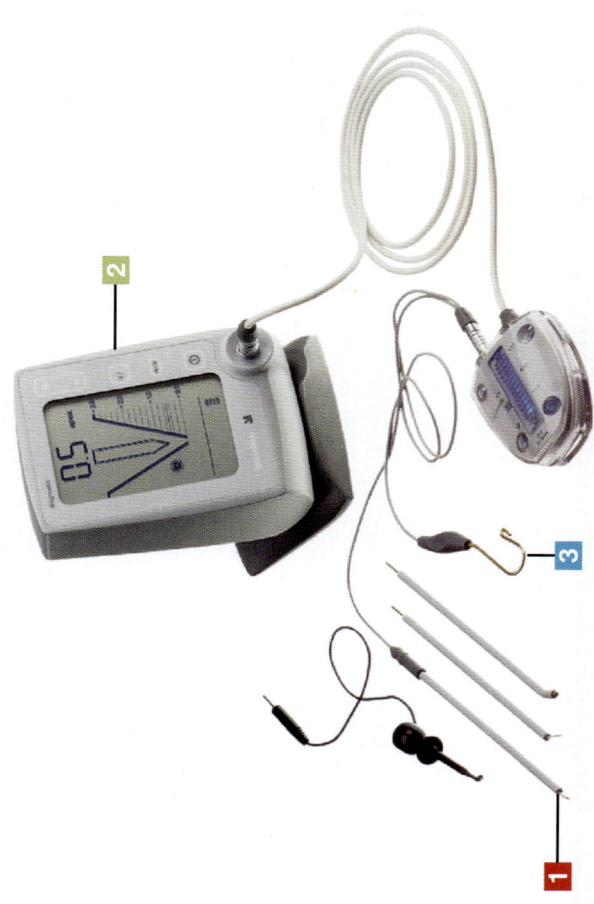

Electronic Apex Locator

Function ▶ To electronically measure length of canal to apex of tooth

Characteristics ▶
1 Attaches to file or reamer and is placed in canal using dry or wet environment
2 Readout indicates length of canal—Tone or digital
3 This device goes under the tongue during the Apex Locator procedure

Practice Note ▶ Electronic Apex Locator is used exclusively with endodontic tray setups.

Sterilization Notes ▶ Electronic Apex Locator devices that enters patient's mouth must be precleaned. Then, place in a sterilizing pouch with an internal process indicator, seal, then sterilize. OR, wrap with an internal process indicator inside and secure on the outside with process indicator tape, then sterilize. Verify appropriate color change has been achieved in external process indicator immediately after removal from sterilizer. Check internal process indicator before treatment. Refer to state regulations for any additional state requirements. Barriers should be used on the unit, or the manufacturer's recommendation for disinfection should be followed.

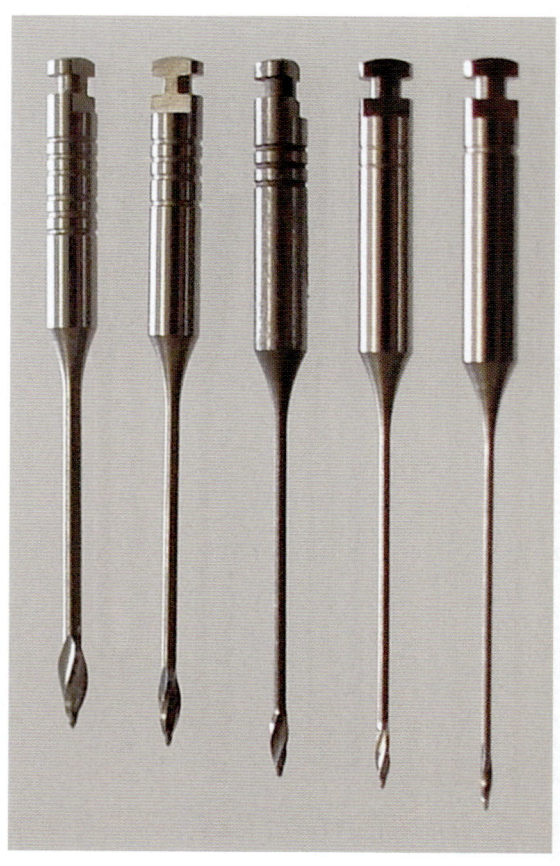

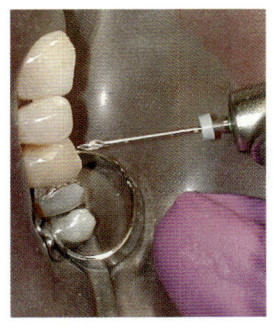

Gates Glidden Bur or Drill

Functions ▶ To enlarge walls of pulp chamber

To open canal orifice

Characteristics ▶ Long-shank bur

Elliptical or flame-shaped cutting edge

Latch Type Bur—Used with slow-speed contra-angle handpiece, air driven or electric

Range of sizes—Size identified by number of grooves on shank

Two lengths—Shorter for posterior teeth, longer for anterior teeth

Practice Note ▶ Gates Glidden Burs are used exclusively on endodontic tray setups.

Sterilization Notes ▶ Gates Glidden Bur or Drill must be precleaned. Then, place in a sterilizing pouch with an internal process indicator, seal, then sterilize. OR, wrap with an internal process indicator inside and secure on the outside with process indicator tape, then sterilize. Verify appropriate color change has been achieved in external process indicator immediately after removal from sterilizer. Check internal process indicator before treatment. Refer to state regulations for any additional state requirements. Or used Gates Glidden Bur must be disposed of in a sharps container.

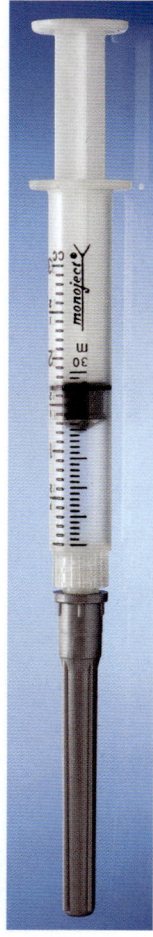

Endodontic Irrigating Syringe

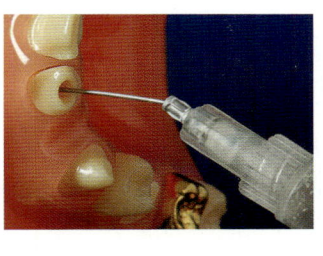

Function ▶ To carry and dispense irrigating solution into canal for cleansing during débridement of canal

Characteristics ▶ Disposable

Two sizes—3 mL (pictured) and 12 mL

Practice Note ▶ Endodontic Irrigating Syringe could be used in areas of dentistry other than on endodontic tray setups.

Sterilization Notes ▶ Endodontic Irrigating Syringe should be disposed of in a sharps container. For single use only.

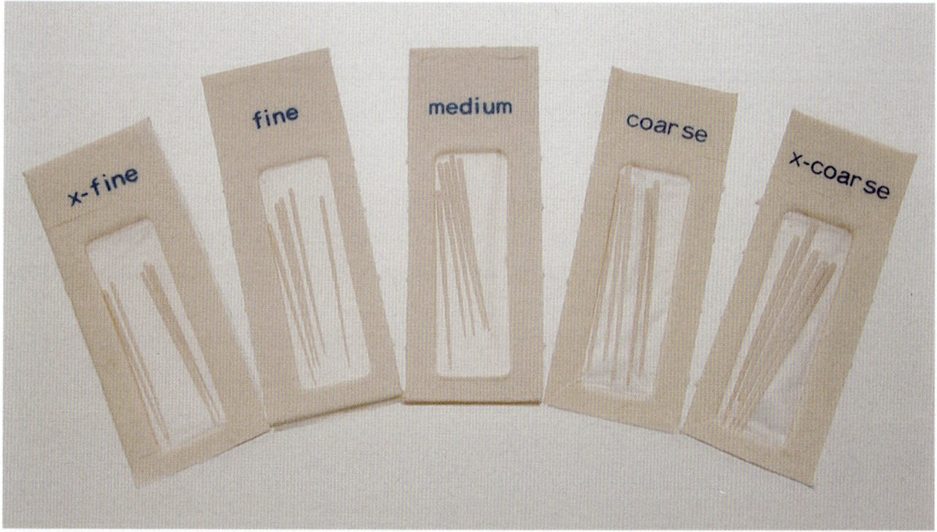
x-fine
fine
medium
coarse
x-coarse

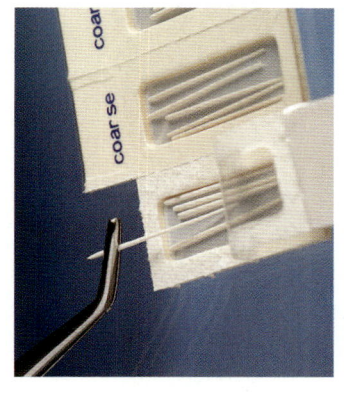

■ INSTRUMENT

Sterile Absorbent Paper Points

Function ▸ To dry pulp chambers of canal—New points inserted repeatedly until pulp chamber is completely dry

Characteristics ▸ Size of point corresponds to width of canal
Range of sizes available

Practice Notes ▸ The length of the paper point is measured to ensure that it corresponds to the length of the canal.
Paper points are used exclusively on endodontic tray setups.

Sterilization Notes ▸ Sterile Absorbent Paper Points should be disposed of in the garbage. Single use only.

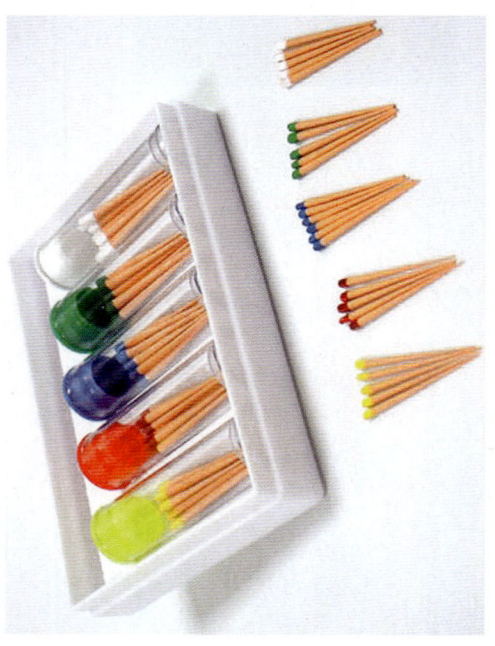

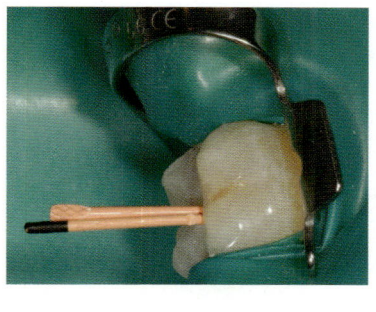

Gutta-Percha

Function ▶ To fill pulp chamber after completion of canal preparation
Called obturation

Characteristics ▶ Solid at room temperature; becomes soft and pliable when
heated
May be heated in a cartridge and then dispensed into canal
Range of sizes—To correspond to size of canal

Practice Notes ▶ Endodontic sealer, a cement material, is used with gutta-
percha for final sealing of the canal.
Gutta-Percha is used exclusively on an endodontic tray setup.

Sterilization Notes ▶ Gutta-Percha should be disposed of in the garbage.

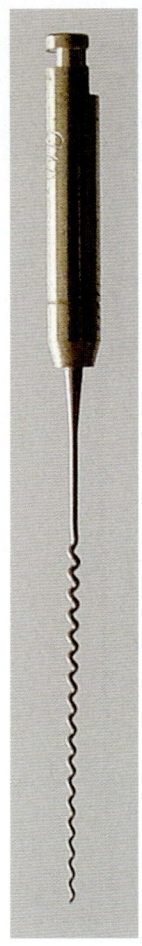

■ INSTRUMENT

Lentulo Spiral

Function ▶ To place endodontic sealer or cement in canal for final seal before placement of gutta-percha

Characteristic ▶ Latch-type shank—Used with slow-speed contra-angled handpiece, air driven or electric

Practice Note ▶ Lentulo Spiral is used exclusively on endodontic tray setups.

Sterilization Notes ▶ Lentulo Spiral must be precleaned. Then, place in a sterilizing pouch with an internal process indicator, seal, then sterilize. OR, wrap with an internal process indicator inside and secure on the outside with process indicator tape, then sterilize. Verify appropriate color change has been achieved in external process indicator immediately after removal from sterilizer. Check internal process indicator before treatment. Refer to state regulations for any additional state requirements. Or used Lentulo spiral must be disposed of in a sharps container.

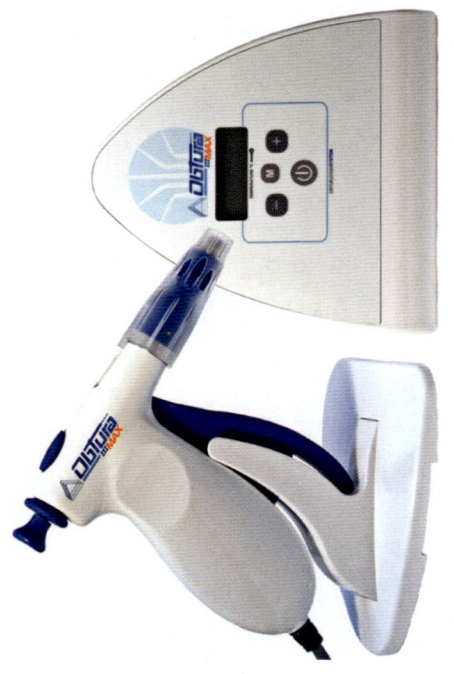

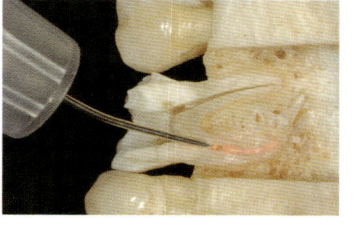

Gutta-Percha Warming Unit

Functions ►
To heat gutta-percha outside the mouth before use
To inject heated gutta-percha in thermoplastic state into prepared canals

Characteristics ►
Gutta-percha pellets—Used to load unit
Delivery system—Needle attaches to gun delivering gutta-percha into canal

Practice Notes ►
Temperature of the gutta-percha in the unit can be adjusted to control the viscosity of the material.
Gutta-Percha Warming Unit is used exclusively with endodontic tray setups.

Sterilization Notes ►
Gutta-Percha Warming Unit needle attached to the gutta-percha warming unit gun must be disposed of in a sharps container. Barriers should be used on Gutta-Percha Warming Unit, OR, unit must be disinfected according to the manufacturer's recommendation.

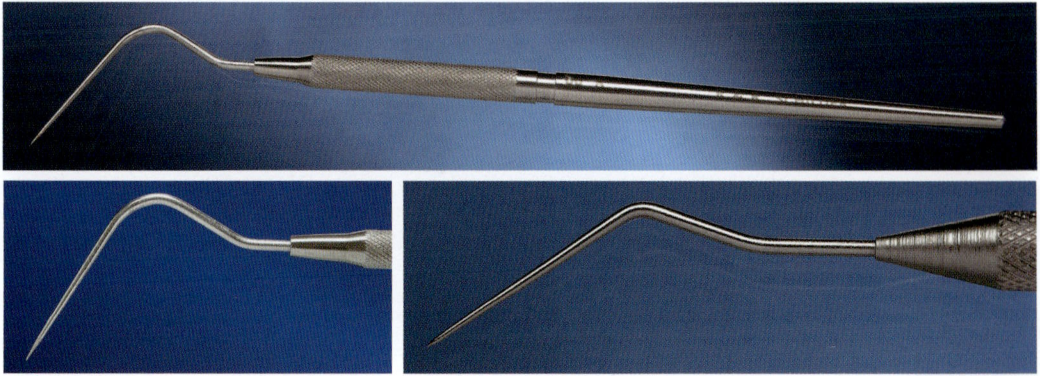

■ INSTRUMENT

Endodontic Spreader

Functions ▶
To help condense gutta-percha laterally in canal
To use for final filling of canal

Characteristics ▶
Pointed tip
Working end—Has rings in millimeter increments
Two handle styles—Conventional (pictured), finger spreader
Range of sizes—To correspond to size of canal

Practice Note ▶
Endodontic Spreader is used exclusively on endodontic tray setups.

Sterilization Notes ▶
Endodontic Spreader must be precleaned. Then, place in a sterilizing pouch with an internal process indicator, seal, then sterilize. OR, wrap with an internal process indicator inside and secure on the outside with process indicator tape, then sterilize. Verify appropriate color change has been achieved in external process indicator immediately after removal from sterilizer. Check internal process indicator before treatment. Refer to state regulations for any additional state requirements.

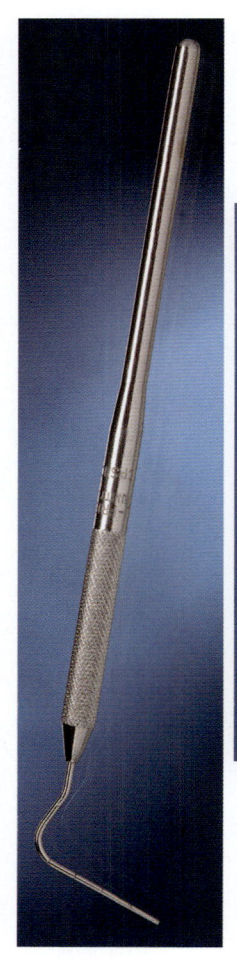

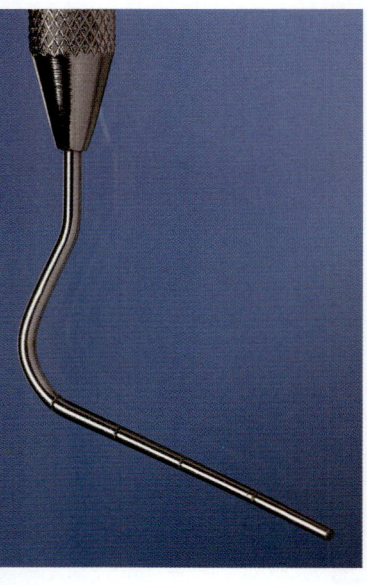

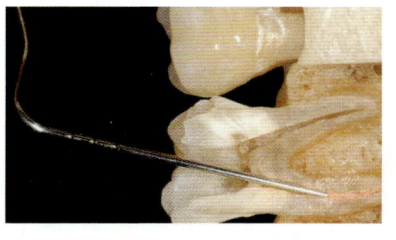

Endodontic Plugger

Functions ▶ To help condense gutta-percha vertically in canal
To use for final filling of canal

Characteristics ▶ Flat tip for condensing gutta-percha
Working end—Has rings in millimeter increments
Two handle styles—Conventional (pictured), finger spreader
Range of sizes—To correspond to size of canal

Practice Note ▶ Endodontic Plugger is used exclusively on endodontic tray setups.

Sterilization Notes ▶ Endodontic Plugger must be precleaned. Then, place in a sterilizing pouch with an internal process indicator, seal, then sterilize. OR, wrap with an internal process indicator inside and secure on the outside with process indicator tape, then sterilize. Verify appropriate color change has been achieved in external process indicator immediately after removal from sterilizer. Check internal process indicator before treatment. Refer to state regulations for any additional state requirements.

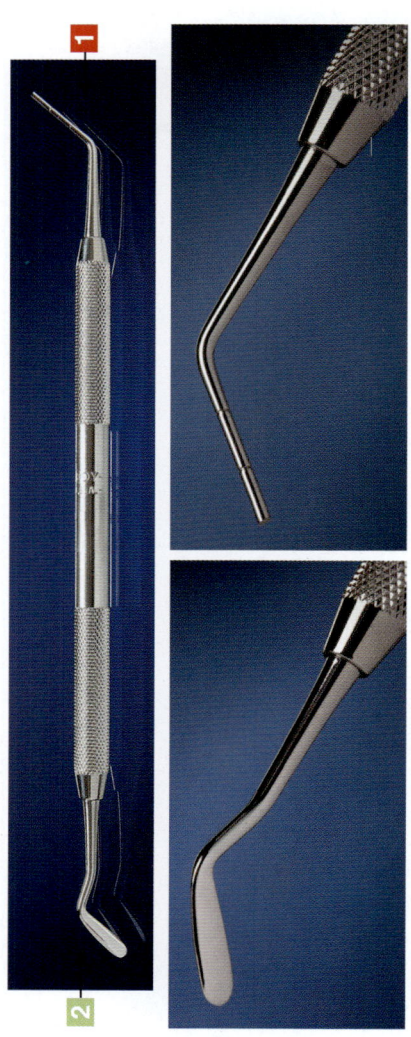

INSTRUMENT

Glick Instrument

Functions ▶ To condense gutta-percha into endodontically prepared teeth, using plugger end

To sever excess gutta-percha after plugger end is heated

To carry and place material into tooth, using paddle end

Characteristics ▶ Double ended:

1 Plugger end—May have rings in millimeter increments

2 Paddle end

Practice Note ▶ Glick Instrument is used exclusively on endodontic tray setups.

Sterilization Notes ▶ Glick Instrument must be precleaned. Then, place in a sterilizing pouch with an internal process indicator, seal, then sterilize. OR, wrap with an internal process indicator inside and secure on the outside with process indicator tape, then sterilize. Verify appropriate color change has been achieved in external process indicator immediately after removal from sterilizer. Check internal process indicator before treatment. Refer to state regulations for any additional state requirements.

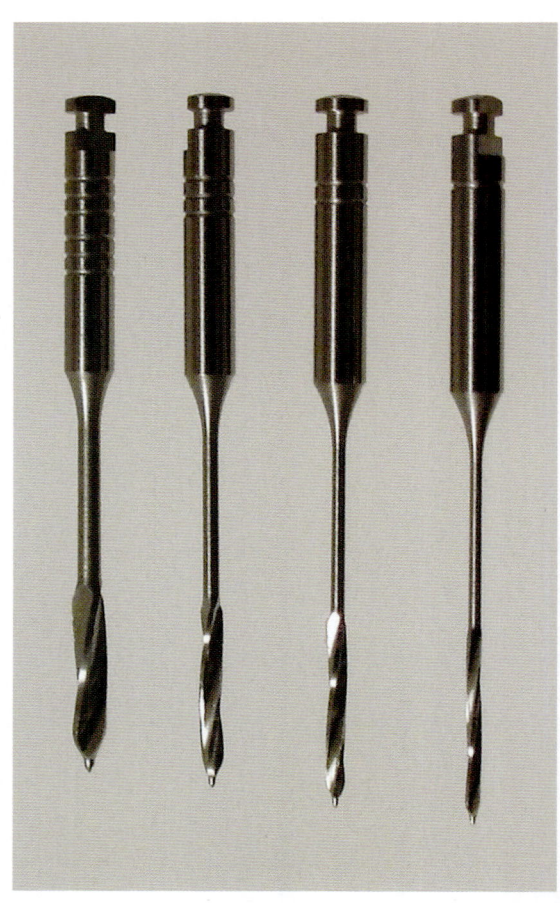

INSTRUMENT

Peso File

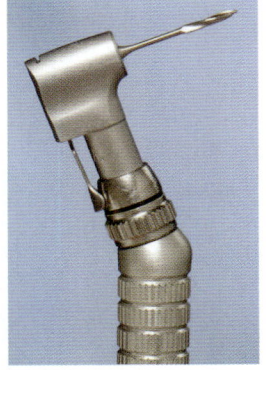

Functions ▶
To prepare canal for endodontic post
To remove portion of gutta-percha sealed in canal to make room for endodontic post

Characteristics ▶
Parallel cutting edges
Latch-type shank—Used with slow-speed contra-angle handpiece, air driven or electric
Range of sizes—Size identified by number of grooves on shank

Practice Note ▶
Peso File is used exclusively on endodontic tray setups.

Sterilization Notes ▶
Peso File must be precleaned. Then, place in a sterilizing pouch with an internal process indicator, seal, then sterilize. OR, wrap with an internal process indicator inside and secure on the outside with process indicator tape, then sterilize. Verify appropriate color change has been achieved in external process indicator immediately after removal from sterilizer. Check internal process indicator before treatment. Refer to state regulations for any additional state requirements. Or used Peso File must be disposed of in a sharps container.

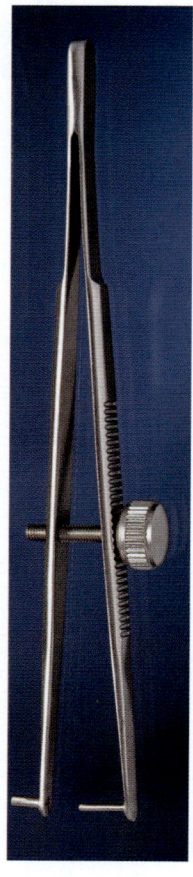

■ INSTRUMENT

Micro Retro Amalgam Carrier

Function ▶ To carry amalgam to surgical site of apicoectomy

Characteristics ▶ Very small—To accommodate retro fills for apicoectomy

Surgical apicoectomy procedure is performed, if needed, after an endodontic procedure is completed.

Practice Note ▶ Micro Retro Amalgam Carrier is used with a surgical tray setup for an apicoectomy.

Sterilization Notes ▶ Micro Retro Amalgam Carrier must be precleaned, open, and unlocked. Then, place in an open and unlocked position in a sterilizing pouch with an internal process indicator, seal, then sterilize. OR, wrap with an internal process indicator inside and secure on the outside with process indicator tape, then sterilize. Verify appropriate color change has been achieved in external process indicator immediately after removal from sterilizer. Check internal process indicator before treatment. Refer to state regulations for any additional state requirements.

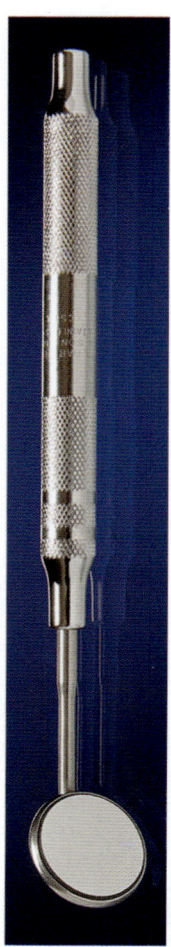

■ INSTRUMENT

Micro Retro Mouth Mirror

Function ▶ To view surgical site of apicoectomy retro fill

Characteristics ▶ Very small—To accommodate retro fills for apicoectomy
Smaller sizes available

Practice Note ▶ Micro Retro Mouth Mirror is used with a surgical tray setup for an apicoectomy.

Sterilization Notes ▶ Micro Retro Mouth Mirror must be precleaned. Then, place in a sterilizing pouch with an internal process indicator, seal, then sterilize. OR, wrap with an internal process indicator inside and secure on the outside with process indicator tape, then sterilize. Verify appropriate color change has been achieved in external process indicator immediately after removal from sterilizer. Check internal process indicator before treatment. Refer to state regulations for any additional state requirements.

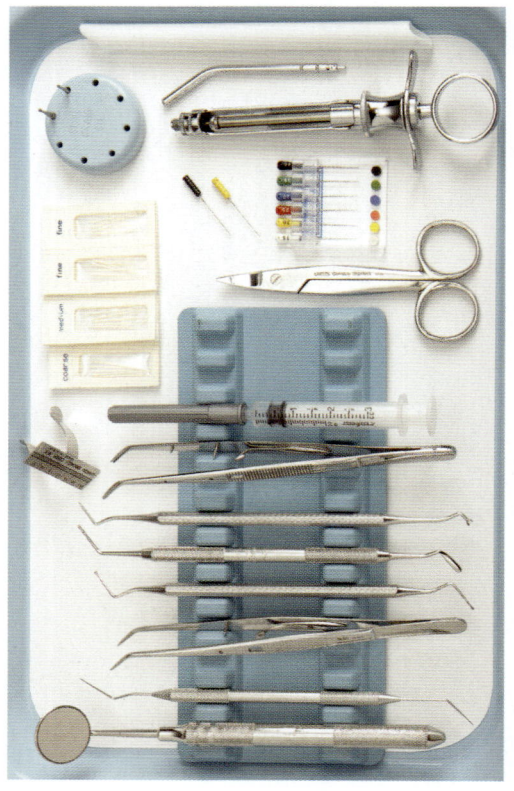

Opening a Tooth for Endodontic Therapy

TOP ROW (LEFT TO RIGHT)

Millimeter ruler with finger ring; coarse, medium, and fine absorbent sterile paper points; burs in bur block

BOTTOM ROW (LEFT TO RIGHT)

Mouth mirror, endodontic explorer, endodontic locking forceps, endodontic long-shank spoon excavator, Glick instrument, Woodson, endodontic locking forceps (extra), irrigating disposable syringe, scissors, broaches, endodontic K-type file with color-coded rubber stops, anesthetic aspirating syringe, air/water syringe tip, high-volume evacuation (HVE) tip

Sterilization Notes ▶ Refer to each picture for correct procedure for instrument sterilization or disposal of instrument or material. Refer to other chapters for additional instruments on this tray setup that are not included in this chapter.

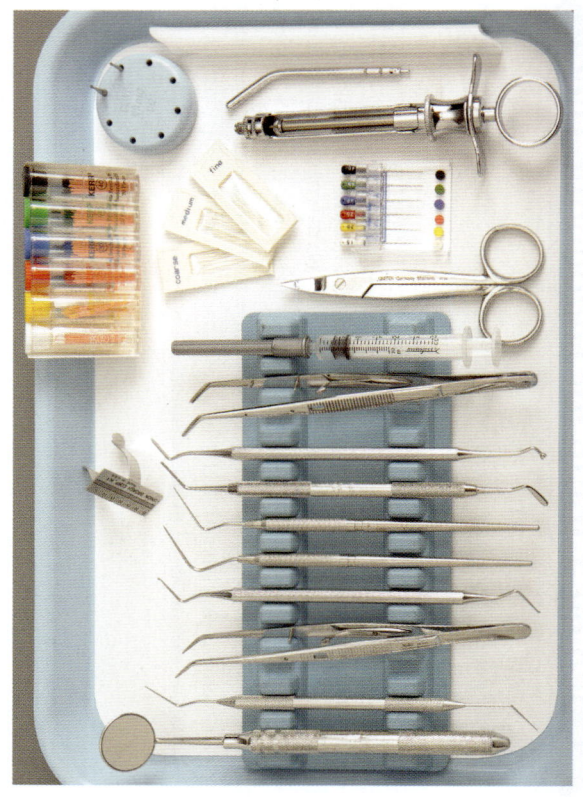

■ TRAY SETUP

Sealing a Tooth for Endodontic Therapy

TOP ROW (LEFT TO RIGHT)

Millimeter ruler with finger ring; gutta-percha in vials—Assorted sizes; coarse, medium, fine absorbent sterile paper points; burs in bur block

BOTTOM ROW (LEFT TO RIGHT)

Mouth mirror, endodontic explorer, endodontic locking forceps, endodontic long-shank spoon excavator, endodontic spreader, endodontic plugger, Glick instrument, Woodson, endodontic locking cotton forceps (extra), irrigating disposable syringe, scissors, endodontic K-type file with color-coded rubber stops, anesthetic aspirating syringe, air/water syringe tip, high-volume evacuation (HVE) tip

Sterilization Notes ▶ Refer to each picture for correct procedure for instrument sterilization or disposal of instrument or material. Refer to other chapters for additional instruments on this tray setup that are not included in this chapter.

12

Hygiene Instruments

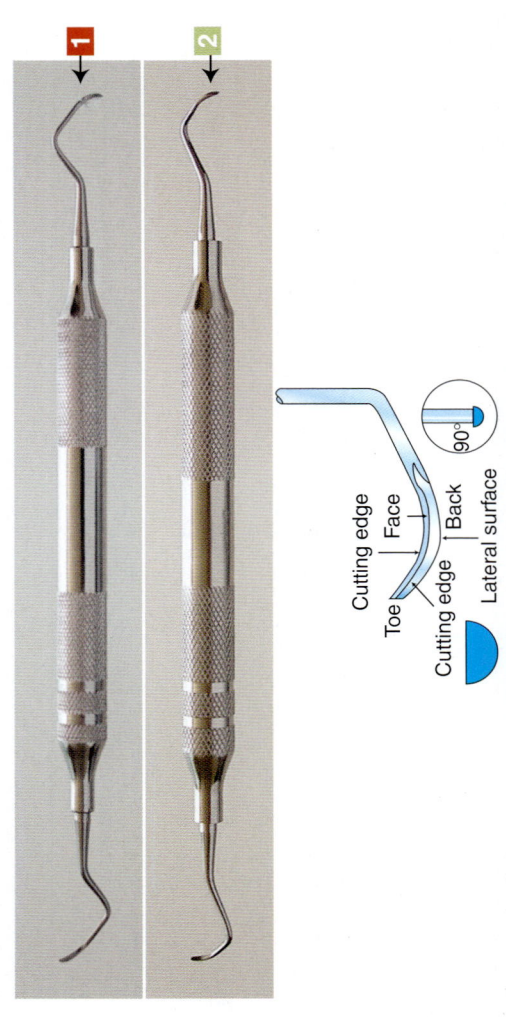

Cutting edge

Face

Toe

Cutting edge

Back

Lateral surface

90°

Universal Curettes (Curets)

INSTRUMENT

Functions ▸
To remove deposits and stains from teeth
To remove soft tissue lining of periodontal pocket and root planing

Characteristics ▸
Blade—Two cutting edges, rounded toe, rounded back; at 90-degree angle to lower shank
Flexible or rigid shank; length varies to accommodate clinical crown of tooth
Single or double ended
Range of sizes
Curette named by designer:

1 Barnhart ½
2 Ratcliff ⅜

Practice Note ▸
Universal Curettes are used on hygiene, periodontal, and operative tray setups.

Sterilization Notes ▸
Universal Curettes must be precleaned. Then, place in a sterilizing pouch with an internal process indicator, seal, then sterilize. OR, wrap with an internal process indicator inside and secure on the outside with process indicator tape, then sterilize. Verify appropriate color change has been achieved in external process indicator immediately after removal from sterilizer. Check internal process indicator before treatment. Refer to state regulations for any additional state requirements.

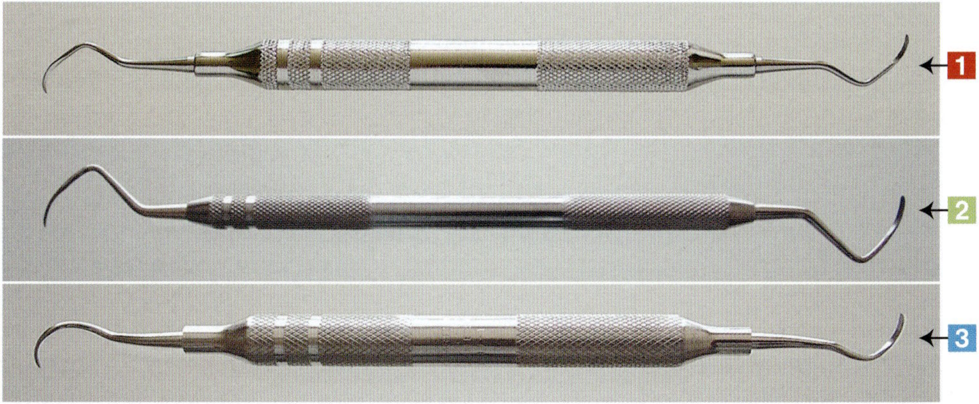
1
2
3

Universal Curettes (Curet)

Functions ▶

To scale supragingival and subgingival surfaces

To remove deposits and stains from teeth

To remove soft tissue lining of periodontal pocket and root planing

Characteristics ▶

Blade—Two cutting edges, rounded toe, rounded back; at 90-degree angle to lower shank

Flexible or rigid shank; length varies to accommodate clinical crown of tooth

Single or double ended

Range of sizes

Curette named by designer:

1 UC/Rule ⅚

2 Loma Linda ¹¹/₁₂

3 McCall ¹⁷/₁₈

Practice Note ▶

Universal Curettes are used on hygiene, periodontal, and operative tray setups.

Sterilization Notes ▶

Universal Curettes must be precleaned. Then, place in a sterilizing pouch with an internal process indicator, seal, then sterilize. OR, wrap with an internal process indicator inside and secure on the outside with process indicator tape, then sterilize. Verify appropriate color change has been achieved in external process indicator immediately after removal from sterilizer. Check internal process indicator before treatment. Refer to state regulations for any additional state requirements.

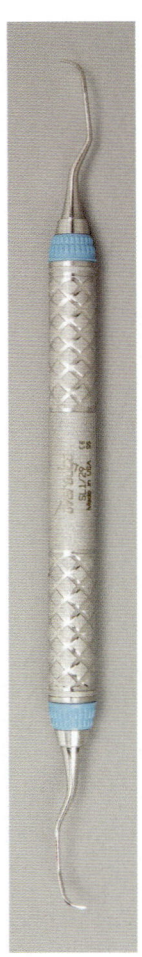

■ INSTRUMENT

Langer Universal Curettes

Functions ▶

To scale supragingival and subgingival surfaces

To remove deposits and stains from teeth

To remove soft tissue lining of periodontal pocket and root planing

Characteristics ▶

Blade—Two cutting edges, with face at 90-degree angle to lower shank

Design function with three bends in the shank, improving posterior access

Langer universal curettes designed with the shank design of a Gracey combined with a universal blade

Single or double ended

Range of sizes

Practice Note ▶

Langer Universal Curettes are used on hygiene and periodontal tray setups.

Sterilization Notes ▶

Langer Universal Curettes must be precleaned. Then, place in a sterilizing pouch with an internal process indicator, seal, then sterilize. OR, wrap with an internal process indicator inside and secure on the outside with process indicator tape, then sterilize. Verify appropriate color change has been achieved in external process indicator immediately after removal from sterilizer. Check internal process indicator before treatment. Refer to state regulations for any additional state requirements.

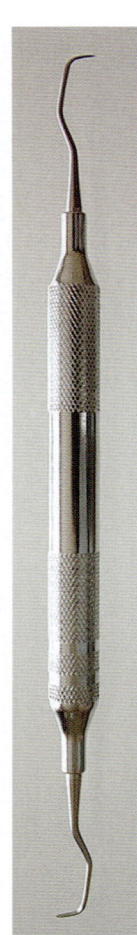

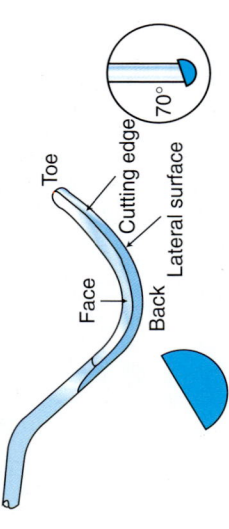

Toe

Cutting edge

Face

Back

Lateral surface

70°

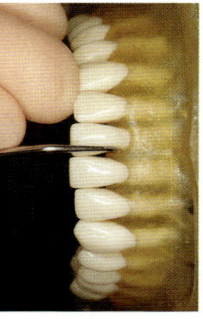

Area-Specific Curettes—Anterior

Functions ▶ To scale and remove deposits from subgingival surfaces of anterior teeth

To use for root planing, periodontal débridement, and soft tissue curettage

Characteristics ▶ Two cutting edges (only lower cutting edge used)

Blade—Rounded back and toe; at 70-degree angle to lower shank; types: standard, rigid, extra rigid

Curvature of blade designed to adapt to specific teeth and surfaces

Range of sizes available: ½, ¾, ⅚

Curette named by designer: Gracey, Kramer–Nevins, Turgeon

Practice Note ▶ Area-Specific Curettes—Anterior are used on hygiene and periodontal tray setups.

Sterilization Notes ▶ Area-Specific Curettes must be precleaned. Then, place in a sterilizing pouch with an internal process indicator, seal, then sterilize. OR, wrap with an internal process indicator inside and secure on the outside with process indicator tape, then sterilize. Verify appropriate color change has been achieved in external process indicator immediately after removal from sterilizer. Check internal process indicator before treatment. Refer to state regulations for any additional state requirements.

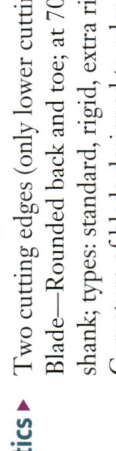

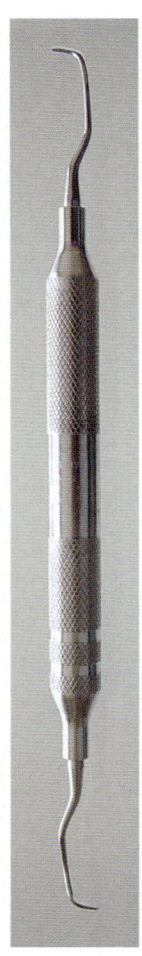

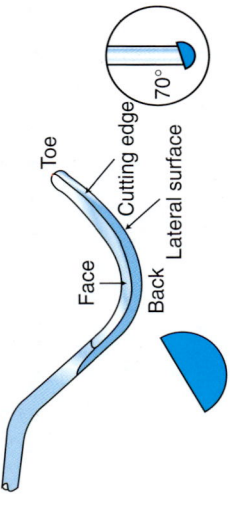

Toe

Face

Cutting edge

Back

Lateral surface

70°

■ INSTRUMENT

Area-Specific Curettes—Posterior

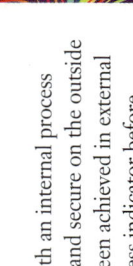

Functions ▶

To scale and remove deposits from subgingival surfaces of posterior teeth

To use for root planing, periodontal débridement, and soft tissue curettage

Characteristics ▶

Two cutting edges (only lower cutting edge used)

Blade—Rounded back and toe; at 70-degree angle to lower shank; types: standard, rigid, extra rigid

Curvature of blade designed to adapt to specific teeth and surfaces

Range of size, shape, and bends in shank

Two bends in shank

Examples: 7/8, 9/10

Three bends in shank

Examples: 11/12, 13/14, 15/16, 17/18

Curette named by designer: Gracey, Kramer-Nevins, Turgeon

Practice Note ▶

Area-Specific Curettes—Posterior are used on hygiene and periodontal tray setups.

Sterilization Notes ▶

Area-Specific Curettes must be precleaned. Then, place in a sterilizing pouch with an internal process indicator, seal, then sterilize. OR, wrap with an internal process indicator inside and secure on the outside with process indicator tape, then sterilize. Verify appropriate color change has been achieved in external process indicator immediately after removal from sterilizer. Check internal process indicator before treatment. Refer to state regulations for any additional state requirements.

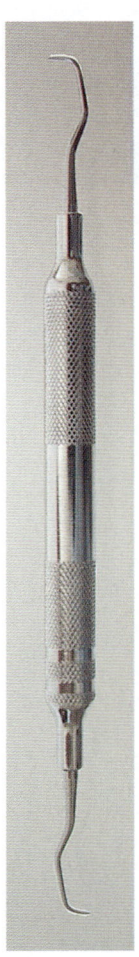

Extended Area-Specific Curettes—Anterior

Function ▶ To scale and remove deposits in deep periodontal pockets 5 mm or deeper

Characteristics ▶ Two cutting edges (only lower cutting edge used)
Blade at 70-degree angle to lower shank; types: standard, rigid, extra rigid
Curvature of blade designed to adapt to anteriors
Terminal shank redesigned—3 mm longer than standard area-specific curette
Manufacturer's trademark name usually follows ½, ¾, ⅚ numbering system
Range of sizes—Commonly used types: ¾, ⅚
Double-ended curettes packaged in sets
Curettes named by designer: Gracey ½

Practice Note ▶ Extended Area-Specific Curettes—Anterior are used on hygiene and periodontal tray setups.

Sterilization Notes ▶ Extended Area-Specific Curettes must be precleaned. Then, place in a sterilizing pouch with an internal process indicator, seal, then sterilize. OR, wrap with an internal process indicator inside and secure on the outside with process indicator tape, then sterilize. Verify appropriate color change has been achieved in external process indicator immediately after removal from sterilizer. Check internal process indicator before treatment. Refer to state regulations for any additional state requirements.

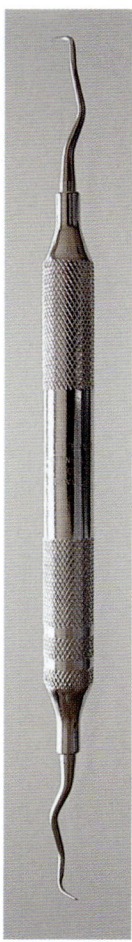

Extended Area-Specific Curettes—Posterior

Function ▶ To scale and remove deposits in deep periodontal pockets (5 mm or deeper)

Characteristics ▶ Two cutting edges (only lower cutting edge used)

Blade at 70-degree angle to lower shank; types: standard, rigid, extra rigid

Curvature of blade designed to adapt to premolars, molars

Terminal shank redesigned—3 mm longer than standard area-specific curette

Range of sizes

Commonly used types: $^{11}/_{12}$, $^{13}/_{14}$, $^{15}/_{16}$, $^{17}/_{18}$

Double-ended curettes packaged in sets

Curettes named by designer: Gracey $^{11}/_{12}$ rigid, Gracey $^{11}/_{12}$

Practice Note ▶ Extended Area-Specific Curettes—Posterior are used on hygiene and periodontal tray setups.

Sterilization Notes ▶ Extended Area-Specific Curettes must be precleaned. Then, place in a sterilizing pouch with an internal process indicator, seal, then sterilize. OR, wrap with an internal process indicator inside and secure on the outside with process indicator tape, then sterilize. Verify appropriate color change has been achieved in external process indicator immediately after removal from sterilizer. Check internal process indicator before treatment. Refer to state regulations for any additional state requirements.

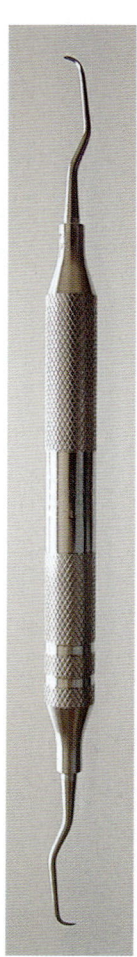

Mini Extended Area-Specific Curettes—Anterior

Function ▸ To scale in deep periodontal pockets (5 mm)

Characteristics ▸ Blade redesigned to be half the length of extended area-specific curette

Designed for narrow roots, pockets, or furcations

Two cutting edges (only lower cutting edge used)

Blade at 70-degree angle to lower shank; types: standard, rigid, extra rigid

Curvature of blade designed to adapt to anteriors

Range of sizes

Manufacturer's trademark name usually follows ½, ¾, ⅚ numbering system

Curettes named by designer: Gracey ½

Practice Note ▸ Mini Extended Area-Specific Curettes—Anterior are used on hygiene and periodontal tray setups.

Sterilization Notes ▸ Mini Extended Area-Specific Curettes must be precleaned. Then, place in a sterilizing pouch with an internal process indicator, seal, then sterilize. OR, wrap with an internal process indicator inside and secure on the outside with process indicator tape, then sterilize. Verify appropriate color change has been achieved in external process indicator immediately after removal from sterilizer. Check internal process indicator before treatment. Refer to state regulations for any additional state requirements.

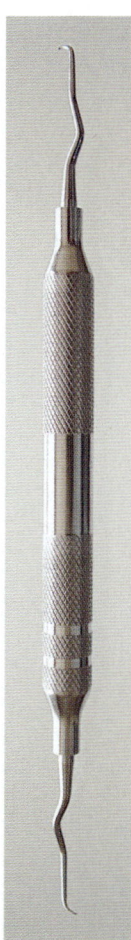

Mini Extended Area-Specific Curettes—Posterior

■ INSTRUMENT

Function ▸ To scale in deep periodontal pockets (5 mm)

Characteristics ▸ Blade redesigned to be half the length of extended area-specific curette

Designed for narrow roots, pockets, or furcations

Two cutting edges (only lower cutting edge used)

Blade at 70-degree angle to lower shank; types: standard, rigid, extra rigid

Curvature of blade designed to adapt to premolars and molars

Range of size, shape, and bends in shank available

Two bends in shank

Examples: 7/8, 9/10

Three bends in shank

Examples: 11/12, 13/14, 15/16, 17/18

Curettes named by designer: Gracey 11/12 mini extender

Practice Note ▸ Mini Extended Area-Specific Curettes—Posterior are used on hygiene and periodontal tray setups.

Sterilization Notes ▸ Mini Extended Area-Specific Curettes—Posterior must be precleaned. Then, place in a sterilizing pouch with an internal process indicator, seal, then sterilize. OR, wrap with an internal process indicator inside and secure on the outside with process indicator tape, then sterilize. Verify appropriate color change has been achieved in external process indicator immediately after removal from sterilizer. Check internal process indicator before treatment. Refer to state regulations for any additional state requirements.

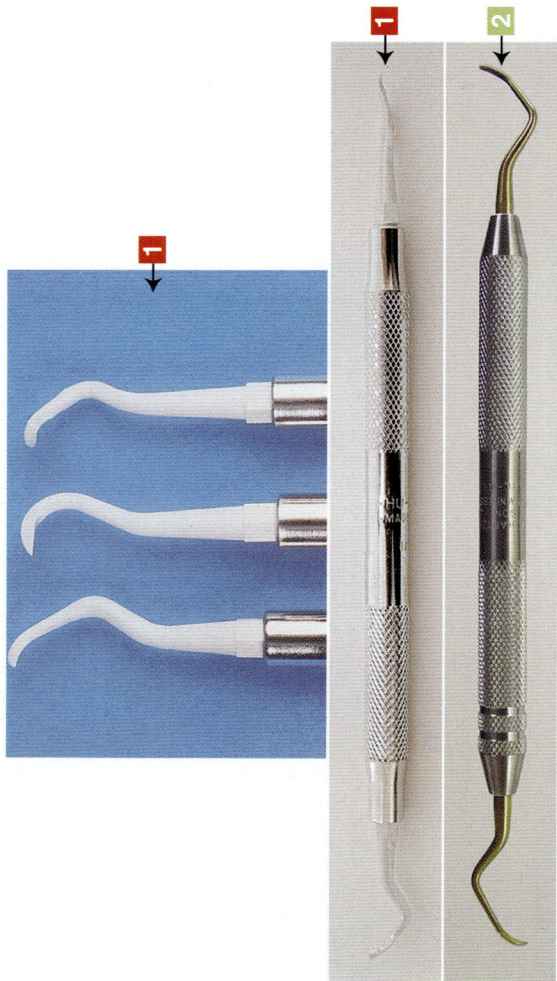

■ INSTRUMENT

Implant Scaler

Function ▶ To remove deposits and stains from surface of implant

Characteristics ▶

1. Disposable tips (each tip should be sterilized before use). Instrument with disposable tip attached.

2. Titanium-coated scaler

Different designs allow scaling without scratching of titanium implants

Some tips are made of Plasteel—A high-grade resin

Practice Note ▶ Implant Scalers are used on hygiene and periodontal tray setups.

Sterilization Notes ▶ Handle and titanium-coated scaler must be precleaned. Then, place in a sterilizing pouch with an internal process indicator, seal, then sterilize. OR, wrap with an internal process indicator inside and secure on the outside with process indicator tape, then sterilize. Verify appropriate color change has been achieved in external process indicator immediately after removal from sterilizer. Check internal process indicator before treatment. Refer to state regulations for any additional state requirements. Or disposable scaler tip should be disposed of in a sharps container.

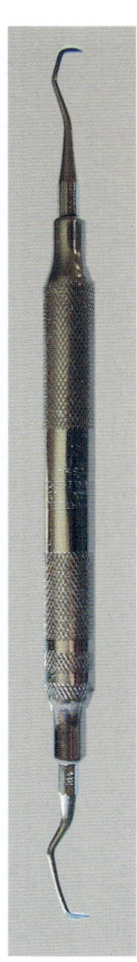

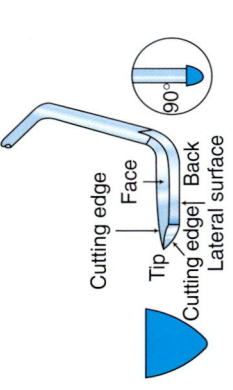

Cutting edge

Face

90°

Tip

Cutting edge | Back

Lateral surface

Straight Sickle Scaler

Function ▶ To remove large amounts of deposits from supragingival surfaces

Characteristics ▶ Two cutting edges on straight blade that ends in sharp point
Long; two bends in shank
Variety of sizes and angles
Single or double ended—Two ends may be shaped differently

Practice Note ▶ Straight Sickle Scaler is used on hygiene and periodontal tray setups.

Sterilization Notes ▶ Straight Sickle Scaler must be precleaned. Then, place in a sterilizing pouch with an internal process indicator, seal, then sterilize. OR, wrap with an internal process indicator inside and secure on the outside with process indicator tape, then sterilize. Verify appropriate color change has been achieved in external process indicator immediately after removal from sterilizer. Check internal process indicator before treatment. Refer to state regulations for any additional state requirements.

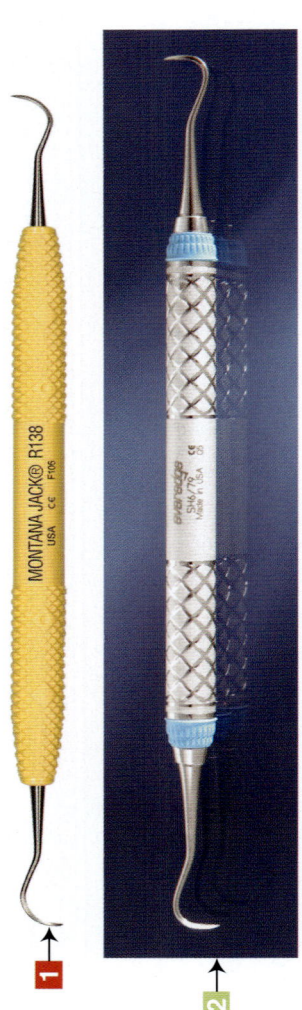

1

2

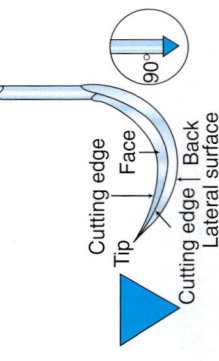

Cutting edge

Face

Tip

Cutting edge ↑ | Back

Lateral surface

90°

Curved Sickle Scaler

Function ▸ To remove large amounts of deposits from supragingival surfaces

Characteristics ▸ Two cutting edges on curved blade that ends in sharp point
Long, straight shank with one gentle bend
Variety of sizes and angles
Single or double ended—Two ends may be shaped differently

1 Montana Jack—Sharper, thinner blades with solid resin handle for comfortable grip.
2 Traditional Curved Sickle Scaler

Practice Note ▸ Curved Sickle Scaler is used on hygiene and periodontal tray setups.

Sterilization Notes ▸ Curved Sickle Scaler must be precleaned. Then, place in a sterilizing pouch with an internal process indicator, seal, then sterilize. OR, wrap with an internal process indicator inside and secure on the outside with process indicator tape, then sterilize. Verify appropriate color change has been achieved in external process indicator immediately after removal from sterilizer. Check internal process indicator before treatment. Refer to state regulations for any additional state requirements.

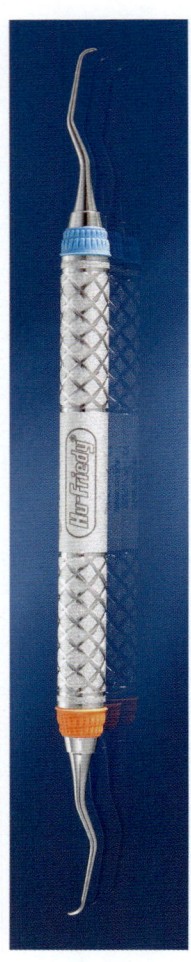

Micro Mini-Five Area-Specific Curette

Function ▶ To scale into periodontal pockets and root surfaces of 5 mm or more

Characteristics ▶ Blade half the length of After Five or standard Gracey curettes

Shank slightly increased rigidity compared with traditional mini five Gracey curettes

Practice Notes ▶ Designed for narrow pockets and furcations

Micro Mini-Five Area-Specific Curette is used on hygiene and periodontal tray setups

Sterilization Notes ▶ Micro Mini-Five Area-Specific Curette must be precleaned. Then, place in a sterilizing pouch with an internal process indicator, seal, then sterilize. OR, wrap with an internal process indicator inside and secure on the outside with process indicator tape, then sterilize. Verify appropriate color change has been achieved in external process indicator immediately after removal from sterilizer. Check internal process indicator before treatment. Refer to state regulations for any additional state requirements.

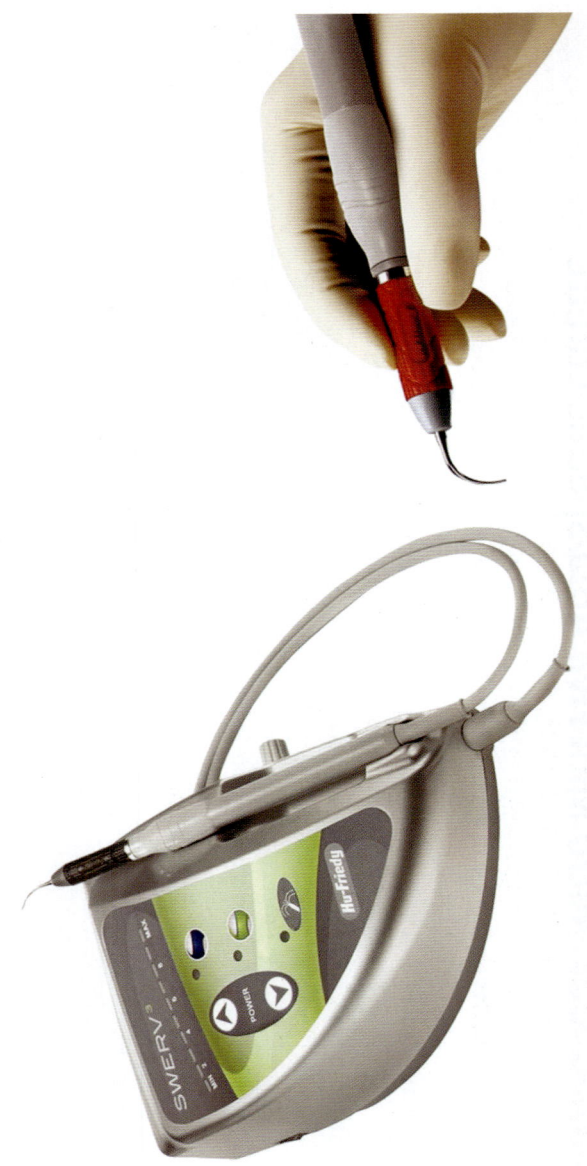

Magnetostrictive Power Scaler

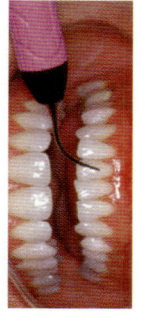

Function ▶ To use with water-cooled ultrasonic inserts vibrating at high frequency

Characteristics ▶ Ultra-high frequency sound waves convert mechanical energy into vibrations (frequency ranges from 18 to 50 kHz).

Some units (depending on manufacturer) have self-contained water reservoirs.
Some units (depending on manufacturer) have an additional air/water/sodium bicarbonate slurry polishing system to remove extrinsic stains and dental plaque.
A variety of sizes and designs are available.

Practice Note ▶ Magnetostrictive Power Scaler/Ultrasonic Scaling Unit is used during a routine prophylaxis appointment or for other appointments for root planing.

Sterilization Notes ▶ Barriers should be used for Power Scaler unit. Refer to the manufacturer's recommendation for disinfecting the unit. Power scaler inserts must be precleaned. Then, place in a sterilizing pouch with an internal process indicator, seal, then sterilize. OR, wrap with an internal process indicator inside and secure on the outside with process indicator tape, then sterilize. Verify appropriate color change has been achieved in external process indicator immediately after removal from sterilizer. Check internal process indicator before treatment. Refer to state regulations for any additional state requirements.

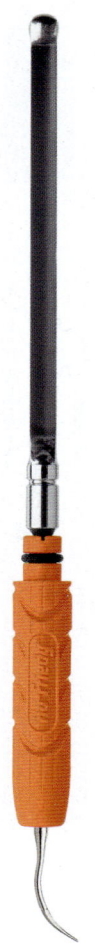

Ultrasonic Scaler Instrument Tip—Supragingival

Functions ▶

To remove supragingival calculus from teeth

To remove bacterial plaque from periodontal pockets

To remove heavy debris and stains from teeth

To remove excess cement from orthodontic bands after cementation and after band removal

Characteristics ▶

Supragingival Tip is inserted into the tubing on the ultrasonic scaling unit

Available in different lengths (called stacks): 25 kHz or 30 kHz, depending on unit

Water-cooled inserts (Water systems vary with internal or external water delivery.)

Variety of shapes, sizes, and designs, depending on designated and varying grips

Example: Original prophy

Tip style: Finely beveled internal water delivery tube

Practice Notes ▶

Ultrasonic Scaler Tip—Supragingival is used on hygiene and periodontal tray setups.

These tips are also known as ultrasonic inserts.

Sterilization Notes ▶

Ultrasonic Scaler Tip—Supragingival must be precleaned. Then, place in a sterilizing pouch with an internal process indicator, seal, then sterilize. OR, wrap with an internal process indicator inside and secure on the outside with process indicator tape, then sterilize. Verify appropriate color change has been achieved in external process indicator immediately after removal from sterilizer. Check internal process indicator before treatment. Refer to state regulations for any additional state requirements.

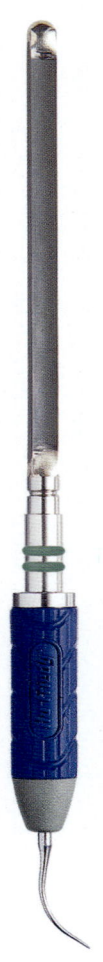

Ultrasonic Scaler Instrument Tip—Subgingival

■ INSTRUMENT

Functions ▶
To remove subgingival calculus from teeth
To remove bacterial plaque from periodontal pockets

Characteristics ▶
Subgingival Scaler Tip is inserted into the tubing on the ultrasonic scaling unit.
Available in different lengths (called stacks): 25 kHz or 30 kHz, depending on unit
Water-cooled inserts (Water systems vary with internal or external water delivery.)
Variety of shapes, sizes, and designs, depending on designated area and varying grips
Example: After Five design for subgingival areas
Tip style: Finely beveled internal water delivery tube (pictured)

Practice Notes ▶
Ultrasonic Scaler Tip—Subgingival is used on hygiene and periodontal tray setups.
These tips are also known as ultrasonic inserts.

Sterilization Notes ▶
Ultrasonic Scaler Tip—Subgingival must be precleaned. Then, place in a sterilizing pouch with an internal process indicator, seal, then sterilize. OR, wrap with an internal process indicator inside and secure on the outside with process indicator tape, then sterilize. Verify appropriate color change has been achieved in external process indicator immediately after removal from sterilizer. Check internal process indicator before treatment. Refer to state regulations for any additional state requirements.

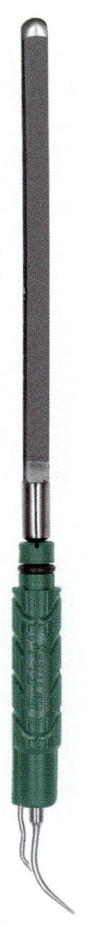

Ultrasonic Scaler Instrument Tip—Furcation

■ INSTRUMENT

Function ▶ To remove bacterial plaque from furcation areas

Characteristics ▶ Furcation Tip is inserted into the tubing on the ultrasonic scaling unit.

Available in different lengths (called stacks): 25 kHz or 30 kHz, depending on unit

Water-cooled inserts (Water systems vary with internal or external water delivery.)

Variety of shapes, sizes, and designs, depending on designated area and varying grips

Example: Furcation Plus design

Tip style: 0.8-mm ball end adapts to furcation, external water delivery tube (pictured)

Practice Notes ▶ Ultrasonic Scaler Tip—Furcation is used on hygiene and periodontal tray setups.

These tips are also known as ultrasonic inserts.

Pictured: Original Prophy

Sterilization Notes ▶ Ultrasonic Scaler Tip—Furcation must be precleaned. Then, place in a sterilizing pouch with an internal process indicator, seal, then sterilize. OR, wrap with an internal process indicator inside and secure on the outside with process indicator tape, then sterilize. Verify appropriate color change has been achieved in external process indicator immediately after removal from sterilizer. Check internal process indicator before treatment. Refer to state regulations for any additional state requirements.

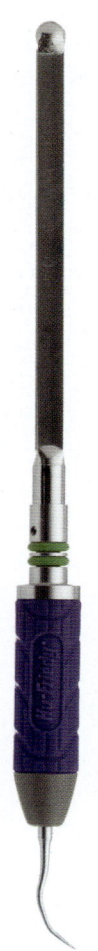

Ultrasonic Scaler Instrument Tip—Universal

Function ▶ To remove bacterial plaque and general deposits

Characteristics ▶ Universal tip is inserted into the tubing on the ultrasonic scaling unit.
Available in different lengths (called stacks): 25 kHz or 30 kHz, depending on unit
Water-cooled inserts (Water systems vary with internal or external water delivery.)
Variety of shapes, sizes, and designs, depending on designated area and varying grips
Example: Streamline design
Tip style: Water delivered directly from base of tip, eliminating need for external water system; efficient at low settings (pictured)

Practice Notes ▶ Ultrasonic Scaler Tip—Universal is used on hygiene and periodontal tray setups.
These tips are also known as ultrasonic inserts.

Sterilization Notes ▶ Ultrasonic Scaler Tip—Universal must be precleaned. Then, place in a sterilizing pouch with an internal process indicator, seal, then sterilize. OR, wrap with an internal process indicator inside and secure on the outside with process indicator tape, then sterilize. Verify appropriate color change has been achieved in external process indicator immediately after removal from sterilizer. Check internal process indicator before treatment. Refer to state regulations for any additional state requirements.

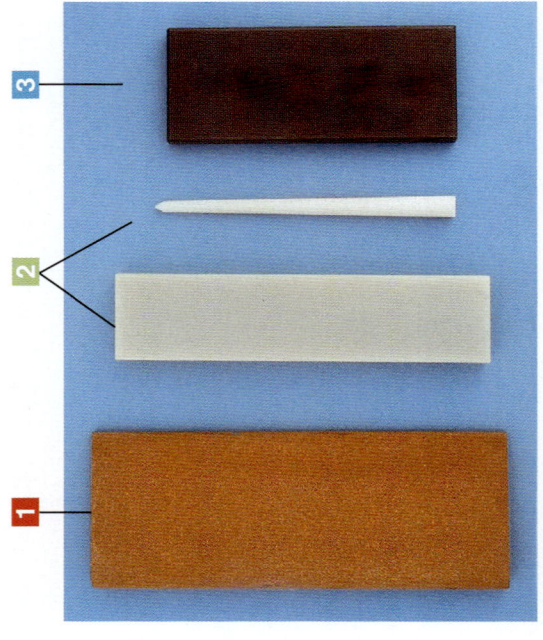

■ INSTRUMENT

Sharpening Stones

Function ▶ To sharpen scalers and curettes

Characteristics ▶ Types of stones:

1 India stones—Remove the most metal when used and should be followed with an Arkansas or ceramic stone

2 Arkansas stones—Provide a polished edge (flat and cone-shaped pictured)

3 Ceramic stones—Provide a polished edge and do not require lubrication

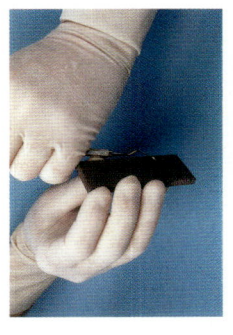

Practice Note ▶ Sharpening Stones are used on hygiene and periodontal tray setups.

Sterilization Notes ▶ Sharpening Stones must be precleaned. Then, place in a sterilizing pouch with an internal process indicator, seal, then sterilize. OR, wrap with an internal process indicator inside and secure on the outside with process indicator tape, then sterilize. Verify appropriate color change has been achieved in external process indicator immediately after removal from sterilizer. Check internal process indicator before treatment. Refer to state regulations for any additional state requirements.

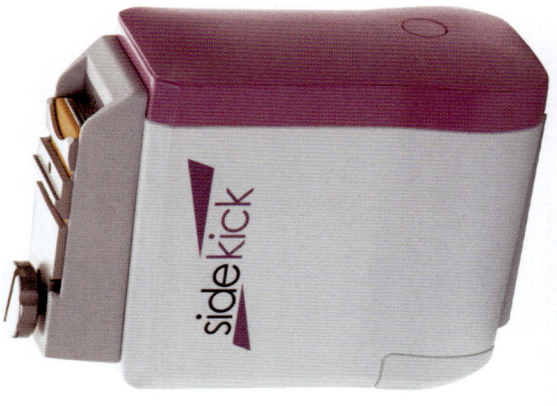

■ INSTRUMENT

Battery-Operated Sharpening Device

Function ▶ To sharpen scalers and curettes

Characteristics ▶ Stone moves underneath a stainless-steel guideplate, which puts the blade at factory angles. Sharpener has a power device with instrument guide channels and a vertical backstop to help control blade angulation. (Pictured: Sidekick Sharpener)

Practice Note ▶ Battery-Operated Sharpening Device should be used with sterile scalers and curettes, and then instruments resterilized after sharpening.

Sterilization Notes ▶ Barrier wrap; disinfect or sterilize certain parts of equipment according to the manufacturer's recommendation. Sharpened Scalers and Curettes must be precleaned. Then, place in a sterilizing pouch with an internal process indicator, seal, then sterilize. OR, wrap with an internal process indicator inside and secure on the outside with process indicator tape, then sterilize. Verify appropriate color change has been achieved in external process indicator immediately after removal from sterilizer. Check internal process indicator before treatment. Refer to state regulations for any additional state requirements.

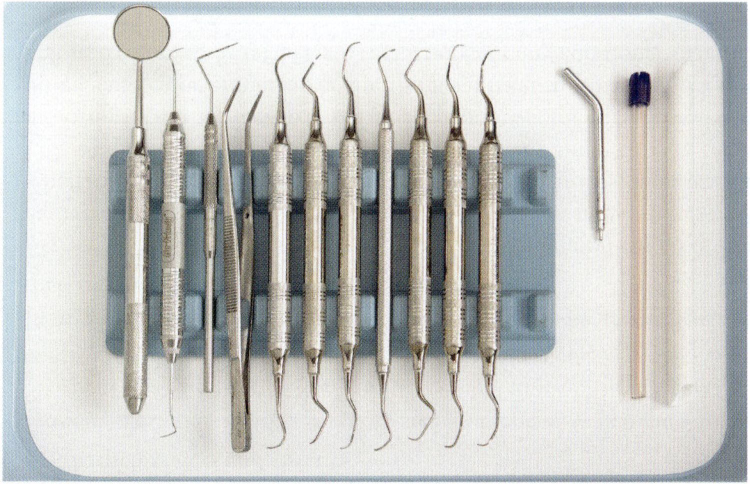

Hygiene

FROM LEFT TO RIGHT

Mouth mirror, explorer, periodontal probe, cotton forceps, curved sickle scaler, 4L/4R universal posterior, universal Langer ½, Ratcliff ¾, Gracey ⅞, Gracey ¹¹/₁₂, Gracey ¹³/₁₄, air/water syringe tip, low-volume saliva ejector, high-volume evacuation (HVE) tip.

Sterilization Notes ▶ Refer to each picture for correct procedure for instrument sterilization or disposal of instrument or material. Refer to other chapters for additional instruments on this tray setup that are not included in this chapter.

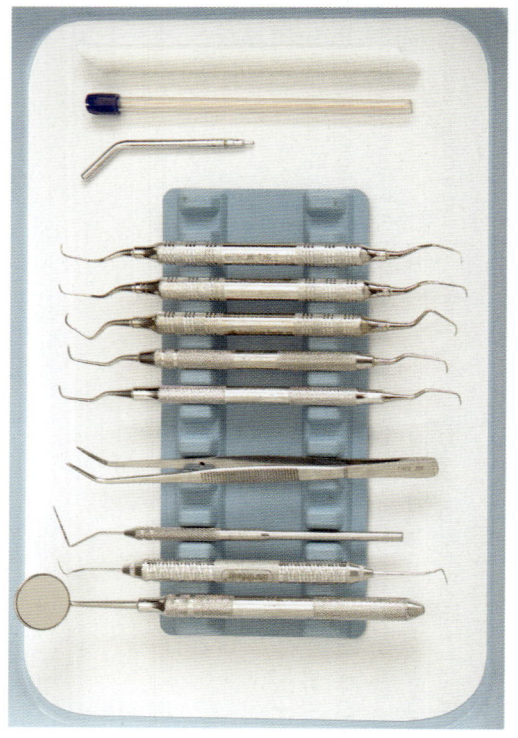

Root Planing

FROM LEFT TO RIGHT

Mouth mirror, explorer, periodontal probe, cotton forceps, Gracey ½, Gracey ¾, Gracey ⁷/₈, Gracey ¹¹/₁₂, Gracey ¹³/₁₄, air/water syringe tip, low-volume saliva ejector, high-volume evacuation (HVE) tip.

Sterilization Notes ▶ Refer to each individual picture for correct procedure for instrument sterilization or disposal of instrument or material. Refer to other chapters for additional instruments on this tray setup that are not included in this chapter.

13

Preventive and Sealant Instruments and Whitening Trays

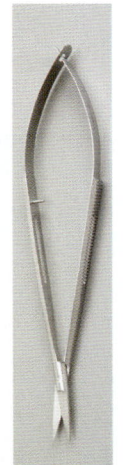

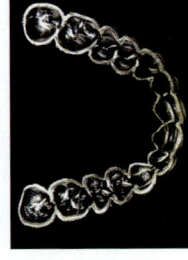

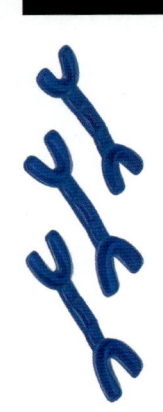

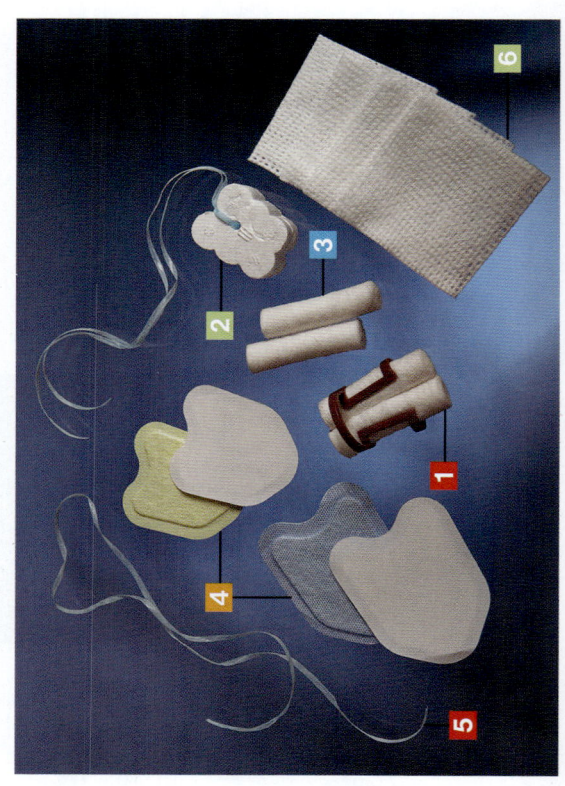

■ INSTRUMENT

Disposables

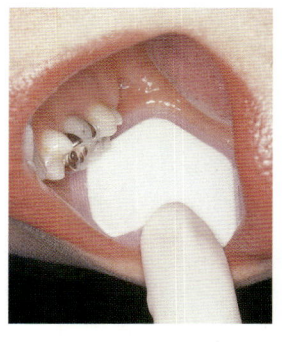

Functions ▶ To use with all types of dental procedures

To use when area in the mouth needs to stay dry

Characteristics ▶

1 Cotton Roll Holder for mandibular arch; one cotton roll is placed on the buccal side of the teeth, and the other is placed on the lingual side of the teeth.

2 Disposable Bite Block with ligature tie for safety so as to retrieve if patient swallows bite block.

3 Cotton Rolls

4 Dry Aids for keeping mouth dry—Small and large

5 Dental floss

6 2 × 2 gauze

Dry Aid is placed on the buccal mucosa—inside the cheek—opposite the maxillary second molar near the Stensen's duct to absorb saliva originating from the parotid gland.

Practice Note ▶ Disposables are used on all dental tray procedures, including sealant and other restorative tray setups.

Sterilization Notes ▶ All Disposables should be disposed of in the garbage. Single use only.

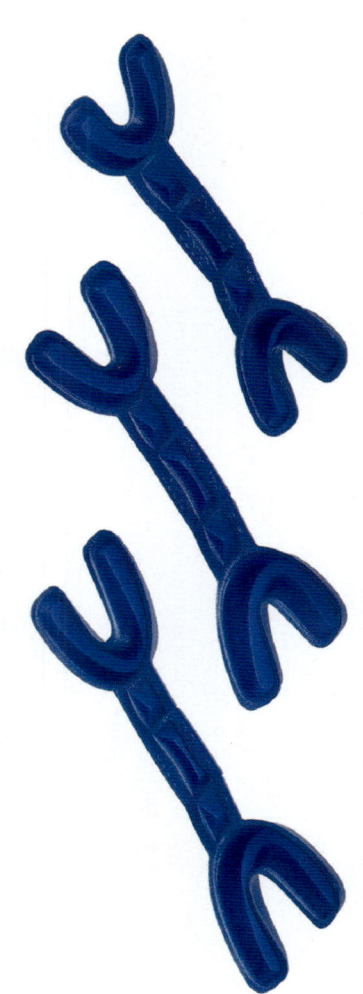

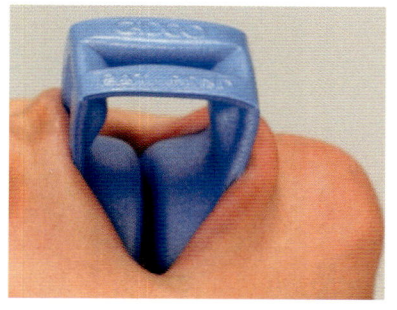

Fluoride Trays—Disposable

Functions ▶ To fill trays with fluoride; remineralizing enamel
To help prevent decay by mineralizing the teeth

Characteristic ▶ Variety of disposable trays are available
Fluoride treatment for trays are in form of gel or foam.
Fluoride Varnish—Applies directly on teeth without trays
Other types of Fluoride available

Practice Note ▶ Fluoride treatment may begin at children's 6-month checkup appointment.
Fluoride Trays are used on fluoride tray setups.

Sterilization Notes ▶ Fluoride Trays should be disposed of in the garbage. Single use only.

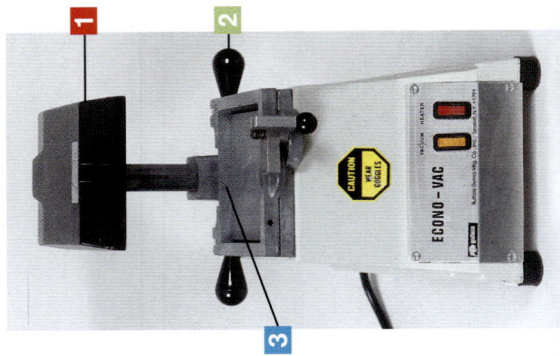

■ INSTRUMENT

Vacuum Former

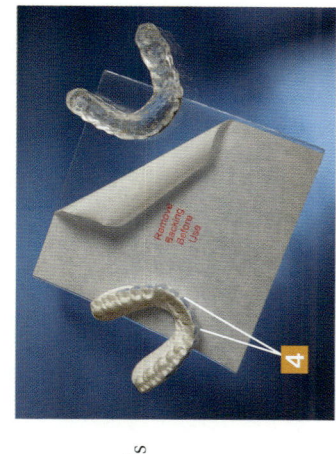
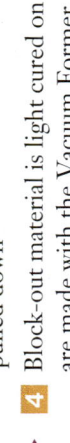
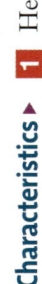

Functions ▶ To make whitening trays, custom temporary crowns, night guards, orthodontic positioners, and mouth guards

To heat plastic square for bleaching trays

To vacuum form the plastic tray over the patient's model to make the bleaching tray and devices as mentioned above

Characteristics ▶
1 Heating element that softens the thermoplastic resin
2 Handles to pull down plastic
3 Vacuum to mold plastic to tray after it is pulled down

Practice Note ▶
4 Block-out material is light cured on the facial side of the model before whitening trays are made with the Vacuum Former.

Sterilization Notes ▶ The manufacturer's recommendation should be followed for disinfecting the Vacuum Former.

1

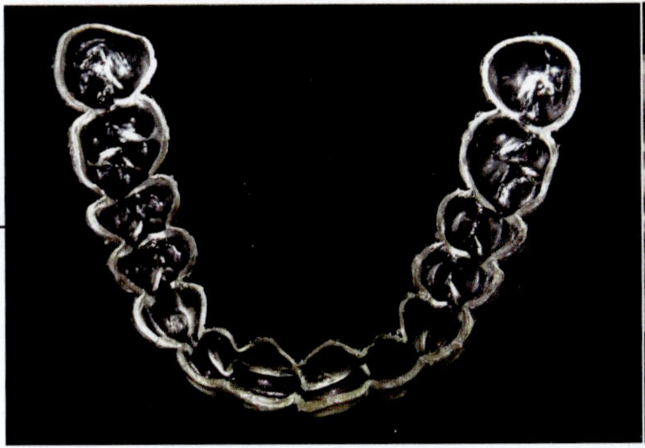

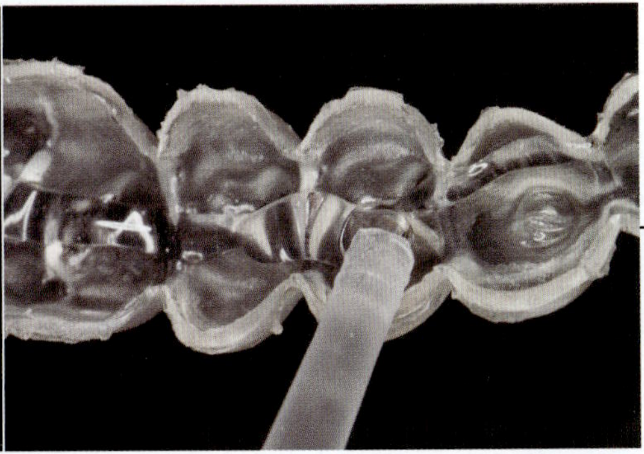

2

Custom-Fitted Whitening Tray

Function ▶ To lighten the color of dark or discolored teeth

Characteristics ▶
1. Custom-fitted trays are made in the dental office with the vacuum former.
2. Trays hold a peroxide-based gel.

Different percentages of gel available

Usage regimens vary according to dentist recommendations

Practice Note ▶ Bleaching Trays should stop short of the gingival margin of the soft tissues to avoid gingival irritation.

Sterilization Notes ▶ Clean and disinfect according to dentist's recommendation.

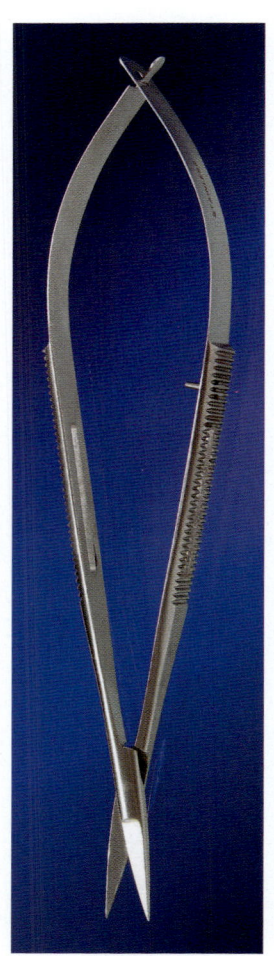

Scissors—Short Blade

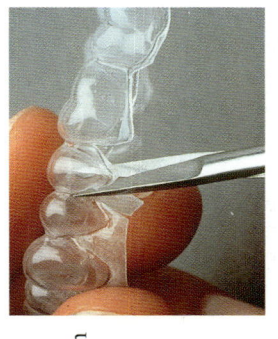

INSTRUMENT

Function ▶ To precisely cut material especially for whitening trays.

Characteristic ▶ Fine cutting blade

Practice Note ▶ Short-Blade Scissors are used on whitening tray setup and on other operative tray setups.

Sterilization Notes ▶ Scissors—Short Blade must be precleaned, open, and unlocked. Then, place in an open and unlocked position in a sterilizing pouch with an internal process indicator, seal, then sterilize. OR, wrap with an internal process indicator inside and secure on the outside with process indicator tape, then sterilize. Verify appropriate color change has been achieved in external process indicator immediately after removal from sterilizer. Check internal process indicator before treatment. Refer to state regulations for any additional state requirements.

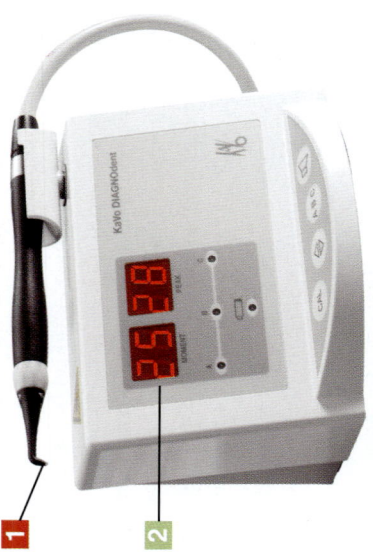

DIAGNOdent

■ INSTRUMENT

Functions ▶ To aid in the detection of caries within the tooth structure

To detect caries in the structure of the tooth before placing sealants

Characteristics ▶ DIAGNOdent accurately diagnoses occlusal caries.

1 Laser detects the caries in the tooth.

2 Digital display is seen on the screen.

Practice Note ▶ DIAGNOdent is used with sealant and occasionally restorative tray setups.

Sterilization Notes ▶ The manufacturer's recommendation should be followed for disinfecting DIAGNOdent unit. Barriers should be placed on wand that is used intraorally. Refer to manufacturer's recommendation for precleaning and sterilization of the DIAGNOdent tips.

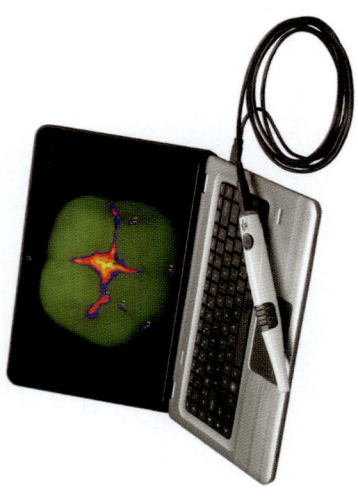

Spectra Fluorescence Caries Detection Aid System

Functions ▶

To aid in the detection of caries

To aid in the detection of caries during the restorative phase to verify that all caries have been removed.

Characteristics ▶

Components

- Lightweight handpiece with high resolution, auto-exposure CCD sensor
- Spacer that maintains an appropriate distance between the lens tip and the tooth surface and blocks stray light during examinations
- Cable to connect handpiece to computer

Uses fluorescence to detect caries in fissures and smooth surfaces

Doppler radar–like images provide both color and numerical indicators; in active mode, carious regions appear red, and healthy enamel appears green

120-degree button ring allows the user to freeze, unfreeze, and capture images with one finger.

Practice Note ▶

The Spectra detects decay hidden between the margins of existing composite and amalgam restorations.

Sterilization Notes ▶

The manufacturer's recommendation should be followed for disinfecting Spectra. Barriers should be placed on camera handpiece that is used intraorally. Spacers are "reusable, however," must be precleaned and sterilized before use.

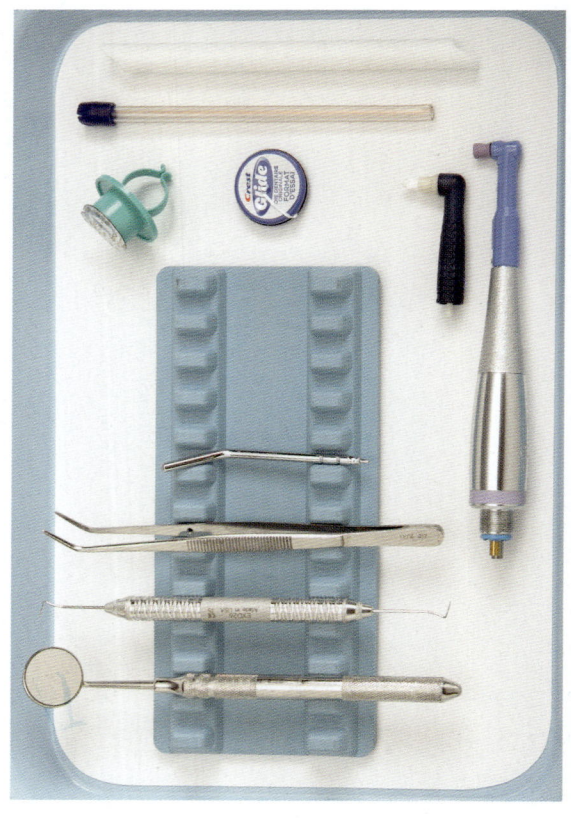

Prophylaxis Polishing

TOP (LEFT TO RIGHT)

Mouth mirror, explorer, cotton forceps, air/water syringe tip, polishing agent without fluoride, dental floss, low-volume saliva ejector, high-volume evacuator (HVE) tip

BOTTOM (LEFT TO RIGHT)

Prophy slow-speed handpiece with disposable prophy angle attachment with polishing cup, disposable prophy angle attachment with tapered brush

Sterilization Notes ▶

Refer to each picture for correct procedure for instrument sterilization or disposal of instrument or material. Refer to other chapters for additional instruments on this tray setup that are not included in this chapter.

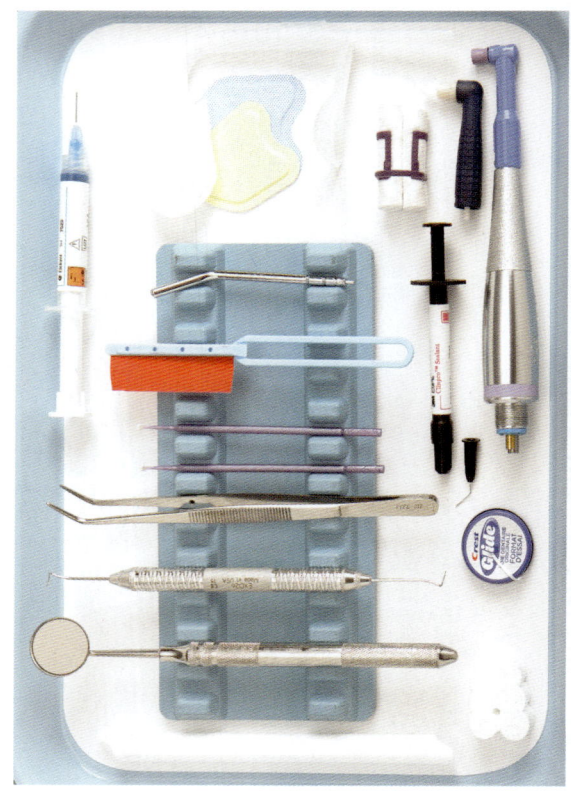

Sealant

VERY TOP OF TRAY

Syringe with etchant

TOP ROW (LEFT TO RIGHT)

High-volume evacuator (HVE) tip mouth mirror, explorer, cotton forceps, microbrushes, disposable articulating paper holder and articulating paper, air/water syringe tip, dry aids, low-volume evacuator for mandibular, cotton rolls in disposable holder

BOTTOM ROW (LEFT TO RIGHT)

Disposable bite block, dental floss, sealant syringe and syringe tip, prophy slow-speed hand-piece with disposable prophy angle attachment with polishing cup, disposable prophy angle attachment with tapered brush

Sterilization Notes ▶ Refer to each picture for correct procedure for instrument sterilization or disposal of instrument or material. Refer to other chapters for additional instruments on this tray setup that are not included in this chapter.

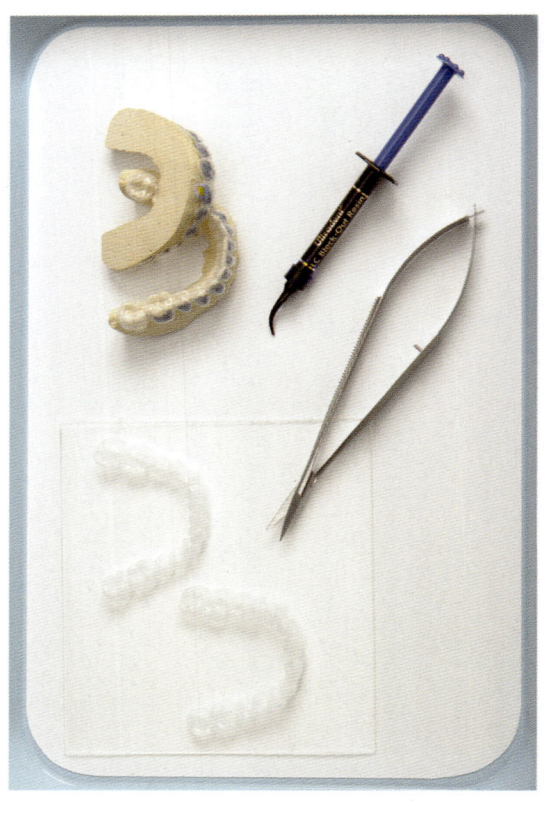

Whitening

LEFT TO RIGHT

Thermoplastic resin square, bleaching trays (maxillary and mandibular), short-blade scissors, block-out material for models, bleaching trays on maxillary and mandibular models

Sterilization Notes ▶ Refer to each picture for correct procedure for instrument sterilization or disposal of instrument or material. Refer to other chapters for additional instruments on this tray setup that are not included in this chapter.

14

Orthodontic Instruments

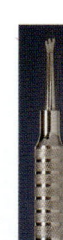

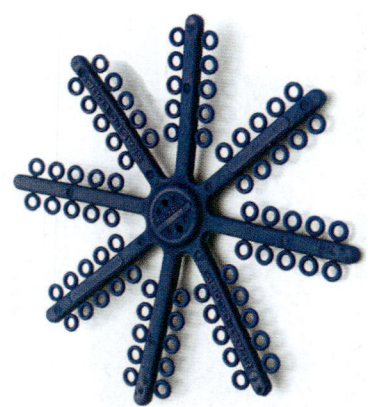

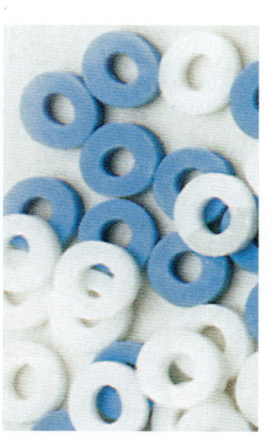

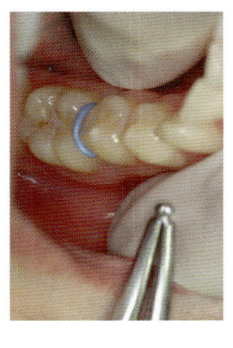

Elastic Separators

Functions ▶ To separate teeth before banding a tooth for orthodontic treatment

To place around contact area of tooth

Characteristic ▶ Elastomeric Separators—Various sizes for different contact areas

Practice Note ▶ Separators are placed on orthodontic separating tray setup.

Sterilization Notes ▶ Elastomeric Separators should be disposed of in the garbage. Single use only.

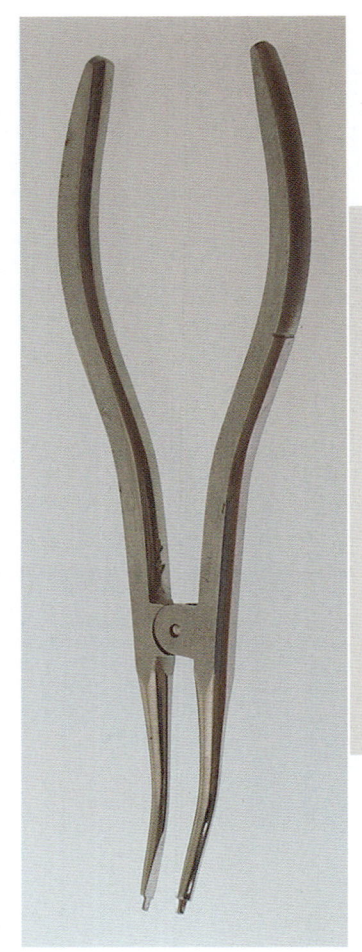

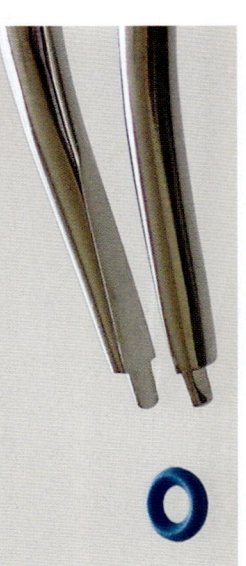

Elastic Separating Pliers

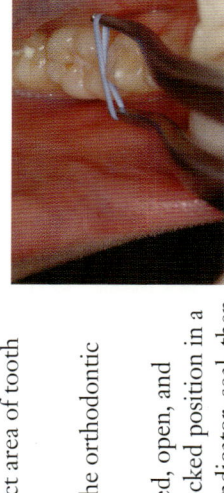

Function ▶ To grip and place separators around contact area of tooth

Characteristic ▶ Single ended

Practice Note ▶ Elastic Separating Pliers are only used on the orthodontic tray setup.

Sterilization Notes ▶ Elastic Separating Pliers must be precleaned, open, and unlocked. Then, place in an open and unlocked position in a sterilizing pouch with an internal process indicator, seal, then sterilize. OR, wrap with an internal process indicator inside and secure on the outside with process indicator tape, then sterilize. Verify appropriate color change has been achieved in external process indicator immediately after removal from sterilizer. Check internal process indicator before treatment. Refer to state regulations for any additional state requirements.

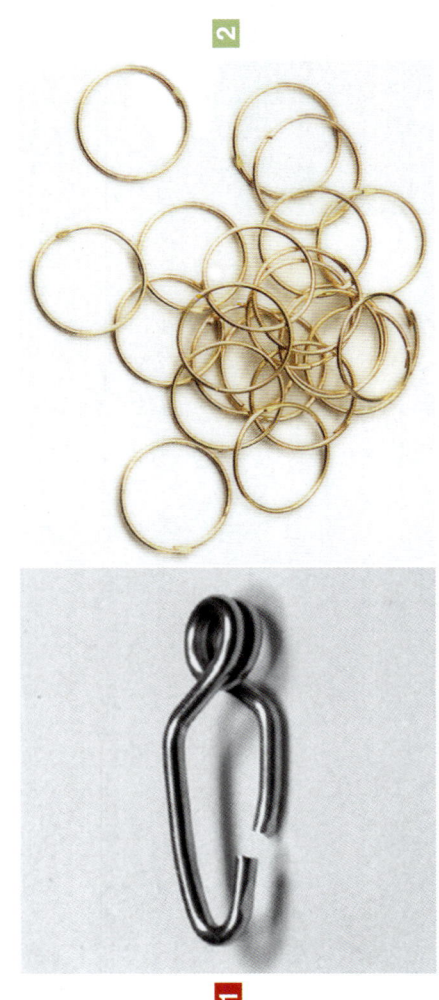

2

1

Steel Spring Separators/Brass Wire Separators

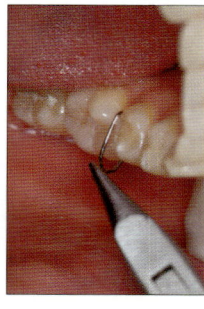 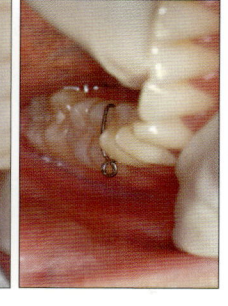

■ INSTRUMENT

Functions ▶
To separate teeth before banding a tooth for orthodontic treatment

To place around contact area of tooth

Characteristics ▶
1 Steel Spring Separators—Various sizes for different-sized contact areas

2 Brass Wire Separators—Placed around contact and twisted clockwise and then cut 3 mm and tucked in order not to impinge on tissue or occlusion

Placed with orthodontic hemostat or bird beak pliers

Practice Note ▶
Separators are placed on orthodontic separating tray setup.

Sterilization Notes ▶
Steel Spring Separators and Brass Wire Separators should be disposed of in a sharps container. Single use only.

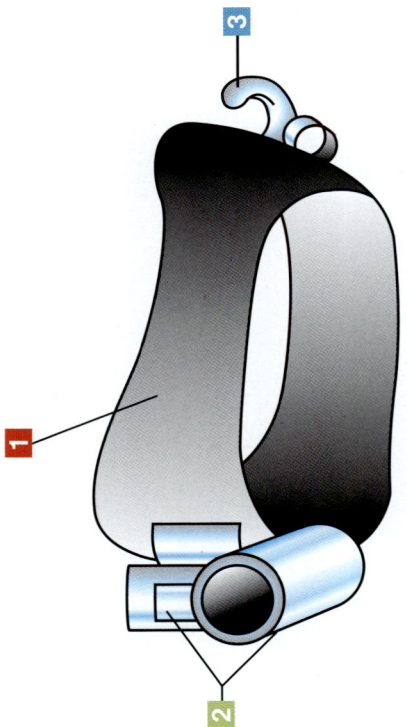

■ INSTRUMENT

Orthodontic Band with Tubing and Hook

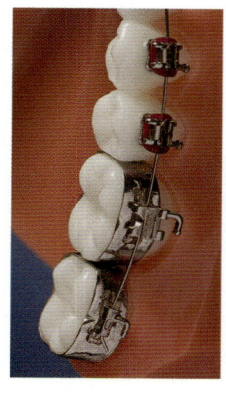

Functions ▶ To fit and cement or bond band around the middle third of the coronal part of the tooth

To hold orthodontic arch wire in place (arch wire moves the teeth, many different shapes and sizes)

To secure headgear in tubing on band

Characteristics ▶

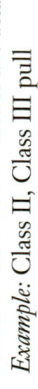

1 Band

2 Tubing:

Arch wire tube (top)—Holds arch wire in place

Headgear tube (bottom)—Holds headgear in place

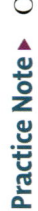

3 Hook—Place where elastics are attached.

Example: Class II, Class III pull

Practice Note ▶ Orthodontic Band is used on orthodontic banding tray setup.

Sterilization Notes ▶ Orthodontic Band should be disposed of in a sharps container. Single use only.

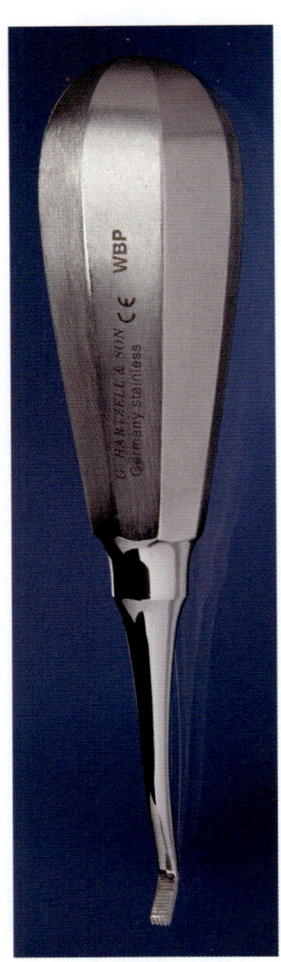

■INSTRUMENT

Band Pusher

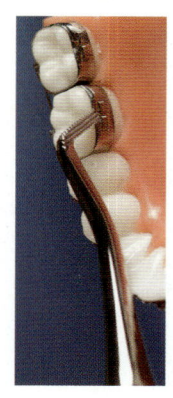

Function ▶ To push orthodontic bands into place during try-in and cementing phases

Characteristic ▶ Single or double ended

Practice Note ▶ Band Pusher is only used on the orthodontic tray setup.

Sterilization Notes ▶ Band Pusher must be precleaned. Then, place in a sterilizing pouch with an internal process indicator, seal, then sterilize. OR, wrap with an internal process indicator inside and secure on the outside with process indicator tape, then sterilize. Verify appropriate color change has been achieved in external process indicator immediately after removal from sterilizer. Check internal process indicator before treatment. Refer to state regulations for any additional state requirements.

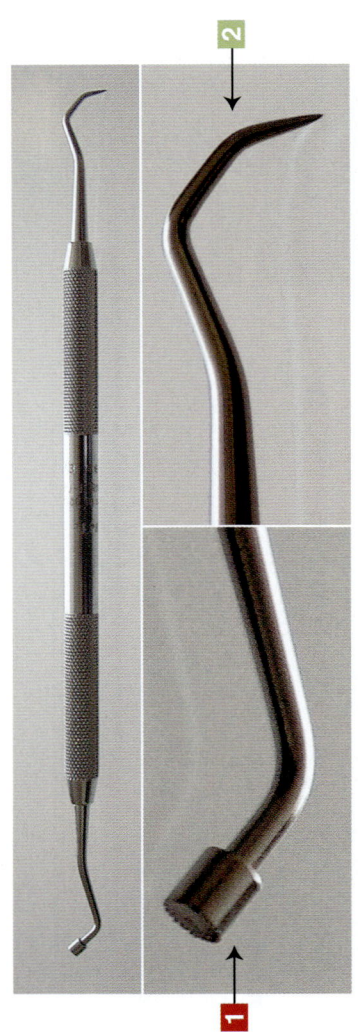

Band Pusher or Plugger with Scaler

Functions ▶ To seat or place orthodontic bands during try-in and cementing phases

To remove excess material after cementation or bonding of bands

Characteristics ▶ Double ended:

1 Band Pusher or Plugger

2 Scaler

Practice Note ▶ Band Pusher with Scaler is used on the orthodontic tray setup.

Sterilization Notes ▶ Band Pusher or Plugger with Scaler must be precleaned. Then, place in a sterilizing pouch with an internal process indicator, seal, then sterilize. OR, wrap with an internal process indicator inside and secure on the outside with process indicator tape, then sterilize. Verify appropriate color change has been achieved in external process indicator immediately after removal from sterilizer. Check internal process indicator before treatment. Refer to state regulations for any additional state requirements.

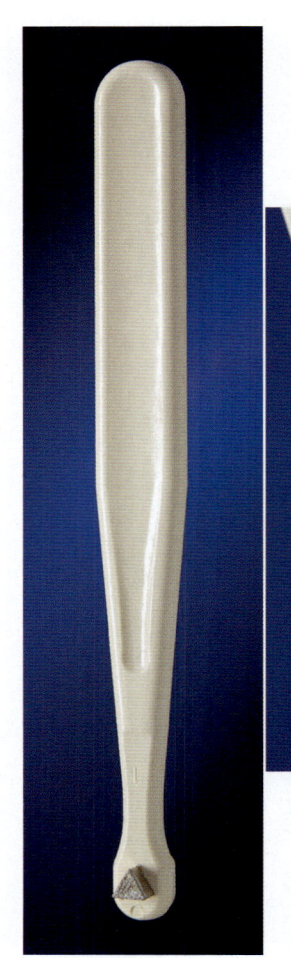
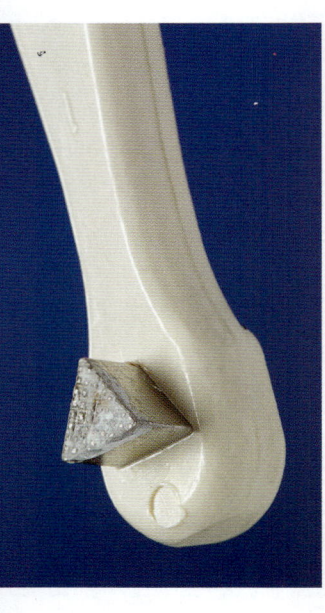

Band Seater—Bite Stick

Function ▶ To assist seating or placing of orthodontic bands for try-in or cementing phase

Characteristics ▶ Single ended
Available in square tip or triangle tip (pictured)

Practice Notes ▶ The patient bites down on the smooth end of the instrument to apply pressure to seat the band.

Band Seater—Bite Stick is only used on the orthodontic tray setup.

Sterilization Notes ▶ Band Seater—Bite Stick must be precleaned. Then, place in a sterilizing pouch with an internal process indicator, seal, then sterilize. OR, wrap with an internal process indicator inside and secure on the outside with process indicator tape, then sterilize. Verify appropriate color change has been achieved in external process indicator immediately after removal from sterilizer. Check internal process indicator before treatment. Refer to state regulations for any additional state requirements.

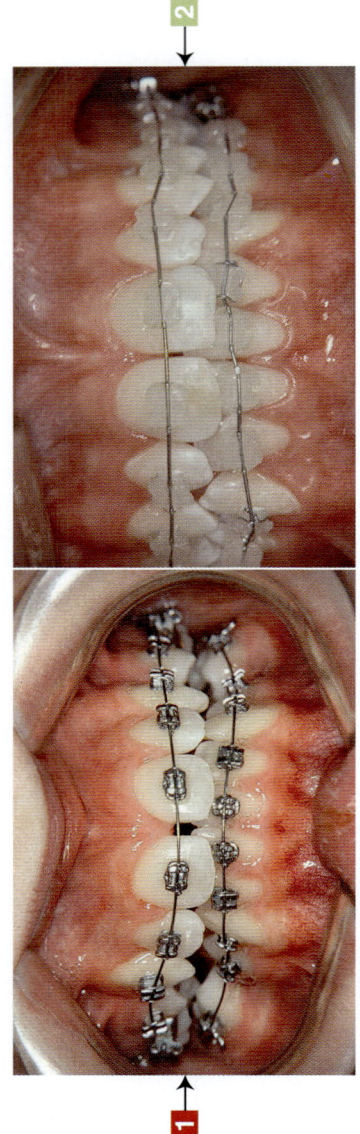

Orthodontic Bracket

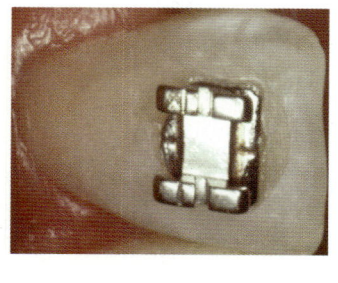

Function ▸ To hold orthodontic arch wire in place (arch wire moves the teeth)

Characteristics ▸ Bracket is bonded to tooth.
Hold arch wire in place
Many different types available:

1 Metal brackets
2 Ceramic brackets (for esthetic purposes)

Practice Note ▸ Orthodontic Brackets are used on orthodontic bonding tray setup.

Sterilization Notes ▸ Orthodontic Brackets should be disposed of in a sharps container. Single use only.

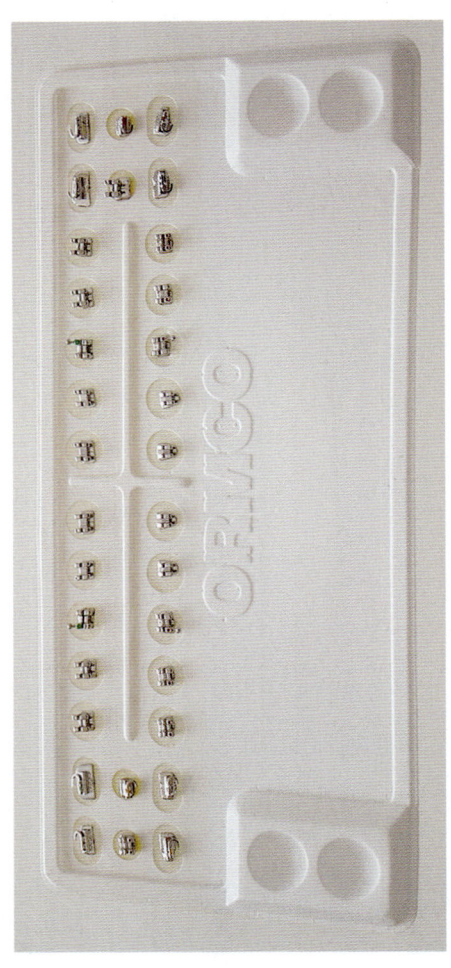

■ INSTRUMENT

Bracket Placement Card

Function ▶ To place each bracket and/or band on card according to tooth placement in mouth

Characteristic ▶ Tape on card holds brackets in place before they are bonded to teeth.

Practice Note ▶ Bracket Placement Card is only used on the orthodontic tray setup.

Sterilization Notes ▶ Bracket Placement Card should be disposed of in the garbage. Single use only.

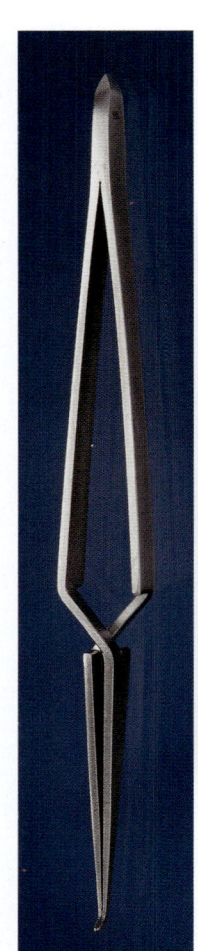

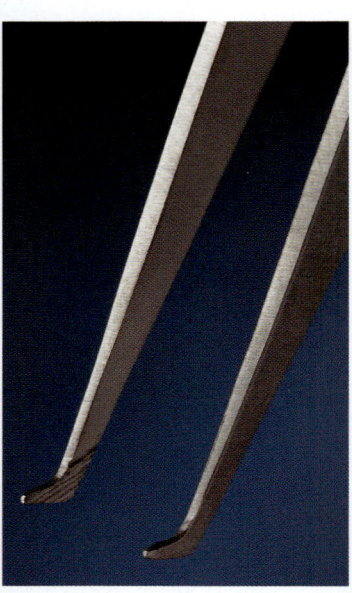

■ INSTRUMENT

Posterior Bracket Placement Pliers

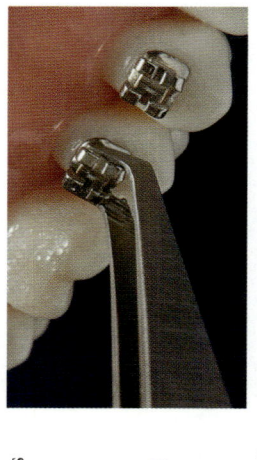

Functions ▶
To hold and carry bracket by placing tip of pliers into slot of bracket

To place bracket on tooth for bonding

Characteristic ▶
Range of sizes

Practice Note ▶
Posterior Bracket Placement Pliers are only used on the orthodontic tray setup.

Sterilization Notes ▶
Posterior Bracket Placement Pliers must be precleaned, open, and unlocked. Then, place in an open and unlocked position in a sterilizing pouch with an internal process indicator, seal, then sterilize. OR, wrap with an internal process indicator inside and secure on the outside with process indicator tape, then sterilize. Verify appropriate color change has been achieved in external process indicator immediately after removal from sterilizer. Check internal process indicator before treatment. Refer to state regulations for any additional state requirements.

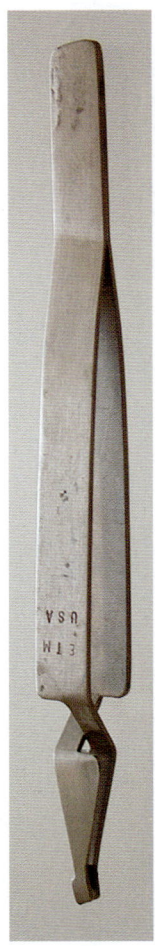

Anterior Bracket Placement Pliers

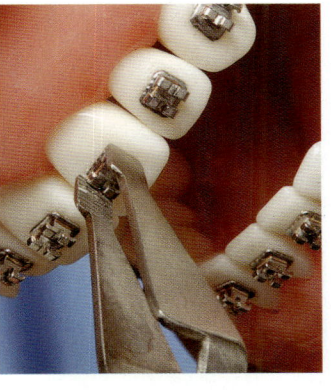

Functions ▶ To hold and carry bracket by placing tip of pliers into slot of bracket
To place bracket on tooth for bonding

Characteristic ▶ Range of sizes

Practice Note ▶ Anterior Bracket Placement Pliers are only used on the orthodontic tray setup.

Sterilization Notes ▶ Anterior Bracket Placement Pliers must be precleaned, open, and unlocked. Then, place in an open and unlocked position in a sterilizing pouch with an internal process indicator, seal, then sterilize. OR, wrap with an internal process indicator inside and secure on the outside with process indicator tape, then sterilize. Verify appropriate color change has been achieved in external process indicator immediately after removal from sterilizer. Check internal process indicator before treatment. Refer to state regulations for any additional state requirements.

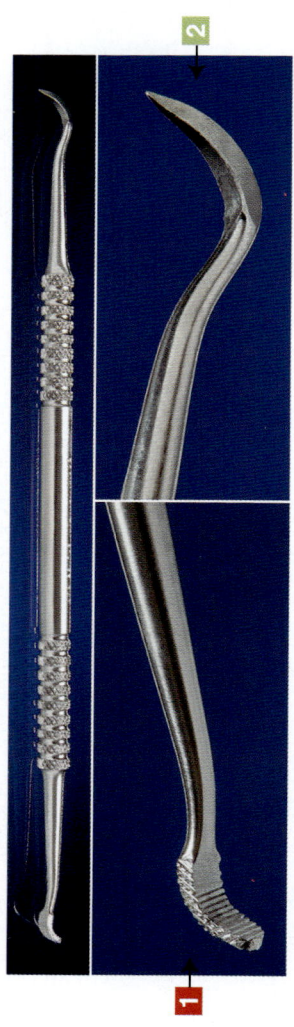

Orthodontic (Shure) Scaler

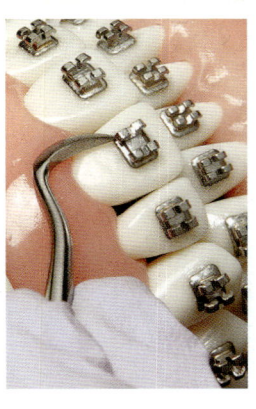

Functions ▶

To place brackets for bonding (both ends)

To remove separators (scaler end)

To remove elastic ligature ties (scaler end)

To remove excess cement or bonding material (scaler end)

To check for loose bands and brackets (both ends)

Characteristics ▶

Universal instrument used for several orthodontic functions

Single ended—Scaler or band pusher

Double ended:

1 Band pusher

2 Orthodontic scaler

Practice Note ▶

Orthodontic Scaler is used on the orthodontic tray setup.

Sterilization Notes ▶

Orthodontic Scaler must be precleaned. Then, place in a sterilizing pouch with an internal process indicator, seal, then sterilize. OR, wrap with an internal process indicator inside and secure on the outside with process indicator tape, then sterilize. Verify appropriate color change has been achieved in external process indicator immediately after removal from sterilizer. Check internal process indicator before treatment. Refer to state regulations for any additional state requirements.

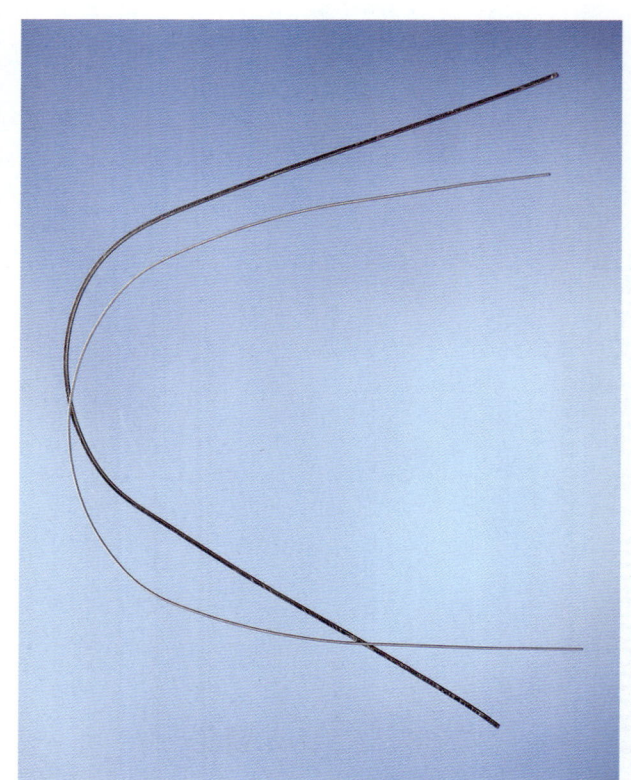

■ INSTRUMENT

Arch Wire

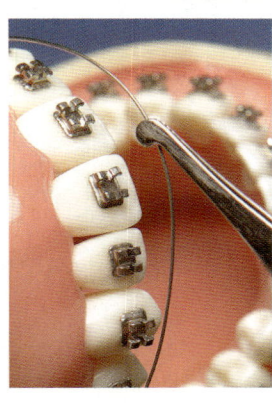

Function ▸
To place into slots of each bracket and secure with a wire or elastomeric ligature tie on every bracket

To move teeth with the force of the arch wire

Characteristics ▸
Different types of arch wire available according to stage of the orthodontic treatment

Nickel titanium—Flexible wire

Stainless steel wire—Stiff and stronger than other types of wire

Beta titanium—Combination of flexibility, strength, and memory

Optiflex—Made from composite material for light force (initial stages) and esthetic purposes

Different shapes and thickness in diameter available according to initial, intermediate, and advanced treatment:

Round wire—Initial and intermediate stages of treatment

Square, rectangular—Final stages of treatment

Practice Note ▸
Arch Wire is used during all phases of orthodontic treatment when brackets and bands are placed on the teeth.

Sterilization Notes ▸
Arch Wire must be disposed of in a sharps container.

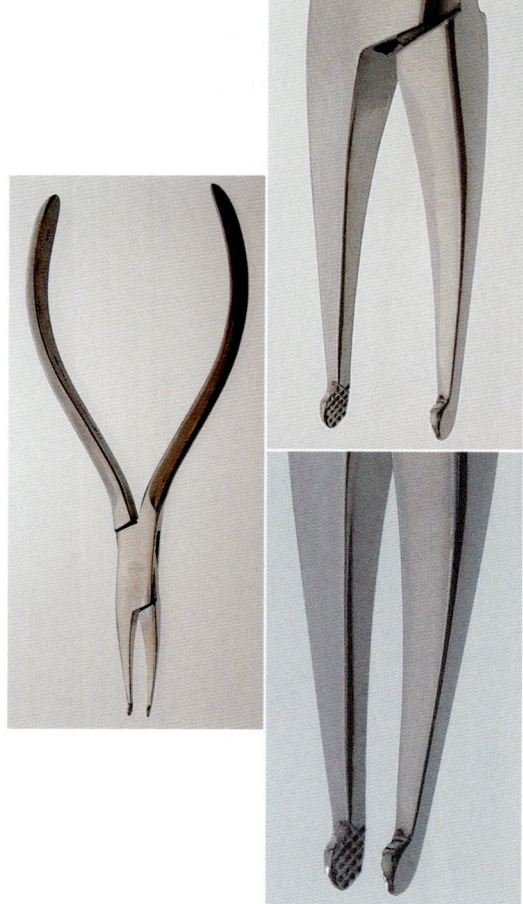

How (or Howe) Pliers

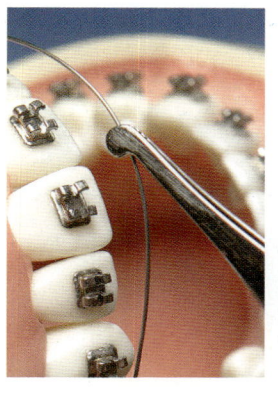

INSTRUMENT

Functions ▶ To place and remove arch wires
To check for loose bands

Characteristics ▶ All-purpose pliers for orthodontic procedures
Serrated tips for better grip on wire
Straight or curved beaks

Practice Note ▶ How Pliers are only used on the orthodontic tray setup.

Sterilization Notes ▶ How Pliers must be precleaned open and unlocked. Then, place in an open and unlocked position in a sterilizing pouch with an internal process indicator, seal, then sterilize. OR, wrap with an internal process indicator inside and secure on the outside with process indicator tape, then sterilize. Verify appropriate color change has been achieved in external process indicator immediately after removal from sterilizer. Check internal process indicator before treatment. Refer to state regulations for any additional state requirements.

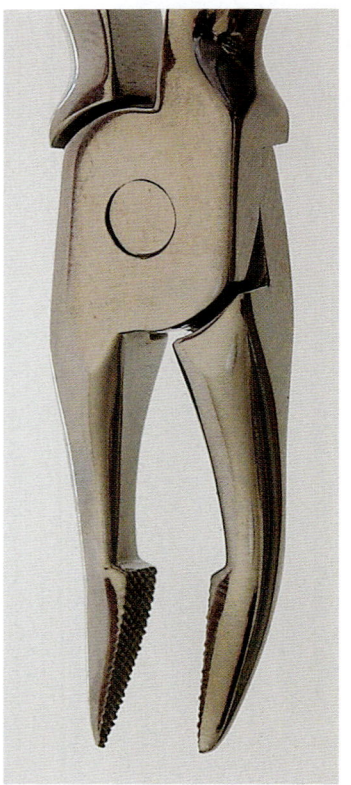

■ INSTRUMENT Weingart Utility Pliers

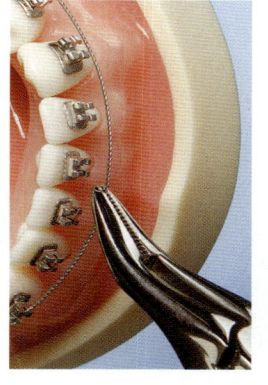

Functions ▸ To place and remove arch wires

To aid a variety of functions for orthodontic procedures

To remove bonded brackets by squeezing bracket

Characteristic ▸ Working ends—Tapered, slim tips to allow pliers to fit between brackets for ease of arch wire placement

Practice Note ▸ Weingart Utility Pliers are only used on the orthodontic tray setup.

Sterilization Notes ▸ Weingart Utility Pliers must be precleaned, open, and unlocked. Then, place in an open and unlocked position in a sterilizing pouch with an internal process indicator, seal, then sterilize. OR, wrap with an internal process indicator inside and secure on the outside with process indicator tape, then sterilize. Verify appropriate color change has been achieved in external process indicator immediately after removal from sterilizer. Check internal process indicator before treatment. Refer to state regulations for any additional state requirements.

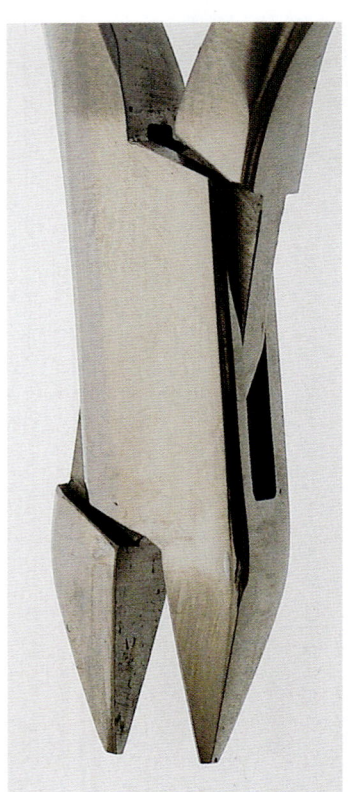

Arch-Bending Pliers

■ INSTRUMENT

Function ▶ To bend arch wires

Characteristic ▶ Variety of styles, depending on type of arch wire used—Round, square, or rectangular

Practice Note ▶ Arch-Bending Pliers are only used on the orthodontic tray setup.

Sterilization Notes ▶ Arch-Bending Pliers must be precleaned, open, and unlocked. Then, place in an open and unlocked position in a sterilizing pouch with an internal process indicator, seal, then sterilize. OR, wrap with an internal process indicator inside and secure on the outside with process indicator tape, then sterilize. Verify appropriate color change has been achieved in external process indicator immediately after removal from sterilizer. Check internal process indicator before treatment. Refer to state regulations for any additional state requirements.

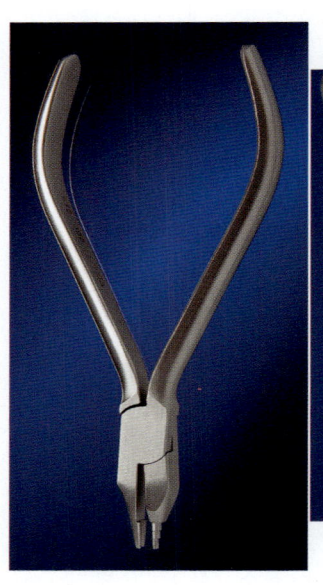
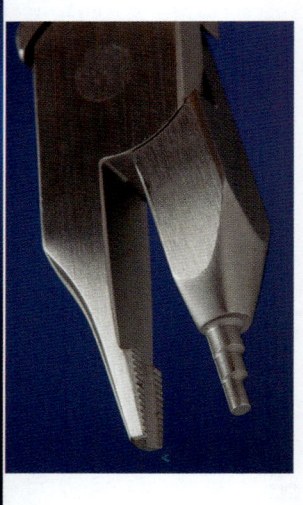

Tweed Loop-Forming Pliers (Jarabak Pliers)

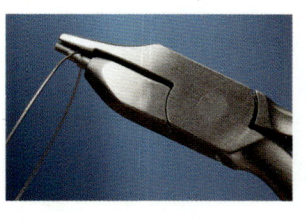

■ **INSTRUMENT**

Functions ▶
To bend and form loops in arch wire
To bend wires for removable appliances

Characteristics ▶
Grooves in beak—Help to bend and form loops in wire
Variety of styles

Practice Note ▶
Tweed Loop-Forming Pliers are only used on the orthodontic tray setup.

Sterilization Notes ▶
Tweed Loop-Forming Pliers must be precleaned, open, and unlocked. Then, place in an open and unlocked position in a sterilizing pouch with an internal process indicator, seal, then sterilize. OR, wrap with an internal process indicator inside and secure on the outside with process indicator tape, then sterilize. Verify appropriate color change has been achieved in external process indicator immediately after removal from sterilizer. Check internal process indicator before treatment. Refer to state regulations for any additional state requirements.

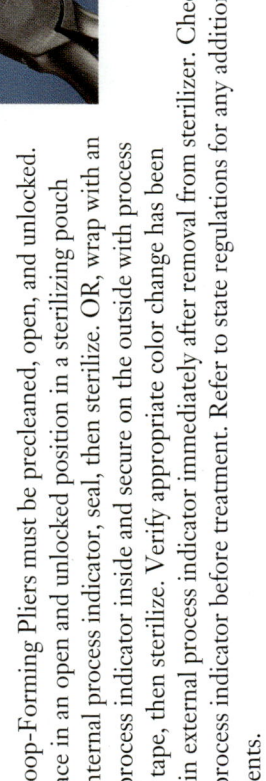

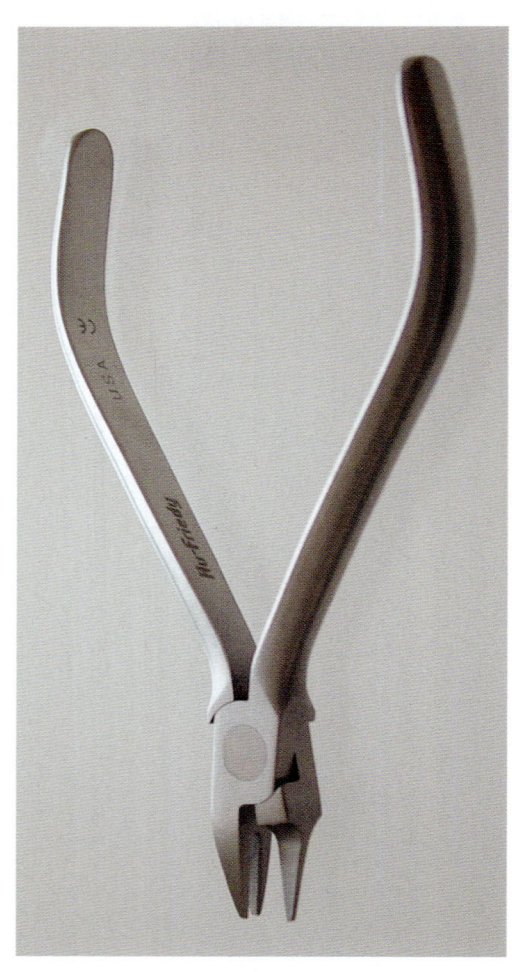

Three-Prong Pliers

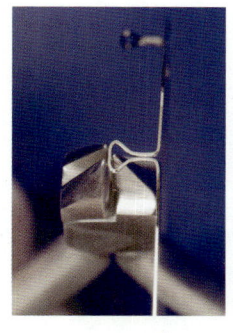

Function ▶ To contour and bend light wire

Characteristic ▶ Range of sizes available

Practice Note ▶ Three-Prong Pliers are only used on the orthodontic tray setup.

Sterilization Notes ▶ Three-Prong Pliers must be precleaned, open, and unlocked. Then, place in an open and unlocked position in a sterilizing pouch with an internal process indicator, seal, then sterilize. OR, wrap with an internal process indicator inside and secure on the outside with process indicator tape, then sterilize. Verify appropriate color change has been achieved in external process indicator immediately after removal from sterilizer. Check internal process indicator before treatment. Refer to state regulations for any additional state requirements.

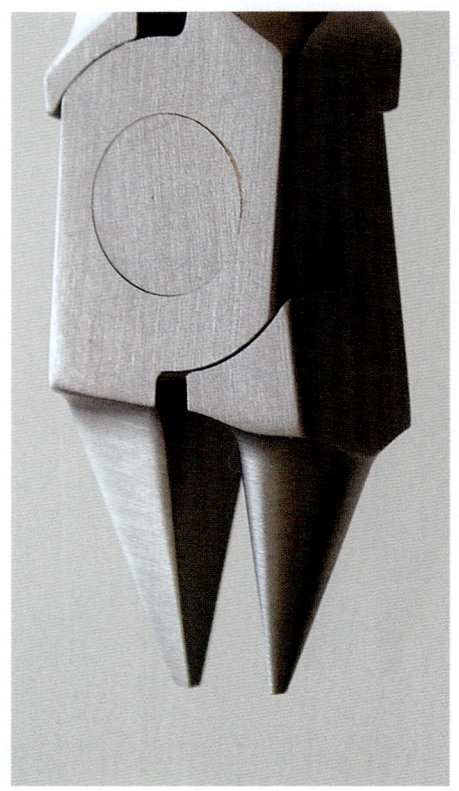

INSTRUMENT

Bird Beak Pliers

Functions ▶
To bend and form orthodontic wire
To remove bonded bracket by squeezing bracket

Characteristics ▶
Versatile wire-bending pliers
Beaks on working end meet very precisely

Practice Note ▶
Bird Beak Pliers are only used on the orthodontic tray setup.

Sterilization Notes ▶
Bird Beak Pliers must be precleaned, open, and unlocked. Then, place in an open and unlocked position in a sterilizing pouch with an internal process indicator, seal, then sterilize. OR, wrap with an internal process indicator inside and secure on the outside with process indicator tape, then sterilize. Verify appropriate color change has been achieved in external process indicator immediately after removal from sterilizer. Check internal process indicator before treatment. Refer to state regulations for any additional state requirements.

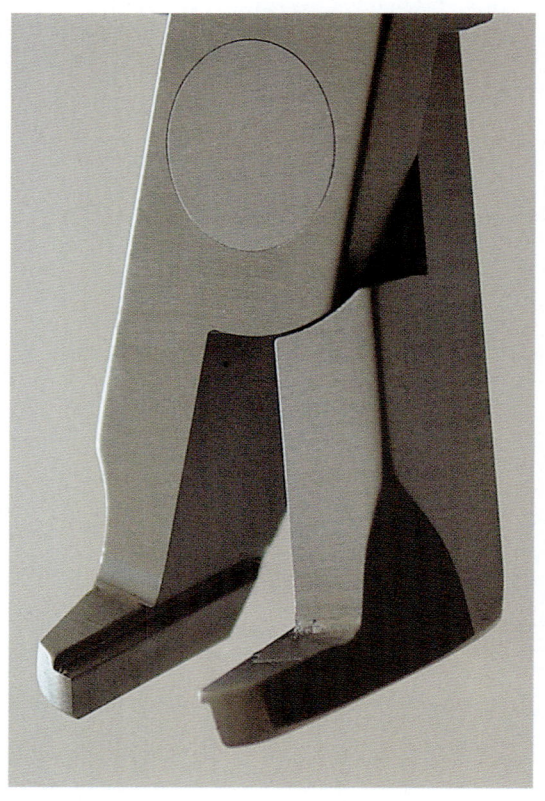

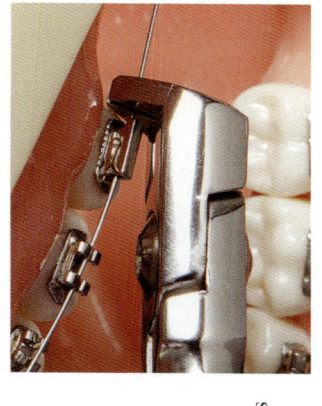

Distal End-Cutting Pliers

Function ▶ To cut distal end of arch wire after placement in brackets and buccal tubes

Characteristic ▶ Catch and hold excess wire after wire has been cut

Practice Note ▶ Distal End-Cutting Pliers are only used on the orthodontic tray setup.

Sterilization Notes ▶ Distal End-Cutting Pliers must be precleaned, open, and unlocked. Then, place in an open and unlocked position in a sterilizing pouch with an internal process indicator, seal, then sterilize. OR, wrap with an internal process indicator inside and secure on the outside with process indicator tape, then sterilize. Verify appropriate color change has been achieved in external process indicator immediately after removal from sterilizer. Check internal process indicator before treatment. Refer to state regulations for any additional state requirements.

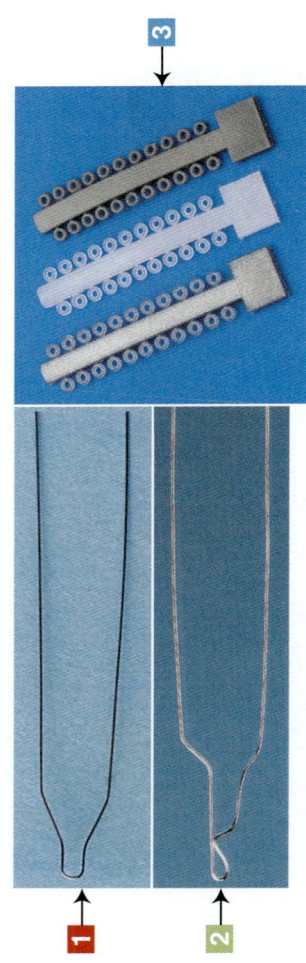

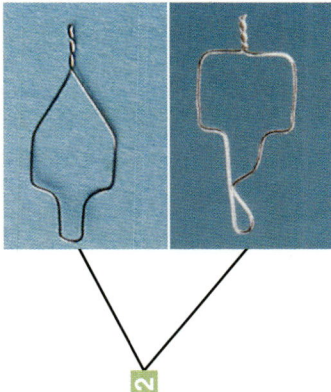

2

INSTRUMENT

Ligatures Ties

Function ▶ To secure the arch wire to the band or bracket

Characteristics ▶

1 Wire Ligature Ties
Thin, flexible wire
Comes in precut length or spools

2 Kobayashi Ties
Preformed hook for Class II and Class II elastic pulls

3 Elastic Ligature Ties
Available in different colors
Comes on a stick (pictured), canes, and chains

Practice Note ▶ Ligature Ties are used on the orthodontic archwire placement tray setup.

Sterilization Notes ▶ Wire Ligature Ties must be disposed of in a sharps container. Elastic ligature ties should be disposed of in garbage.

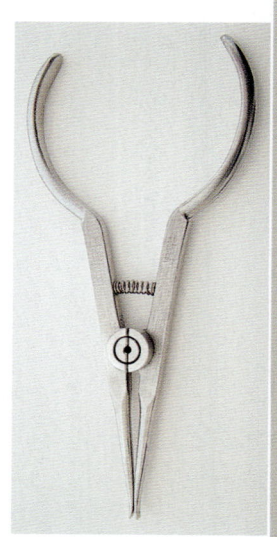

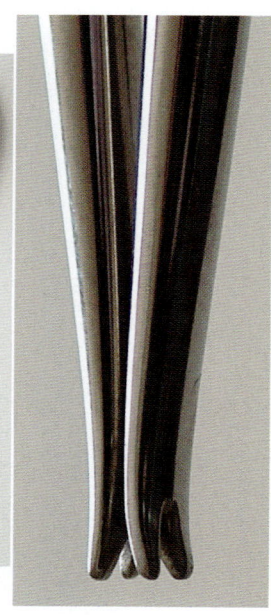

Ligature-Tying (Coon) Pliers

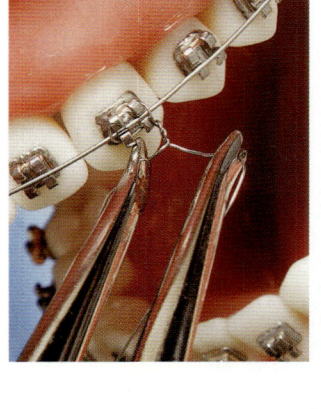

Function ▶ To tie in ligature to arch wire

Characteristics ▶ Channel on pliers—Locks wire ends in place as tips spread

Variety of styles

Practice Note ▶ Ligature-Tying Pliers are only used on the orthodontic tray setup.

Sterilization Notes ▶ Ligature-Tying Pliers must be precleaned, open, and unlocked. Then, place in an open and unlocked position in a sterilizing pouch with an internal process indicator, seal, then sterilize. OR, wrap with an internal process indicator inside and secure on the outside with process indicator tape, then sterilize. Verify appropriate color change has been achieved in external process indicator immediately after removal from sterilizer. Check internal process indicator before treatment. Refer to state regulations for any additional state requirements.

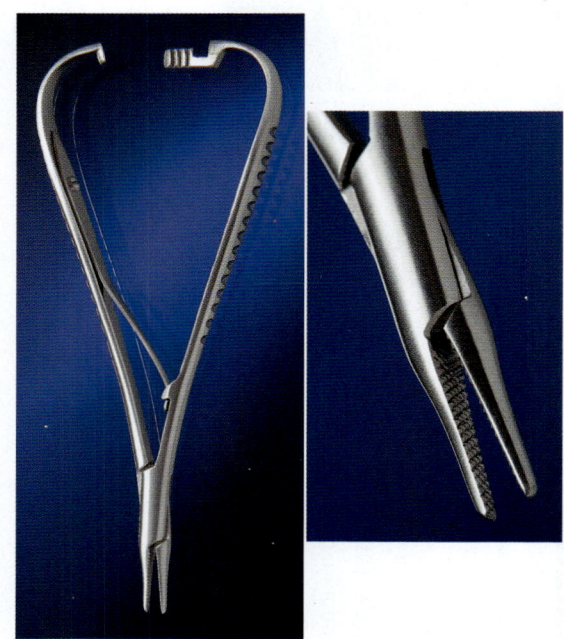

INSTRUMENT

Orthodontic Hemostat

Functions ▸ To hold and place separators

To hold, place, and/or tie ligatures to arch wire

Characteristic ▸ Multifunctional instrument for orthodontic procedures

Example: Mathieu pliers

Practice Note ▸ Orthodontic Hemostat is used on the orthodontic tray setup.

Sterilization Notes ▸ Orthodontic Hemostat must be precleaned, open, and unlocked. Then, place in an open and unlocked position in a sterilizing pouch with an internal process indicator, seal, then sterilize. OR, wrap with an internal process indicator inside and secure on the outside with process indicator tape, then sterilize. Verify appropriate color change has been achieved in external process indicator immediately after removal from sterilizer. Check internal process indicator before treatment. Refer to state regulations for any additional state requirements.

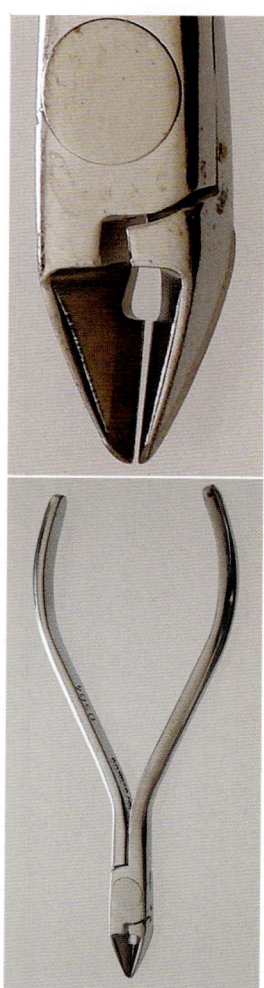

Ligature/Wire Cutters

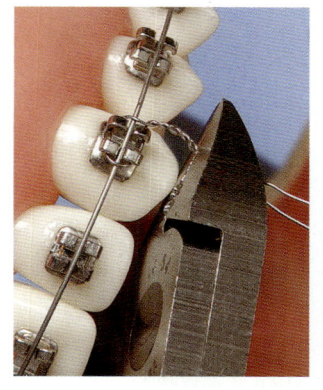

Functions ▶ To cut ligature after it has been tied to arch wire
To cut ligature tie to allow removal of arch wire

Characteristic ▶ Range of sizes available

Practice Note ▶ Ligature/Wire Cutters are used on the orthodontic tray setup.

Sterilization Notes ▶ Ligature/Wire Cutters must be precleaned, open, and unlocked. Then, place in an open and unlocked position in a sterilizing pouch with an internal process indicator, seal, then sterilize. OR, wrap with an internal process indicator inside and secure on the outside with process indicator tape, then sterilize. Verify appropriate color change has been achieved in external process indicator immediately after removal from sterilizer. Check internal process indicator before treatment. Refer to state regulations for any additional state requirements.

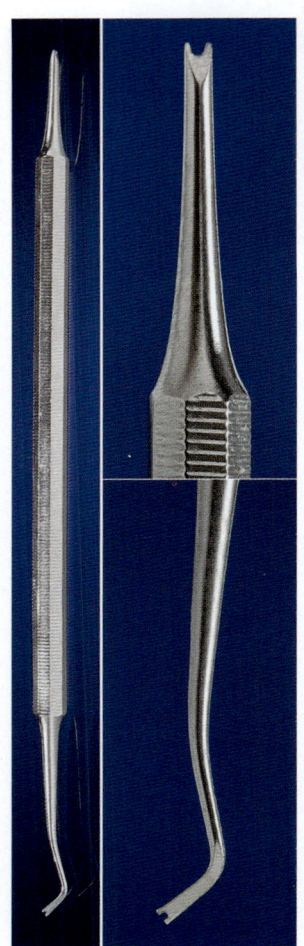

Ligature Director

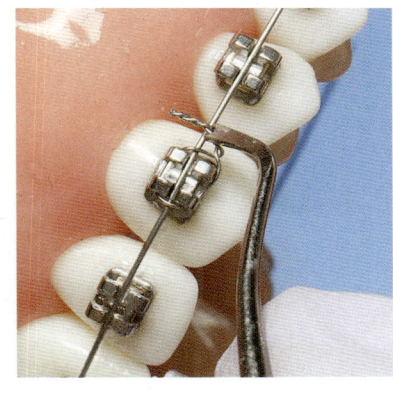

INSTRUMENT

Function ▶ To place ligature wire around brackets after it has been tied to arch wire

Characteristics ▶ Single or double ended
Ends of instrument—Have notches to assist placement of ligature tie around brackets

Practice Note ▶ Ligature Director is used on the orthodontic archwire placement tray setup.

Sterilization Notes ▶ Ligature Director must be precleaned. Then, place in a sterilizing pouch with an internal process indicator, seal, then sterilize. OR, wrap with an internal process indicator inside and secure on the outside with process indicator tape, then sterilize. Verify appropriate color change has been achieved in external process indicator immediately after removal from sterilizer. Check internal process indicator before treatment. Refer to state regulations for any additional state requirements.

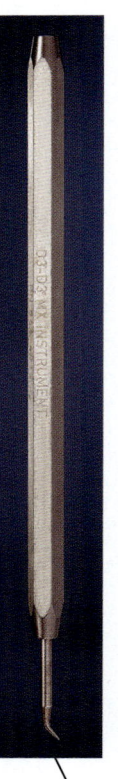

1

Bracket Placement Card for Damon Self-Ligating Brackets with Self-Ligating Instrument

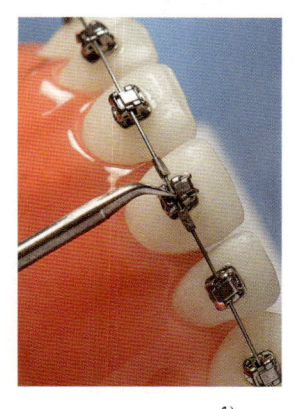

Functions ▶ To place each bracket on card according to tooth placement in mouth

1 Self-Ligating Instrument—To close bracket around arch wire; ligature tie not needed

Characteristic ▶ Tape on card holds brackets in place before they are bonded to teeth.

Practice Note ▶ Bracket Placement Card and Self-Ligating Instrument are used only on orthodontic bonding bracket tray setup.

Sterilization Notes ▶ Bracket Placement Card should be disposed of in the garbage. Single use only. Self-Ligating Instrument must be precleaned. Then, place in a sterilizing pouch with an internal process indicator, seal, then sterilize. OR, wrap with an internal process indicator inside and secure on the outside with process indicator tape, then sterilize. Verify appropriate color change has been achieved in external process indicator immediately after removal from sterilizer. Check internal process indicator before treatment. Refer to state regulations for any additional state requirements.

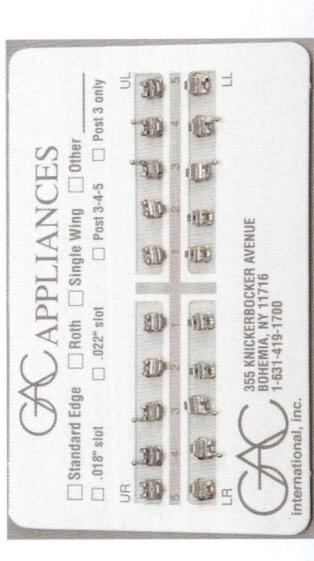

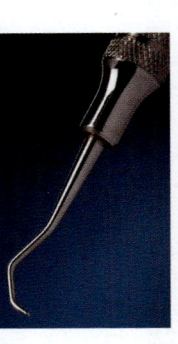

Self-Ligating Brackets with Self-Ligating Instrument

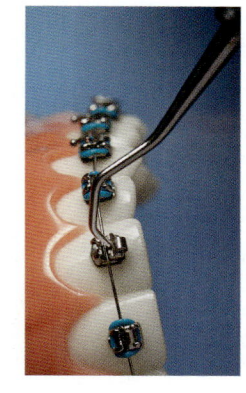

■ INSTRUMENT

Functions ▶ To place each bracket on card according to tooth placement in mouth
Instrument—To open and close bracket around arch wire; ligature tie not needed

Characteristic ▶ Tape on card holds brackets in place before they are bonded to teeth.

Practice Note ▶ Bracket Placement Card and Self-Ligating Instrument are used only on orthodontic
bonding bracket tray setup.

Sterilization Notes ▶ Bracket Placement Card should be disposed of in the garbage. Single use only. Self-Ligating
Instrument must be precleaned. Then, place in a sterilizing pouch with an internal process
indicator, seal, then sterilize. OR, wrap with an
internal process indicator inside and secure on the
outside with process indicator tape, then sterilize.
Verify appropriate color change has been achieved in
external process indicator immediately after removal
from sterilizer. Check internal process indicator before
treatment. Refer to state regulations for any additional
state requirements.

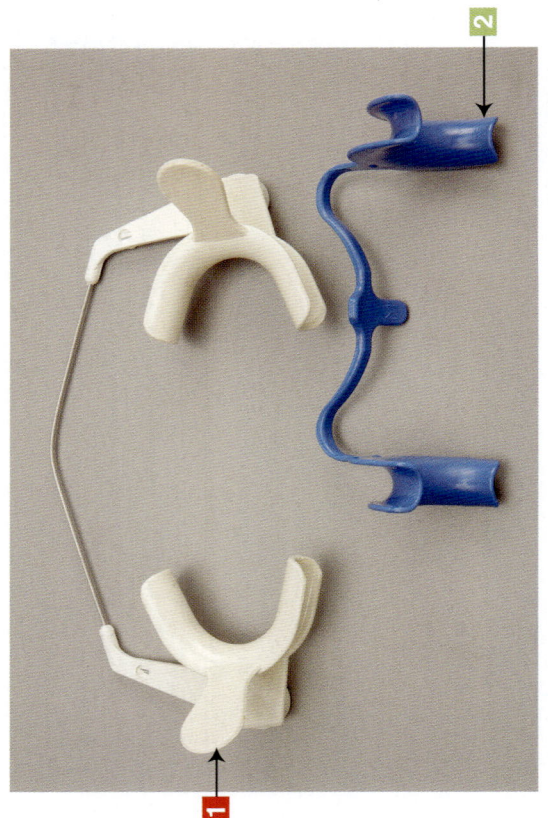

Lip Retractors

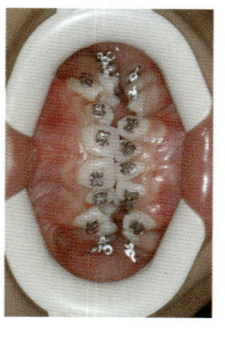

■ INSTRUMENT

Functions ▶ To retract lips, allowing for intraoral access for bonding brackets
To retract lips for intraoral orthodontic photographs

Characteristics ▶
1 Reusable Lip Retractors
2 Disposable Lip Retractors

Practice Note ▶ Lip Retractors are used with orthodontic procedures and other tray setups that include taking intraoral photographs.

Sterilization Notes ▶ Reusable Lip Retractors must be precleaned. Then, place in a sterilizing pouch with an internal process indicator, seal, then sterilize. OR, wrap with an internal process indicator inside and secure on the outside with process indicator tape, then sterilize. Verify appropriate color change has been achieved in external process indicator immediately after removal from sterilizer. Check internal process indicator before treatment. Refer to state regulations for any additional state requirements. Disposable Lip Retractors should be disposed of in garbage.

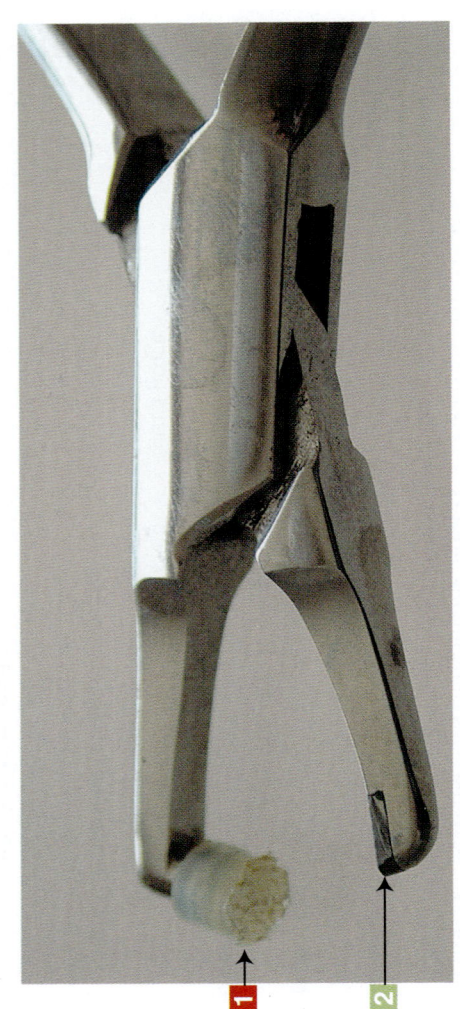

1

2

▪ INSTRUMENT

Posterior Band Remover

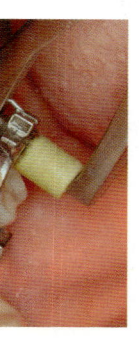

Function ▸ To remove orthodontic bands from teeth

Characteristics ▸ Two beak types:

1 One beak has round cover to place on occlusal surface of tooth to prevent damage during removal of band. Cover can be replaced.

2 Opposite beak is curved and is placed on gingival side of bracket to apply pressure and remove band from tooth.

Practice Note ▸ Posterior Band Remover is used on the orthodontic tray setup.

Sterilization Notes ▸ Posterior Band Remover must be precleaned, open, and unlocked. Then, place in an open and unlocked position in a sterilizing pouch with an internal process indicator, seal, then sterilize. OR, wrap with an internal process indicator inside and secure on the outside with process indicator tape, then sterilize. Verify appropriate color change has been achieved in external process indicator immediately after removal from sterilizer. Check internal process indicator before treatment. Refer to state regulations for any additional state requirements.

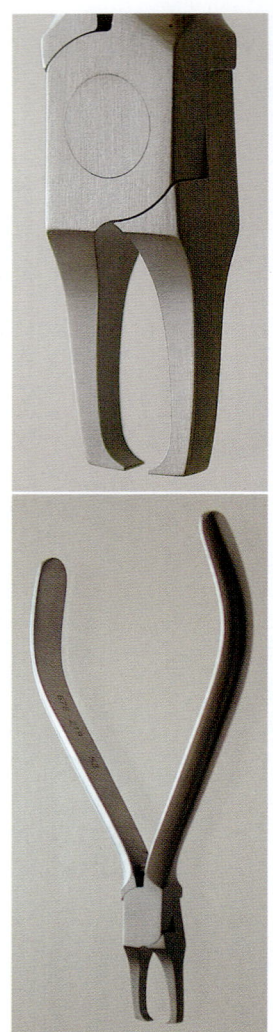

■ INSTRUMENT

Bracket Remover

Function ▶ To remove anterior or posterior brackets from teeth

Characteristic ▶ Grasp bracket to remove it from tooth.

Practice Note ▶ Bracket Remover is used on the orthodontic tray setup.

Sterilization Notes ▶ Bracket Remover must be precleaned, open, and unlocked. Then, place in an open and unlocked position in a sterilizing pouch with an internal process indicator, seal, then sterilize. OR, wrap with an internal process indicator inside and secure on the outside with process indicator tape, then sterilize. Verify appropriate color change has been achieved in external process indicator immediately after removal from sterilizer. Check internal process indicator before treatment. Refer to state regulations for any additional state requirements.

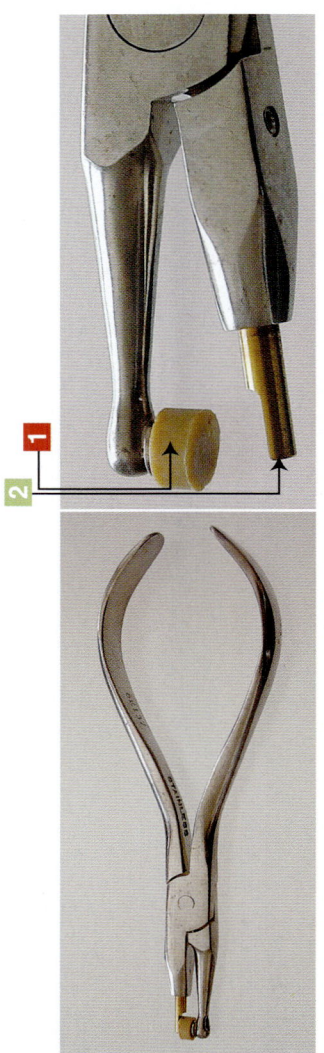

Adhesive-Removing Pliers

Function ▶ To remove excess adhesive after debonding of brackets

Characteristics ▶

1 Plastic pad on round end (pad can be changed)

2 Carbide-inserted tip on short beak—Used to remove the bulk of composite material after debonding

Practice Note ▶ Adhesive-Removing Pliers are used on the orthodontic tray setup.

Sterilization Notes ▶ Adhesive-Removing Pliers must be precleaned, open, and unlocked. Then, place in an open and unlocked position in a sterilizing pouch with an internal process indicator, seal, then sterilize. OR, wrap with an internal process indicator inside and secure on the outside with process indicator tape, then sterilize. Verify appropriate color change has been achieved in external process indicator immediately after removal from sterilizer. Check internal process indicator before treatment. Refer to state regulations for any additional state requirements.

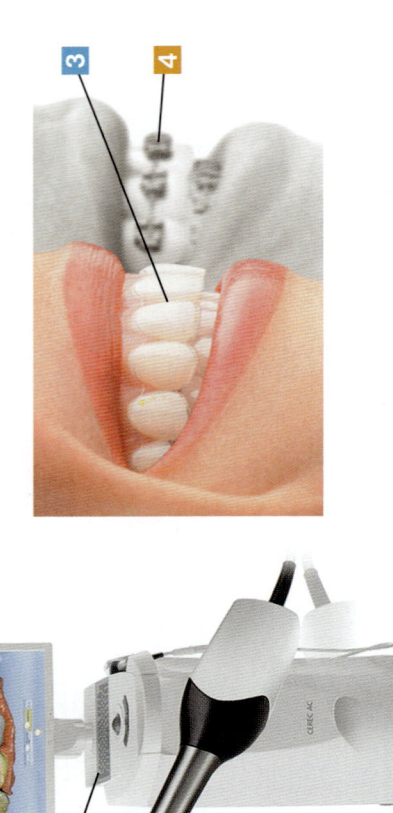

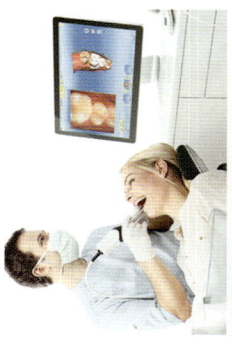
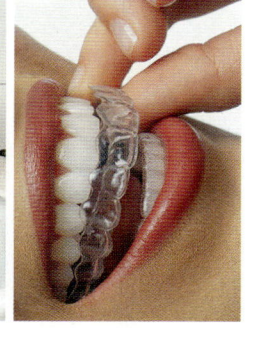

■ INSTRUMENT

Invisalign and CEREC Omnicam

Function ► To take images with an intraoral Wand/Camera of the maxillary and mandibular arches. Images are sent to the computer.

To send images to a lab to manufacture Invisalign appliances and diagnostic images

Characteristics ►

1. Wand/Camera that captures images connected to the computer

2. Cerec Omnicam captures the images of teeth in the maxillary and mandibular arches for Invisalign orthodontic appliances that move teeth for Orthodontic procedures.

3. Invisalign appliance

4. Traditional orthodontics

Images are send to the lab to manufacture a series of Invisalign appliances for Orthodontic movement of the teeth.

Practice Note ► The CEREC Omnicam is used mainly for Orthodontic Invisalign appliances.

Sterilization Notes ► Barriers should be used for the intraoral Wand/Camera. Barriers or overgloves should be used for manipulating the computer on the CEREC Omnicam. Otherwise, refer to the manufacturer's recommendation for disinfecting.

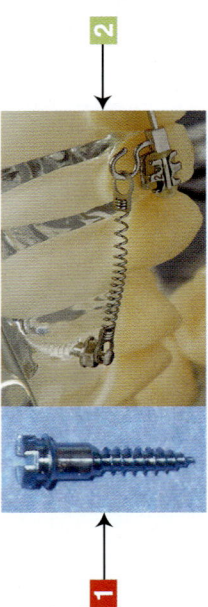

Temporary Anchorage Device (TAD)

Function ▸ To aid in the movement of teeth with skeletal anchorage assisting in orthodontic treatment

Some examples of TAD:

Closure of space between teeth

Tooth uprighting

Open bite correction

To provide an anchor point to move teeth

Characteristics ▸ **1** TAD

2 TAD (arrow) inserted for movement of teeth. TADs are small titanium anchors also referred to as mini implants or mini screws. Before placement, chlorhexidine solution (an antibacterial solution) is placed on the area before anesthesia.

TAD surgery procedure is referred by the orthodontist to a periodontist or a maxillofacial surgeon.

Practice Note ▸ TADs are used with periodontal and maxillofacial surgery setups, oral surgery or periodontal surgery setup, and orthodontic tray setups.

Sterilization Notes ▸ TADs must be disposed of in sharps container. Single use only. Refer to state regulations for any additional state requirements.

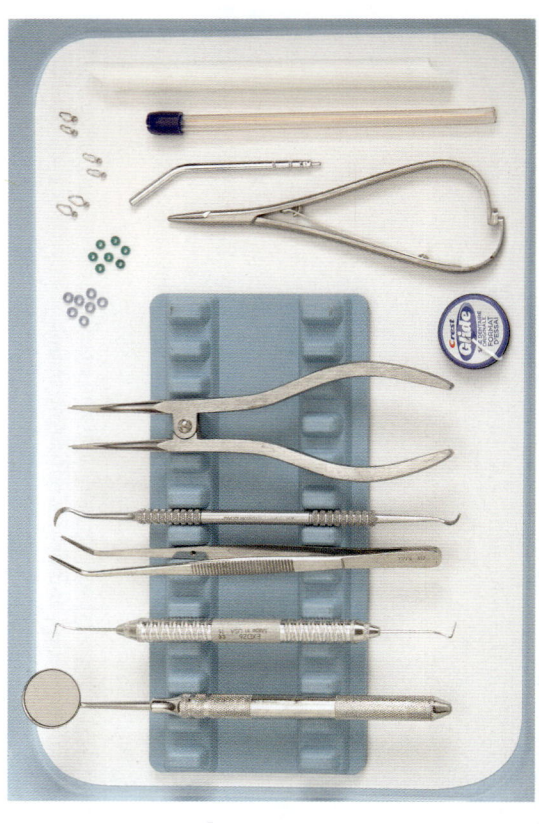

Orthodontic Tooth Separating

TOP

Elastic separators, spring coil separators

BOTTOM (LEFT TO RIGHT)

Mouth mirror, explorer, cotton forceps (pliers), orthodontic (Shure) scaler, elastic separating pliers, floss, orthodontic hemostat (Mathieu pliers), air/water syringe tip, low-volume saliva ejector tip, high-volume evacuation (HVE) tip

Sterilization Notes ▶ Refer to each individual picture for correct procedure for instrument sterilization or disposal of instrument or material. Refer to other chapters for additional instruments on this tray setup that are not included in this chapter.

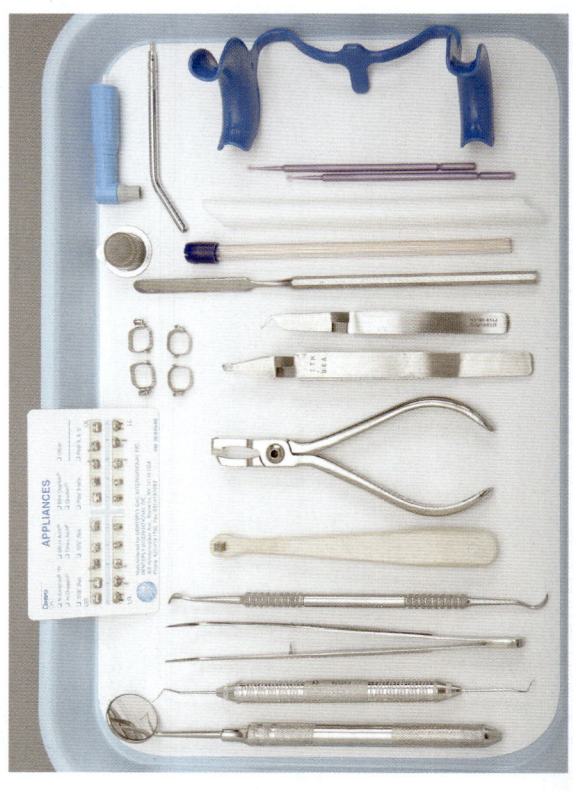

Orthodontic Cementing and Bonding Brackets

TOP ROW (LEFT TO RIGHT)

Bracket placement card with brackets, orthodontic bands, polishing agent without fluoride or glycerin, disposable prophy angle with polishing cup, air/water syringe tip

BOTTOM ROW (LEFT TO RIGHT)

Mouth mirror, explorer, cotton forceps, orthodontic scaler (Shure scaler), band seater-bite stick, posterior band remover, anterior bracket placement pliers, posterior bracket placement pliers, flexible cement spatula, low-volume saliva ejector, high-volume evacuation (HVE) tip, microbrushes, disposable cheek retractors

Sterilization Notes ▶ Refer to each individual picture for correct procedure for instrument sterilization or disposal of instrument or material. Refer to other chapters for additional instruments on this tray setup that are not included in this chapter.

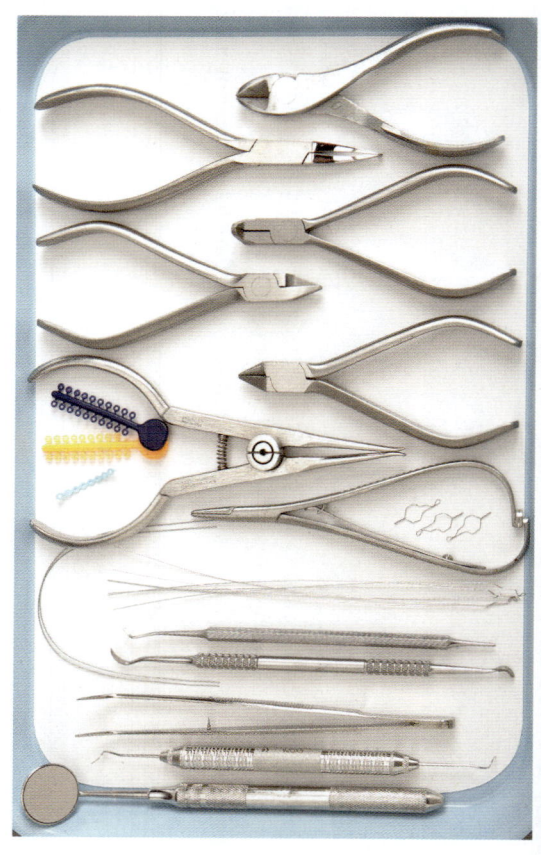

■ TRAY SETUP

Orthodontic Tying-In Arch Wire

TOP (LEFT TO RIGHT)
Preformed archwire, elastic ligature ties

BOTTOM (LEFT TO RIGHT)
Mouth mirror, explorer, cotton forceps, orthodontic (Shure) scaler, ligature director, wire ligature ties, orthodontic hemostat (Mathieu pliers), (under orthodontic hemostat, short wire ligature ties), ligature-tying (Coon) pliers, bird beak pliers, arch-bending pliers, distal-end cutting pliers, How (Howe) pliers, ligature/wire cutters

Sterilization Notes ▸ Refer to each picture for correct procedure for instrument sterilization or disposal of instrument or material. Refer to other chapters for additional instruments on this tray setup that are not included in this chapter.

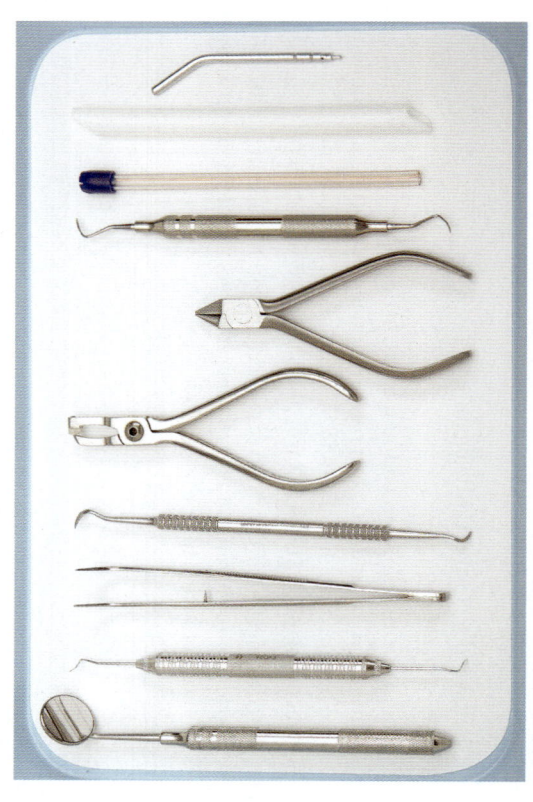

Orthodontic Removing Bands and Brackets

LEFT TO RIGHT

Mouth mirror, explorer, cotton forceps, orthodontic (Shure) scaler, posterior band remover, bird beak pliers, universal curette, low-volume saliva ejector, high-volume evacuation (HVE) tip, air/water syringe tip

Sterilization Notes ▶ Refer to each picture for correct procedure for instrument sterilization or disposal of instrument or material. Refer to other chapters for additional instruments on this tray setup that are not included in this chapter.

Universal Surgical Instruments

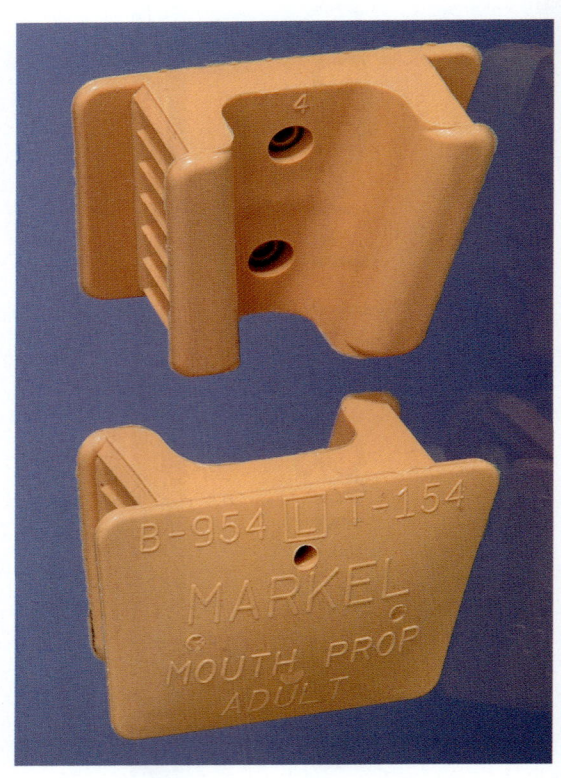

■ INSTRUMENT

Mouth Prop

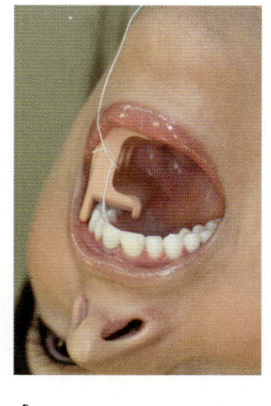

Function ▶ To hold patient's mouth open during dental procedures

Characteristics ▶ Placed in posterior part of mouth while patient bites down

Often used for sedated patients

Disposable mouth props available

Range of sizes—Pediatric to large adult

Practice Notes ▶ Mouth Prop could be used with any dental procedure, including but not exclusive to operative or surgical.

Ligate with floss for safety of patient choking.

Sterilization Notes ▶ Mouth Prop must be precleaned. Then, place in a sterilizing pouch with an internal process indicator, seal, then sterilize. OR, wrap with an internal process indicator inside and secure on the outside with process indicator tape, then sterilize. Verify appropriate color change has been achieved in external process indicator immediately after removal from sterilizer. Check internal process indicator before treatment. Refer to state regulations for any additional state requirements. Disposable Mouth Props should be disposed of in garbage. Single use only.

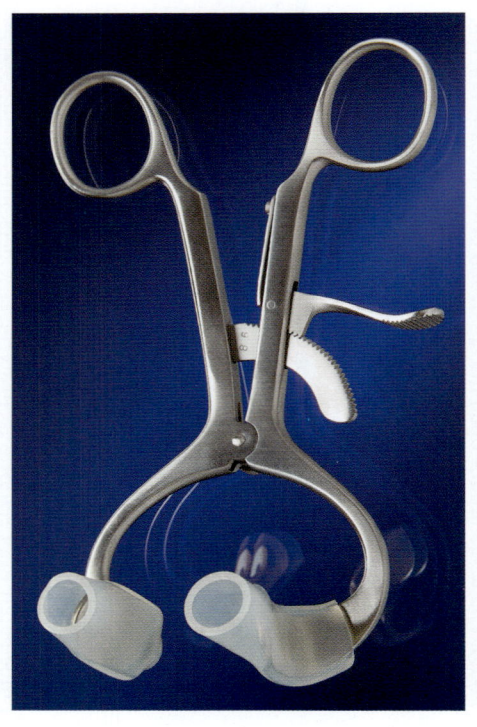

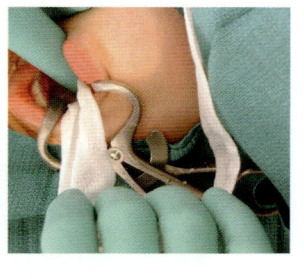

▪ INSTRUMENT

Mouth Gag

Function ▸ To hold patient's mouth open during dental procedures

Characteristics ▸ Often used for sedated patients

Locking device

Range of sizes available

Practice Note ▸ Mouth Gag is mostly used for oral surgery and periodontal surgical procedures when patient is sedated.

Sterilization Notes ▸ Mouth Gag must be precleaned, open, and unlocked. Then, place in an open and unlocked position in a sterilizing pouch with an internal process indicator, seal, then sterilize. OR, wrap with an internal process indicator inside and secure on the outside with process indicator tape, then sterilize. Verify appropriate color change has been achieved in external process indicator immediately after removal from sterilizer. Check internal process indicator before treatment. Refer to state regulations for any additional state requirements.

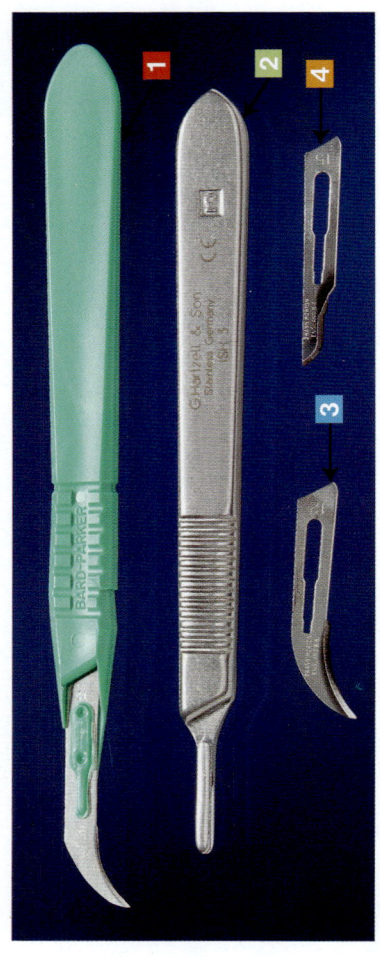

Scalpel Handle with Blades

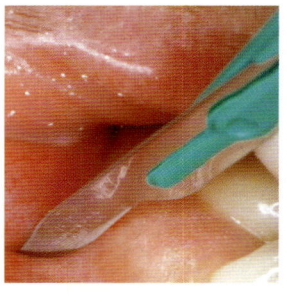

Functions ▶

Handle:

To hold blade in place

Blades:

To cut tissue with blade

To trim interproximal restorations

Characteristics ▶

1 Disposable Handle/Blade in one unit

2 Scalpel Handle

Blades—Disposable, variety of shapes and sizes:

3 #12 Blade

4 #15 Blade

Practice Note ▶

Scalpel with Blades mostly used on oral surgery and periodontal surgical tray setups and occasionally used with composite tray setups for removing flash material and interproximal carving.

Sterilization Notes ▶

Scalpel Handle must be precleaned. Then, place in a sterilizing pouch with an internal process indicator, seal, then sterilize. OR, wrap with an internal process indicator inside and secure on the outside with process indicator tape, then sterilize. Verify appropriate color change has been achieved in external process indicator immediately after removal from sterilizer. Check internal process indicator before treatment. Refer to state regulations for any additional state requirements. Scalpel blade must be disposed of in a sharps container. Disposable handle and blade in one unit must be disposed of in a sharps container.

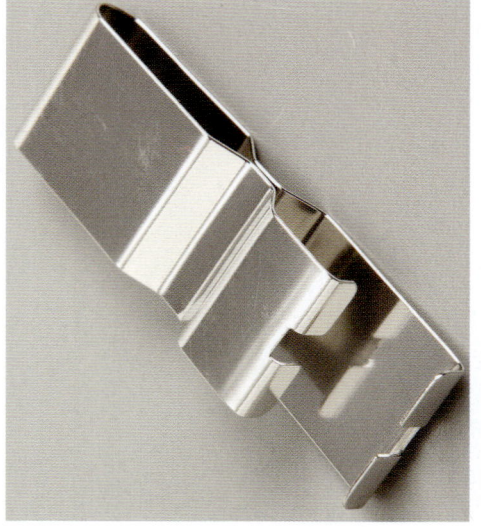

■ INSTRUMENT

Scalpel Blade Remover

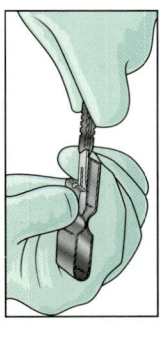

Function ▶ To safely remove blade from scalpel handle

Characteristics ▶ Removes all sizes of blades

Autoclavable

Practice Notes ▶ Steps for removing blade:

1 Insert blade with blade side up; align to notch.

2 Press down on blade remover.

3 Pull handle away from blade.

Scalpel Blade Remover is mostly used on oral surgery and periodontal surgical tray setups.

Sterilization Notes ▶ Scalpel Blade Remover must be precleaned. Then, place in a sterilizing pouch with an internal process indicator, seal, then sterilize. OR, wrap with an internal process indicator inside and secure on the outside with process indicator tape, then sterilize. Verify appropriate color change has been achieved in external process indicator immediately after removal from sterilizer. Check internal process indicator before treatment. Refer to state regulations for any additional state requirements. Scalpel Blade must be disposed of in a sharps container.

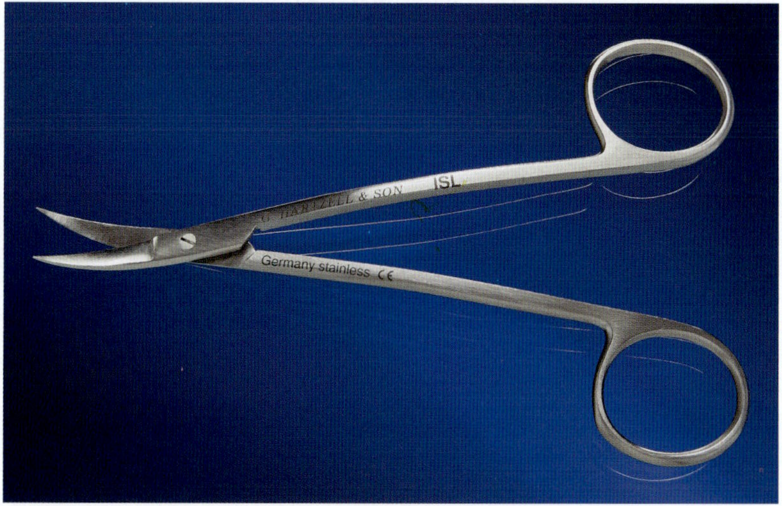
ISL
& SON
Germany stainless CE

■ INSTRUMENT

Tissue Scissors

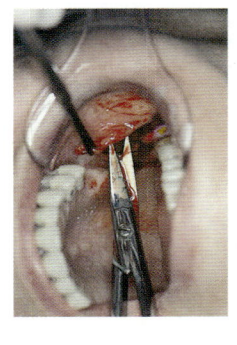

Function ▶ To cut tissue

Characteristics ▶ Straight or curved
Variety of shapes and sizes
Variety of uses

Practice Note ▶ Tissue Scissors are mostly used on oral surgery and periodontal surgical tray setups.

Sterilization Notes ▶ Tissue Scissors must be precleaned, open, and unlocked. Then, place in an open and unlocked position in a sterilizing pouch with an internal process indicator, seal, then sterilize. OR, wrap with an internal process indicator inside and secure on the outside with process indicator tape, then sterilize. Verify appropriate color change has been achieved in external process indicator immediately after removal from sterilizer. Check internal process indicator before treatment. Refer to state regulations for any additional state requirements.

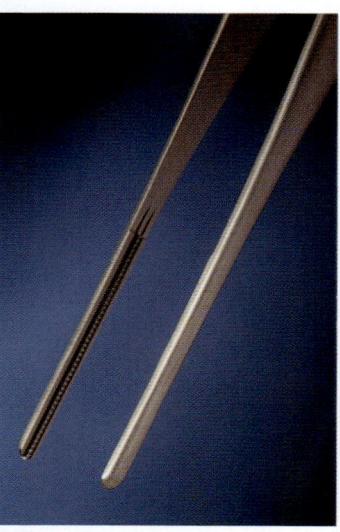

Tissue Forceps

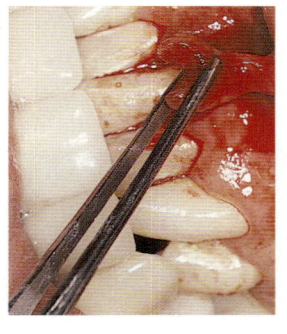

INSTRUMENT	
Function ▶	To hold tissue during surgical procedures
Characteristics ▶	Serrated or rat-tooth tips Range of sizes available
Practice Note ▶	Tissue Forceps are mostly used on oral surgery and periodontal surgical tray setups.
Sterilization Notes ▶	Tissue Forceps must be precleaned, open, and unlocked. Then, place in an open and unlocked position in a sterilizing pouch with an internal process indicator, seal, then sterilize. OR, wrap with an internal process indicator inside and secure on the outside with process indicator tape, then sterilize. Verify appropriate color change has been achieved in external process indicator immediately after removal from sterilizer. Check internal process indicator before treatment. Refer to state regulations for any additional state requirements.

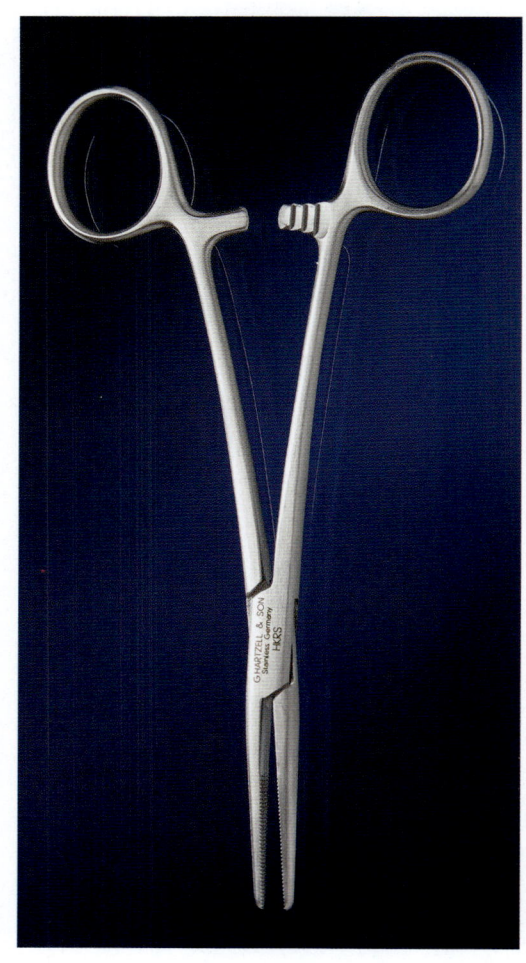

Hemostat

Function ▶
To grasp tissue or bone fragments
To hold and grasp material in and out of the oral cavity

Characteristics ▶
Straight or curved
Working end—Serrated and/or locking
Variety of functions in other dental procedures
Range of sizes available

Practice Notes ▶
Hemostat is mostly used on oral surgery and periodontal surgical tray setups.
Hemostat is also used on restorative and many other tray setups.

Sterilization Notes ▶
Hemostat must be precleaned, open, and unlocked. Then, place in an open and unlocked position in a sterilizing pouch with an internal process indicator, seal, then sterilize. OR, wrap with an internal process indicator inside and secure on the outside with process indicator tape, then sterilize. Verify appropriate color change has been achieved in external process indicator immediately after removal from sterilizer. Check internal process indicator before treatment. Refer to state regulations for any additional state requirements.

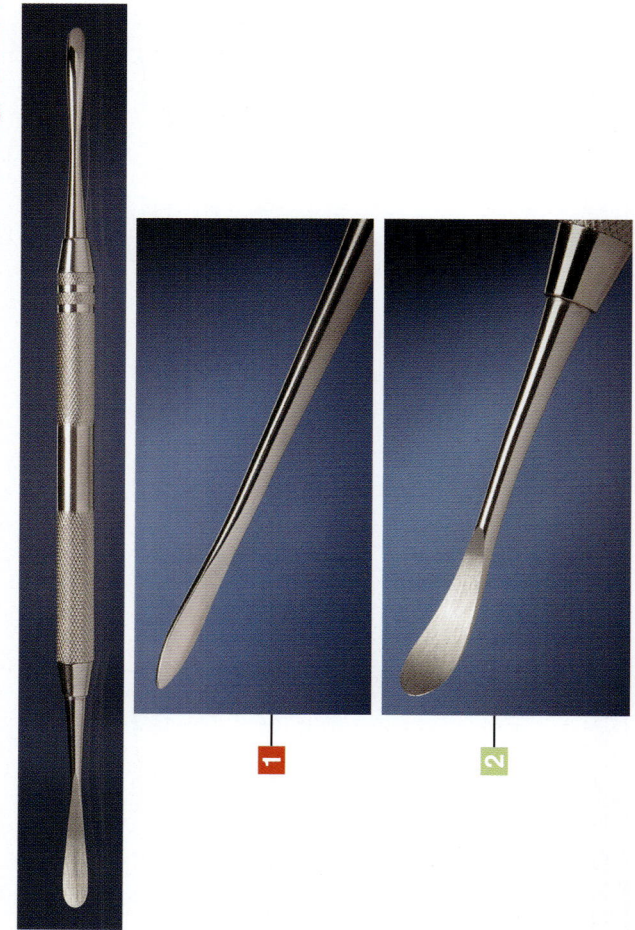

1

2

■ INSTRUMENT

Periosteal Elevator

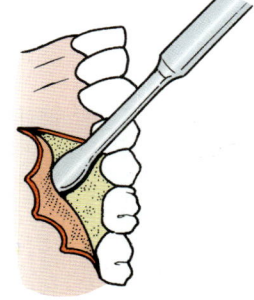

Functions ▸ To separate tissue from tooth or bone
To hold tissue away from surgical site

Characteristics ▸ Working end—Pointed or round
1 Pointed Periosteal Elevator
2 Round Periosteal Elevator
Range of sizes available

Practice Note ▸ Periosteal Elevator is used on oral surgery and periodontal surgical tray setups.

Sterilization Notes ▸ Periosteal Elevator must be precleaned. Then, place in a sterilizing pouch with an internal process indicator, seal, then sterilize. OR, wrap with an internal process indicator inside and secure on the outside with process indicator tape, then sterilize. Verify appropriate color change has been achieved in external process indicator immediately after removal from sterilizer. Check internal process indicator before treatment. Refer to state regulations for any additional state requirements.

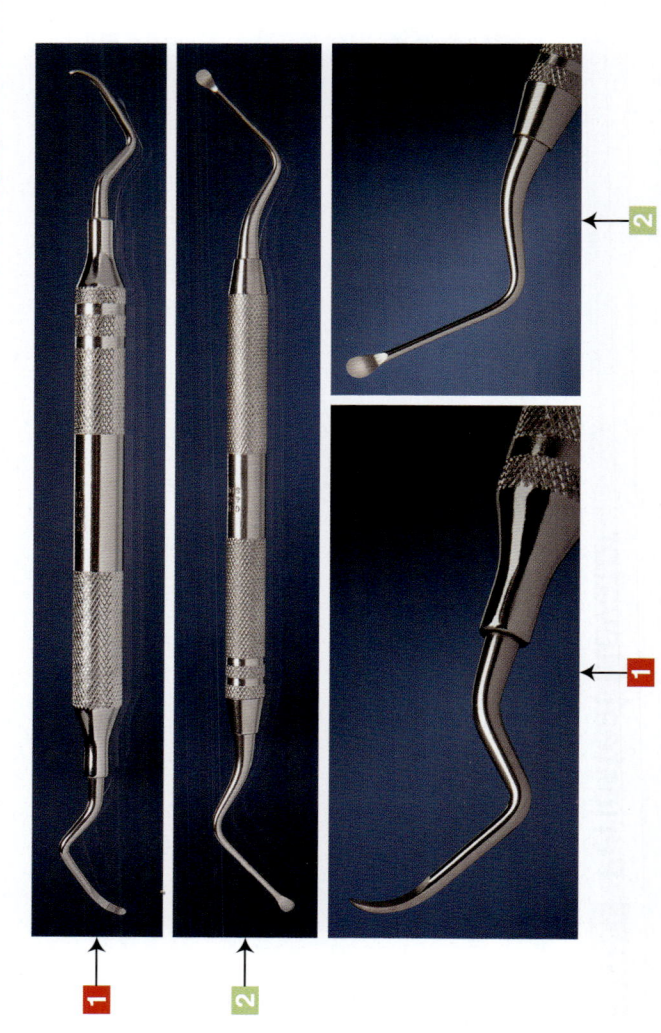

■ INSTRUMENT Surgical Curette

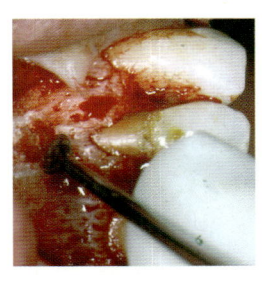

Functions ▶
To remove debris or granulation tissue from surgical site
To remove cyst from extraction site or surgical site
To perform gross tissue débridement

Characteristics ▶
Single or double ended
Variety of sizes and shapes
Examples of commonly used types:

1 Prichard
2 Miller

Practice Note ▶ Surgical Curette is mostly used on oral surgery and periodontal surgical tray setups.

Sterilization Notes ▶ Surgical Curette must be precleaned. Then, place in a sterilizing pouch with an internal process indicator, seal, then sterilize. OR, wrap with an internal process indicator inside and secure on the outside with process indicator tape, then sterilize. Verify appropriate color change has been achieved in external process indicator immediately after removal from sterilizer. Check internal process indicator before treatment. Refer to state regulations for any additional state requirements.

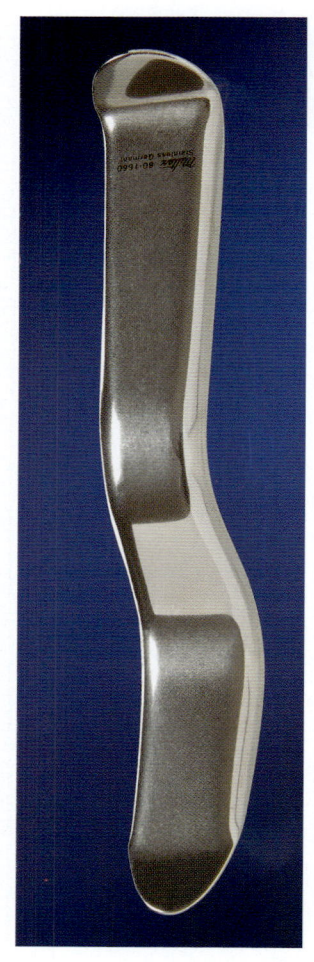

Tongue and Cheek Retractor

■ INSTRUMENT

Function ▶ To hold and retract tongue or cheek during surgery

Characteristic ▶ Variety of styles and sizes
Example of commonly used type: Minnesota—pictured

Practice Note ▶ Tongue and Cheek Retractor is mostly used on oral surgery and periodontal surgical tray setups.

Sterilization Notes ▶ Tongue and Cheek Retractor must be precleaned. Then, place in a sterilizing pouch with an internal process indicator, seal, then sterilize. OR, wrap with an internal process indicator inside and secure on the outside with process indicator tape, then sterilize. Verify appropriate color change has been achieved in external process indicator immediately after removal from sterilizer. Check internal process indicator before treatment. Refer to state regulations for any additional state requirements.

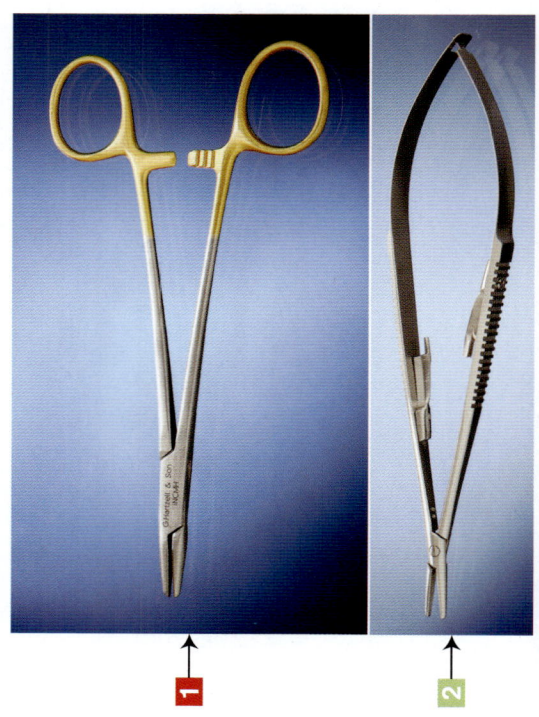

1

2

Surgical Needle Holder

Function ▶ To grasp and manipulate suture needle during use

Characteristics ▶ Working end—Different lengths, curved or straight

Notched ends available (to accommodate needle)

Range of sizes—Micro for microsurgery to large

Variety of styles:

1 Universal
2 Castroviejo

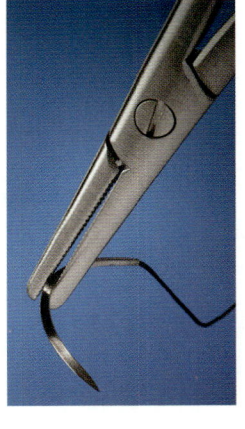

Practice Note ▶ Needle Holder is mostly used on oral surgery and periodontal surgical tray setups.

Sterilization Notes ▶ Needle Holder must be precleaned, open, and unlocked. Then, place in an open and unlocked position in a sterilizing pouch with an internal process indicator, seal, then sterilize. OR, wrap with an internal process indicator inside and secure on the outside with process indicator tape, then sterilize. Verify appropriate color change has been achieved in external process indicator immediately after removal from sterilizer. Check internal process indicator before treatment. Refer to state regulations for any additional state requirements.

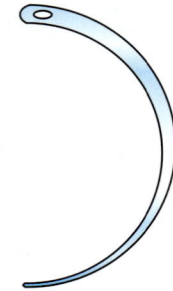

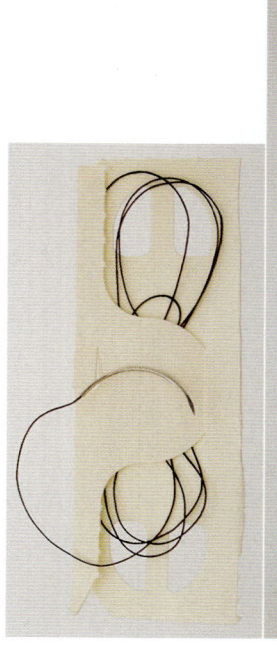

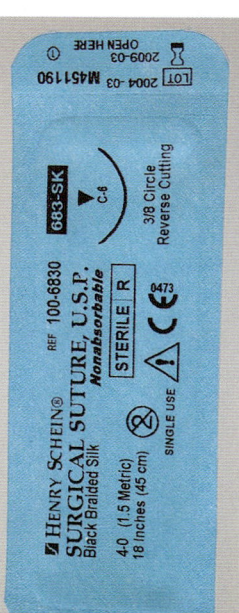

Suture Needle and Sutures

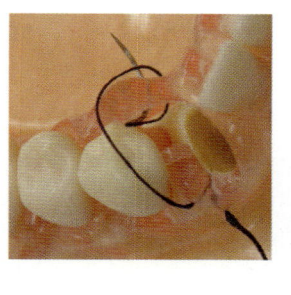

Function ▶ To suture surgical site

Characteristics ▶ Resorbable sutures—Gut plain, chromic gut, polyglycolic acid (PGA)

Nonresorbable sutures—Silk, nylon, polyester, polypropylene

Available in sterile package

Variety of suture needle sizes available with different sutures

Practice Note ▶ Suture Needle and Sutures are mostly used on oral surgery and periodontal surgical tray setups.

Sterilization Notes ▶ Suture Needle and Sutures must be disposed of in a sharps container.

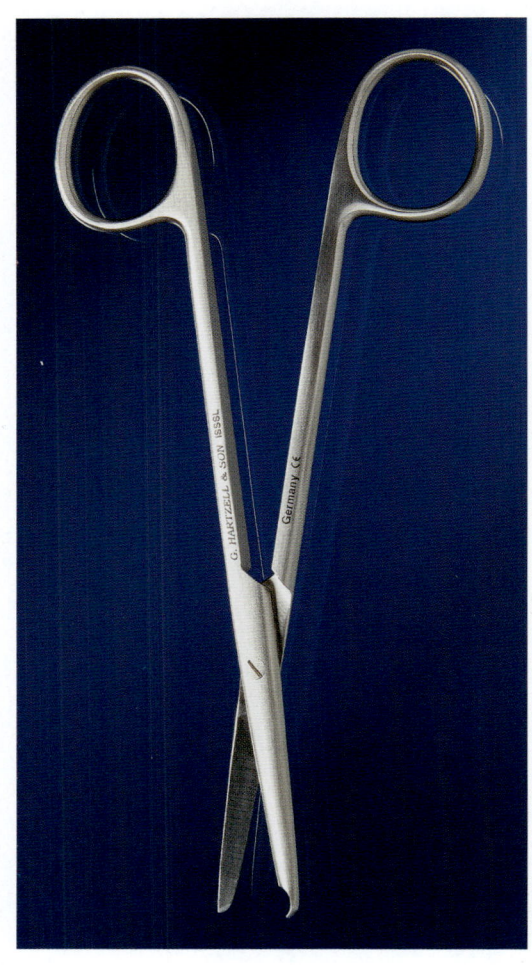

■ INSTRUMENT

Suture Scissors

Function ▶ To cut sutures

Characteristics ▶ Cutting edges—Straight or angled
May have notch on end of cutting edge (shown in picture)
Range of sizes

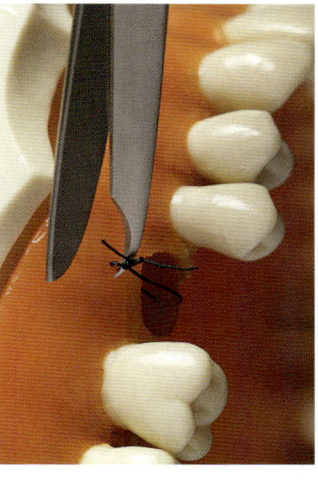

Practice Note ▶ Suture Scissors are mostly used on oral surgery and periodontal surgical tray setups.

Sterilization Notes ▶ Suture Scissors must be precleaned, open, and unlocked. Then, place in an open and unlocked position in a sterilizing pouch with an internal process indicator, seal, then sterilize. OR, wrap with an internal process indicator inside and secure on the outside with process indicator tape, then sterilize. Verify appropriate color change has been achieved in external process indicator immediately after removal from sterilizer. Check internal process indicator before treatment. Refer to state regulations for any additional state requirements.

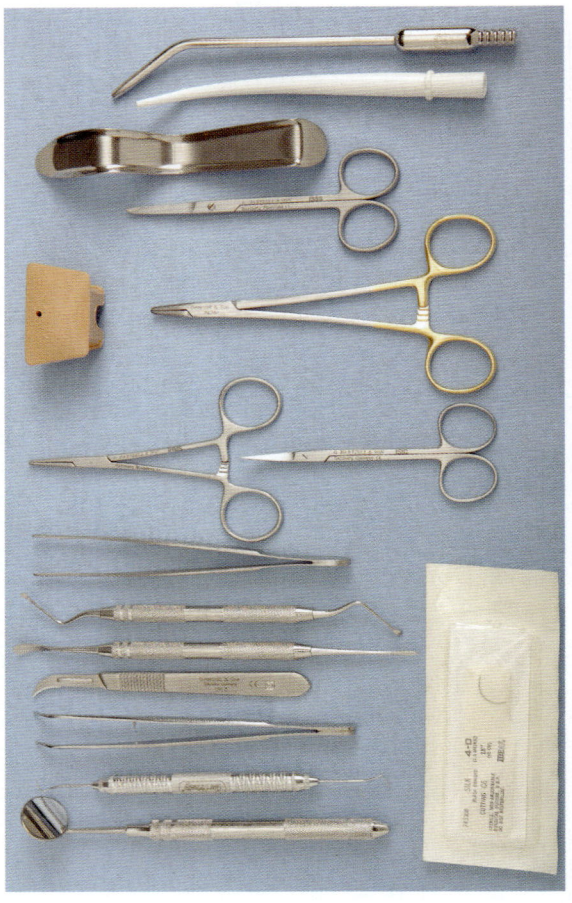

■TRAY SETUP

Universal Surgical

TOP ROW (LEFT TO RIGHT)

Mouth mirror, explorer, cotton forceps (pliers), scalpel with #12 blade, periosteal elevator, surgical curette (Prichard), tissue forceps, hemostat, tissue scissors, mouth prop, needle holder, suture scissors, tongue and cheek retractor, disposable high-volume surgical evacuation tip, high-volume surgical evacuation tip

BOTTOM ROW

Silk suture with needle in sterile package

Sterilization Notes ▶ Refer to each picture for correct procedure for instrument sterilization or disposal of instrument or material. Refer to other chapters for additional instruments on this tray setup that are not included in this chapter.

Periodontal Instruments and Periodontal Surgical Instruments

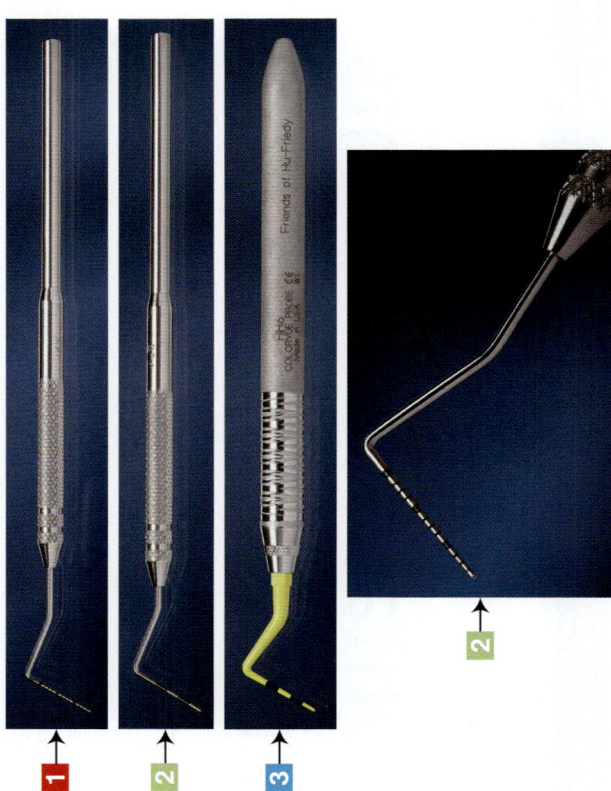

Periodontal Probes

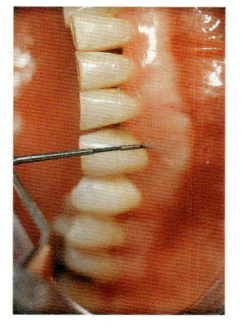

Function ▶ To measure periodontal pocket depth in millimeter increments

Characteristics ▶ Flat or rounded ends

Millimeter-increment markings vary for each style:

1 Color coded—Black markings for millimeter measurements

2 Other styles—Indentations in metal for millimeter measurements-each indentation represents a millimeter.

3 Color-ended probe with black visible markings—Replaceable tip, different tip designs, plastic tip safe for implant probing

Double-ended style available with probe on one end and explorer on the other

Computerized probes available

Practice Note ▶ Periodontal Probe is used on basic setup, dental hygiene, and periodontal tray setups.

Sterilization Notes ▶ Periodontal Probes must be precleaned. Then, place in a sterilizing pouch with an internal process indicator, seal, then sterilize. OR, wrap with an internal process indicator inside and secure on the outside with process indicator tape, then sterilize. Verify appropriate color change has been achieved in external process indicator immediately after removal from sterilizer. Check internal process indicator before treatment. Refer to state regulations for any additional state requirements.

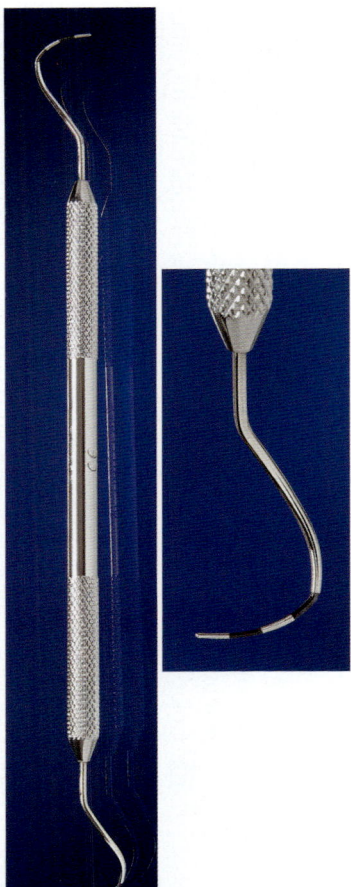

Furcation Probe

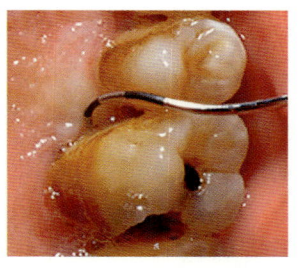

Function ▶ To measure horizontal and vertical pocket depth of multirooted teeth in furcation areas

Characteristics ▶ Flat or rounded ends

Single or double ended

Millimeter-increment markings vary for each style:

- Color coded—Black markings for millimeter measurements
- Other styles—Indentations in metal for millimeter measurements

Example: Nabors probe—Color coded markings for millimeter measurements.

Practice Note ▶ Furcation Probe is used on basic, dental hygiene, and periodontal tray setups.

Sterilization Notes ▶ Furcation Probes must be precleaned. Then, place in a sterilizing pouch with an internal process indicator, seal, then sterilize. OR, wrap with an internal process indicator inside and secure on the outside with process indicator tape, then sterilize. Verify appropriate color change has been achieved in external process indicator immediately after removal from sterilizer. Check internal process indicator before treatment. Refer to state regulations for any additional state requirements.

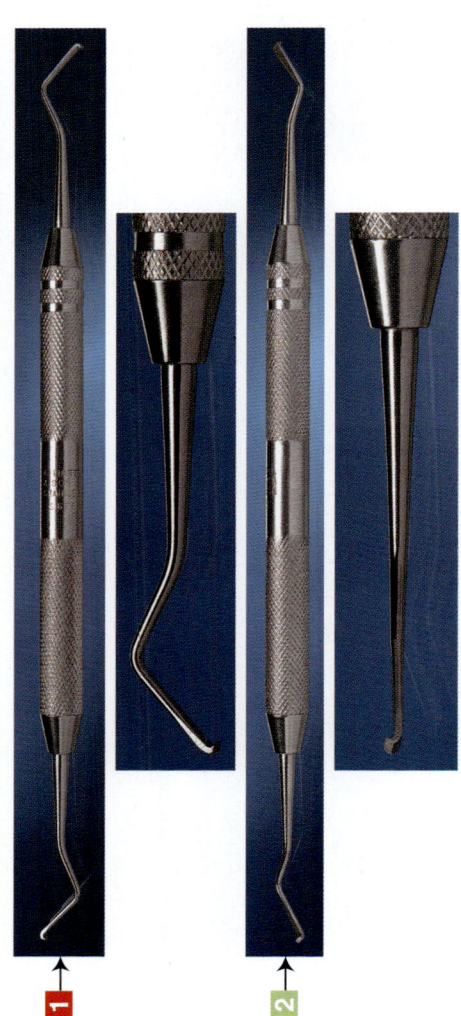

1

2

Hoe Scaler—Mesial/Distal and Buccal/Lingual

Function ▶ To remove subgingival and supragingival calculus

Characteristics ▶
1 Mesial/Distal Hoe
2 Buccal/Lingual Hoe scaler
Used with pulling motion
Straight cutting edge
Single or double ended
Designed to function in anterior or posterior locations
  • Anterior—Shorter, straighter shanks
  • Posterior—Longer, angled shanks

Practice Note ▶ Mesial/Distal and Buccal/Lingual Hoe scalers, according to procedure performed, could be used on dental hygiene and periodontal tray setups.

Sterilization Notes ▶ Mesial/Distal and Buccal/Lingual Hoes Scalers must be precleaned. Then, place in a sterilizing pouch with an internal process indicator, seal, then sterilize. OR, wrap with an internal process indicator inside and secure on the outside with process indicator tape, then sterilize. Verify appropriate color change has been achieved in external process indicator immediately after removal from sterilizer. Check internal process indicator before treatment. Refer to state regulations for any additional state requirements.

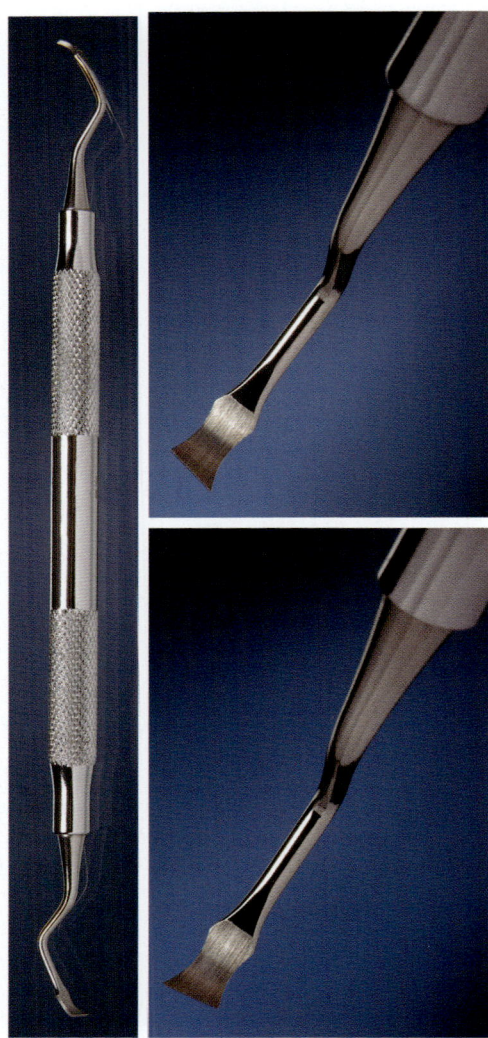

Back-Action Hoe

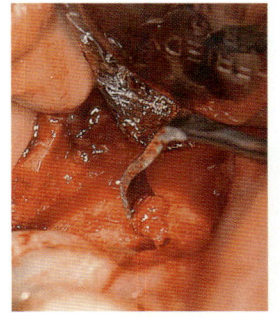

INSTRUMENT	
Function ▸	To remove bone adjacent to teeth without causing trauma
Characteristics ▸	Double ended Variety of sizes and shapes
Practice Note ▸	Back-Action Hoe, according to procedure performed, could be used on dental hygiene and periodontal tray setups.
Sterilization Notes ▸	Back-Action Hoe must be precleaned. Then, place in a sterilizing pouch with an internal process indicator, seal, then sterilize. OR, wrap with an internal process indicator inside and secure on the outside with process indicator tape, then sterilize. Verify appropriate color change has been achieved in external process indicator immediately after removal from sterilizer. Check internal process indicator before treatment. Refer to state regulations for any additional state requirements.

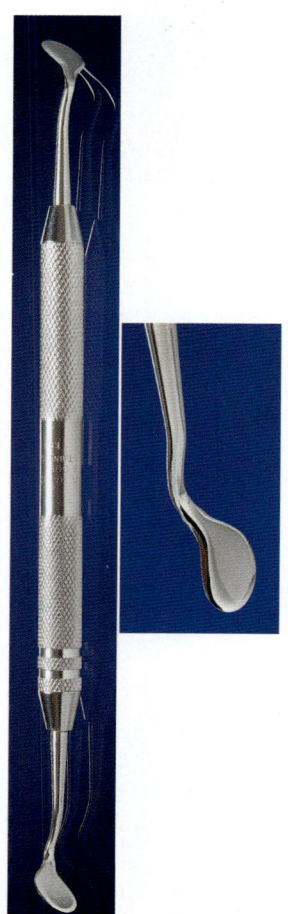

Periodontal Knife—Kidney Shaped

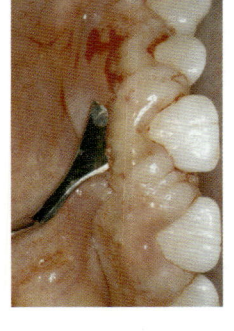

Functions ▶ To use for bevel incision for gingivectomy
To use for gingivoplasty

Characteristics ▶ Variety of sizes and shapes
Named by designer: Kirkland, Goldman-Fox, Buck, Solt

Practice Note ▶ Periodontal Knife—Kidney Shaped is used on periodontal surgical tray setups.

Sterilization Notes ▶ Periodontal Knife—Kidney Shaped must be precleaned. Then, place in a sterilizing pouch with an internal process indicator, seal, then sterilize. OR, wrap with an internal process indicator inside and secure on the outside with process indicator tape, then sterilize. Verify appropriate color change has been achieved in external process indicator immediately after removal from sterilizer. Check internal process indicator before treatment. Refer to state regulations for any additional state requirements.

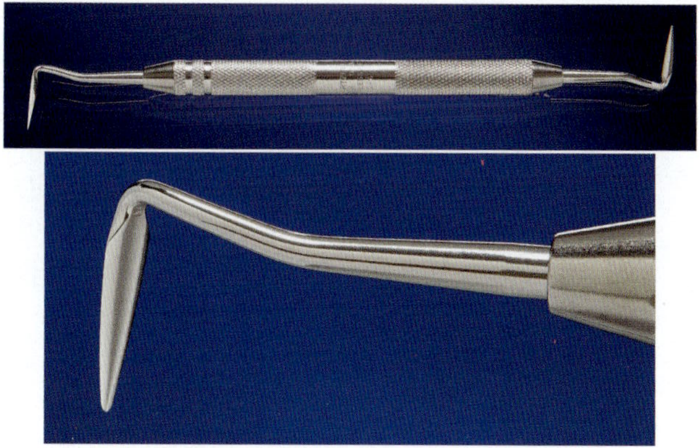

Interdental Knife—Spear Point

Functions ▸

To use for interdental cutting of gingiva

To remove tissue

Characteristics ▸

Blade angulated for easier use

Named by designer: Orban, Goldman-Fox, Buck, Sanders

Single or double ended

Range of sizes

Example: Buck ⅚

Practice Note ▸

Interdental Knife—Spear Point is used on periodontal surgical tray setups.

Sterilization Notes ▸

Interdental Knife—Spear Point must be precleaned. Then, place in a sterilizing pouch with an internal process indicator, seal, then sterilize. OR, wrap with an internal process indicator inside and secure on the outside with process indicator tape, then sterilize. Verify appropriate color change has been achieved in external process indicator immediately after removal from sterilizer. Check internal process indicator before treatment. Refer to state regulations for any additional state requirements.

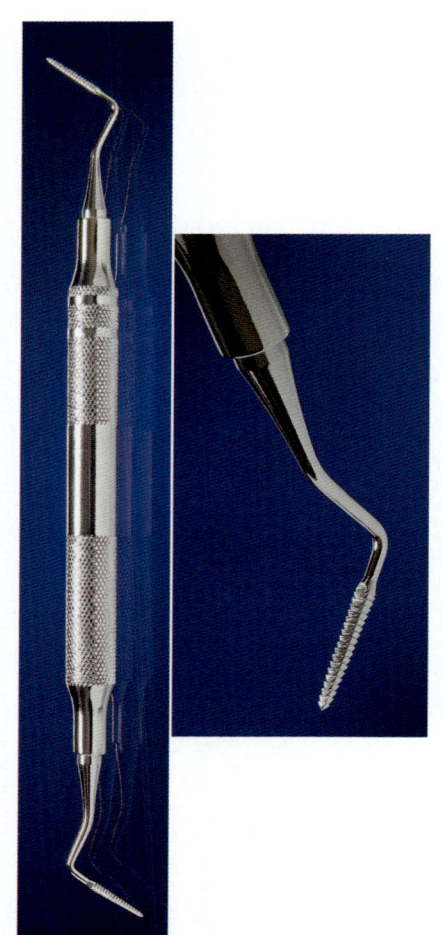

Interdental File

Function ▶ To crush and remove heavy deposits from subgingival and supragingival interproximal areas

Characteristics ▶ Used with push or pull motion

Various angles—Curved, straight, mesial/distal, and buccal/lingual

Examples: Sugarman, Schluger, Buck

Range of sizes available

Practice Note ▶ Interdental File is used on periodontal surgical tray setups.

Sterilization Notes ▶ Interdental File must be precleaned. Then, place in a sterilizing pouch with an internal process indicator, seal, then sterilize. OR, wrap with an internal process indicator inside and secure on the outside with process indicator tape, then sterilize. Verify appropriate color change has been achieved in external process indicator immediately after removal from sterilizer. Check internal process indicator before treatment. Refer to state regulations for any additional state requirements.

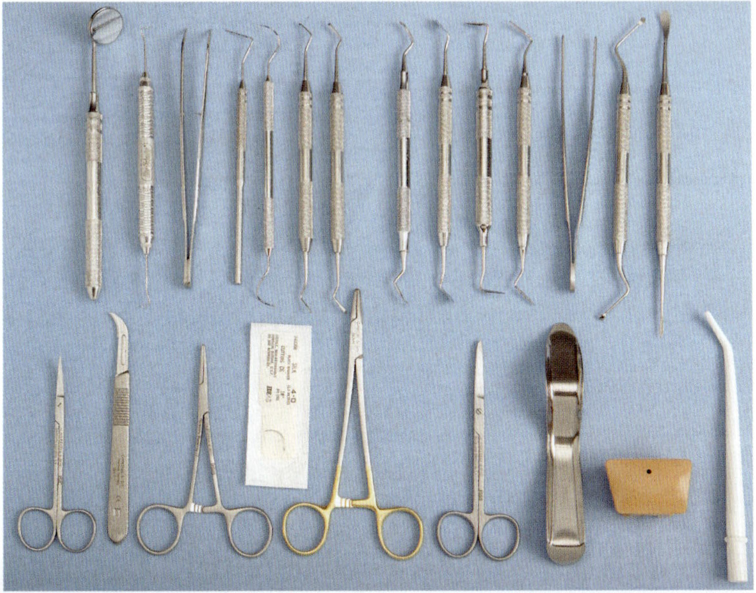

Periodontal Surgical

TOP ROW—LEFT TO RIGHT

Mouth mirror, explorer, cotton forceps (pliers), periodontal probe, furcation probe, mesial/distal hoe, buccal/lingual hoe, back-action hoe, kidney-shaped periodontal knife, interproximal knife, bone file, tissue forceps, surgical curette, periosteal elevator

BOTTOM ROW—LEFT TO RIGHT

Tissue scissors, scalpel with #12 blade, hemostat, silk sutures with needle, needle holder, suture scissors, cheek and tongue retractor (Minnesota), mouth prop, disposable high-volume surgical evacuation tip

Sterilization Notes ▶ Refer to each picture for correct procedure for instrument sterilization or disposal of instrument or material. Refer to Chapter 15 for complete instruments used in periodontal surgery. Also refer to other chapters for additional instruments on tray setup that are not included in this chapter.

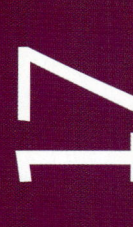

17

Oral Surgery Extraction Instruments

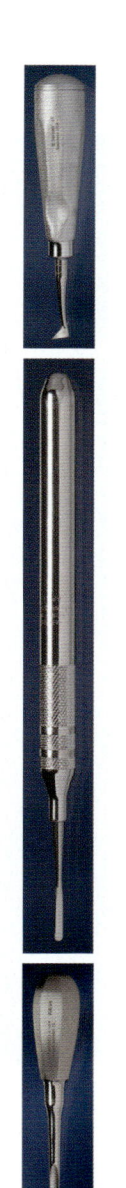

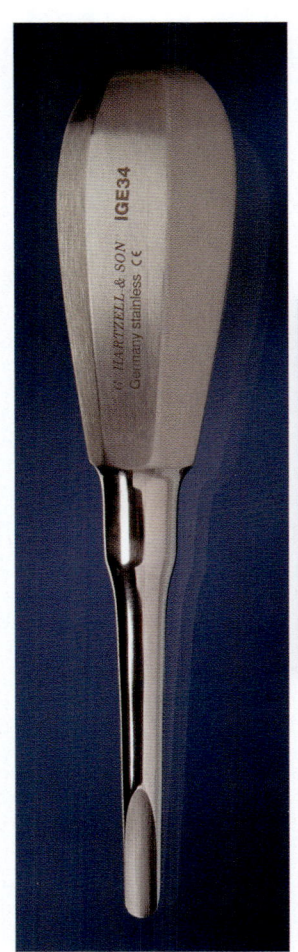

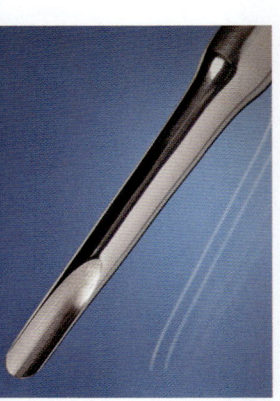

Straight Elevator

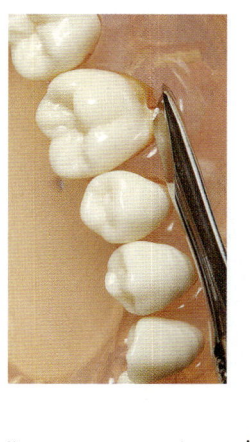

Functions ▶ To loosen tooth from periodontal ligaments before extraction

To separate and lift tooth from socket

Characteristics ▶ Single ended

Range of sizes available

Practice Note ▶ Straight Elevator is used on surgical extraction tray setups.

Sterilization Notes ▶ Straight Elevator must be precleaned. Then, place in a sterilizing pouch with an internal process indicator, seal, then sterilize. OR, wrap with an internal process indicator inside and secure on the outside with process indicator tape, then sterilize. Verify appropriate color change has been achieved in external process indicator immediately after removal from sterilizer. Check internal process indicator before treatment. Refer to state regulations for any additional state requirements.

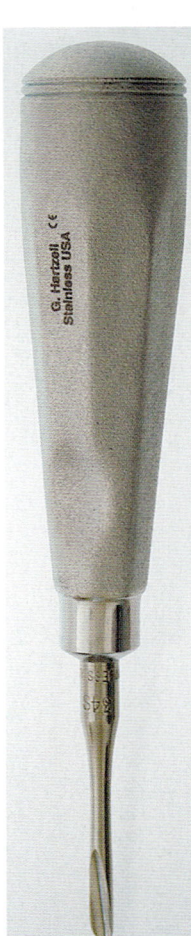

■ INSTRUMENT

Luxating Elevator

Functions ▲ To cut periodontal ligaments before extraction
To rock tooth back and forth before extraction

Characteristics ▲ Single ended
Sharp blade on working end
Blade is serrated
Range of sizes available

Practice Note ▲ Luxating Elevator is used on surgical extraction tray setups.

Sterilization Notes ▲ Luxating Elevator must be precleaned. Then, place in a sterilizing pouch with an internal process indicator, seal, then sterilize. OR, wrap with an internal process indicator inside and secure on the outside with process indicator tape, then sterilize. Verify appropriate color change has been achieved in external process indicator immediately after removal from sterilizer. Check internal process indicator before treatment. Refer to state regulations for any additional state requirements.

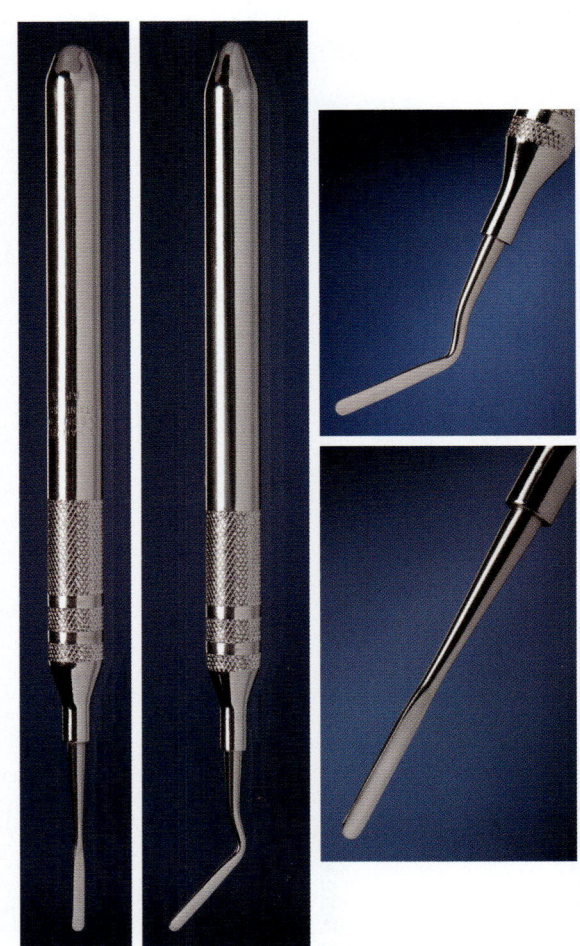

Periotomes

INSTRUMENT

Functions ► To cut periodontal ligaments for atraumatic tooth extraction
To use when dental implant placement is indicated

Characteristics ► Thin, sharp blades—Cause minimal damage to periodontal ligaments and surrounding alveolar bone
Straight or angled blades
Single or double ended
Range of sizes available
Some manufacturers make replaceable tip

Practice Note ► Periotomes are used on surgical extraction tray setups.

Sterilization Notes ► Periotomes must be precleaned. Then, place in a sterilizing pouch with an internal process indicator, seal, then sterilize. OR, wrap with an internal process indicator inside and secure on the outside with process indicator tape, then sterilize. Verify appropriate color change has been achieved in external process indicator immediately after removal from sterilizer. Check internal process indicator before treatment. Refer to state regulations for any additional state requirements.

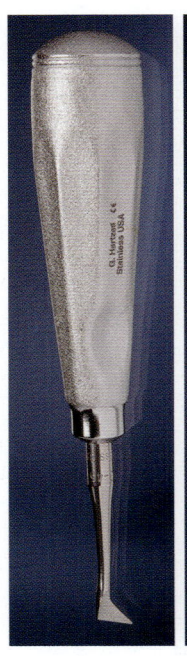
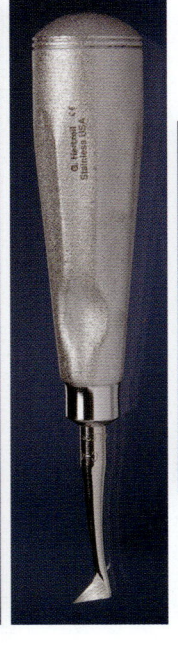
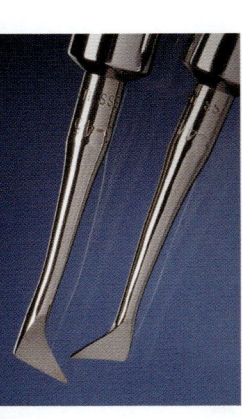

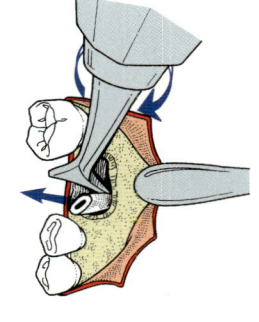

Root Elevators

Functions ▸
To loosen root
To separate and lift root from socket
To use on posterior teeth

Characteristics ▸
Single ended
Right and left pairs
Range of sizes available
Example: Cryer (commonly used type)

Practice Note ▸
Root Elevators are used in surgical extraction tray setups.

Sterilization Notes ▸
Root Elevators must be precleaned. Then, place in a sterilizing pouch with an internal process indicator, seal, then sterilize. OR, wrap with an internal process indicator inside and secure on the outside with process indicator tape, then sterilize. Verify appropriate color change has been achieved in external process indicator immediately after removal from sterilizer. Check internal process indicator before treatment. Refer to state regulations for any additional state requirements.

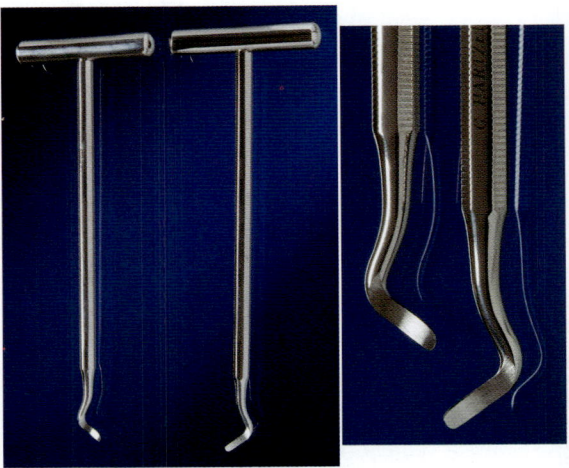

T-Bar Elevators

Functions ▶ To loosen tooth from periodontal ligaments before extraction
To separate tooth from alveolus
To use on posterior teeth

Characteristics ▶ Single ended
Rounded or pointed
Right or left pairs
T-Bar Elevators are available with different style handles
Range of sizes available

Practice Note ▶ T-Bar Elevators are used on surgical extraction tray setups.

Sterilization Notes ▶ T-Bar Elevators must be precleaned. Then, place in a sterilizing pouch with an internal process indicator, seal, then sterilize. OR, wrap with an internal process indicator inside and secure on the outside with process indicator tape, then sterilize. Verify appropriate color change has been achieved in external process indicator immediately after removal from sterilizer. Check internal process indicator before treatment. Refer to state regulations for any additional state requirements.

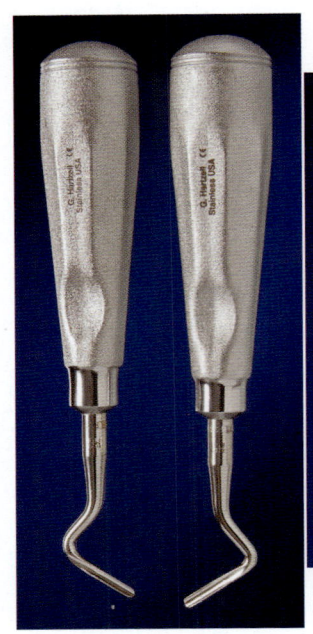
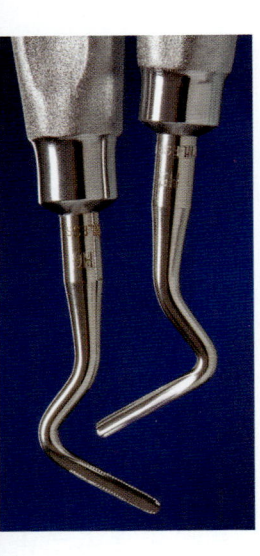

■ INSTRUMENT

Root-Tip Elevators

Function ▶ To lift and remove fragments of root

Characteristics ▶ Single ended
Rounded or pointed
Working ends are serrated
Straight or right and left pairs

Practice Note ▶ Root-Tip Elevators are used on surgical extraction tray setups.

Sterilization Notes ▶ Root-Tip Elevators must be precleaned. Then, place in a sterilizing pouch with an internal process indicator, seal, then sterilize. OR, wrap with an internal process indicator inside and secure on the outside with process indicator tape, then sterilize. Verify appropriate color change has been achieved in external process indicator immediately after removal from sterilizer. Check internal process indicator before treatment. Refer to state regulations for any additional state requirements.

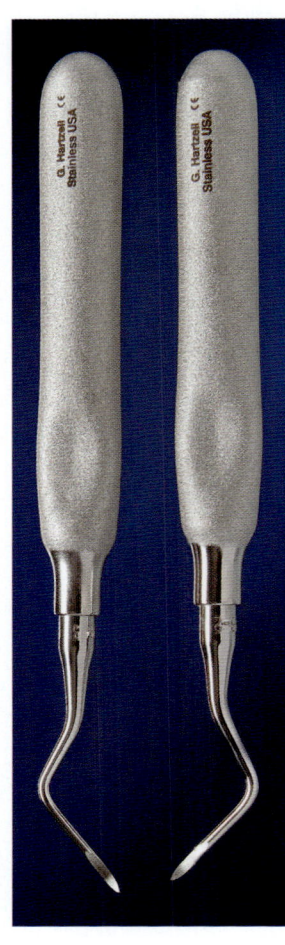

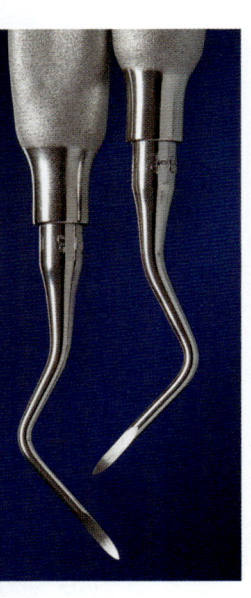

Root-Tip Picks

Function ▸ To lift and remove small root tips in difficult areas

Characteristics ▸ Pointed at working end
Straight or right and left pairs

Practice Note ▸ Root-Tip Picks are used on surgical extraction tray setups.

Sterilization Notes ▸ Root-Tip Picks must be precleaned. Then, place in a sterilizing pouch with an internal process indicator, seal, then sterilize. OR, wrap with an internal process indicator inside and secure on the outside with process indicator tape, then sterilize. Verify appropriate color change has been achieved in external process indicator immediately after removal from sterilizer. Check internal process indicator before treatment. Refer to state regulations for any additional state requirements.

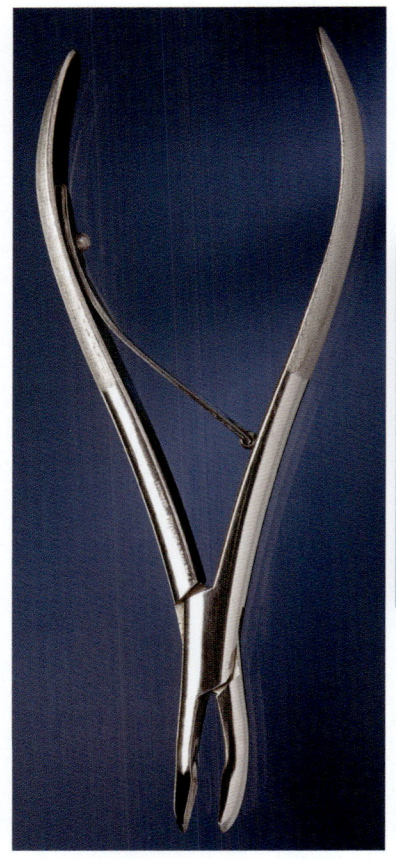
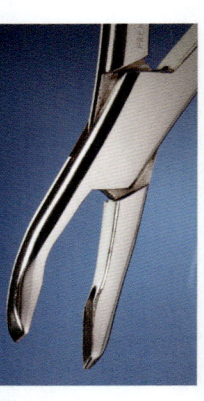

■ INSTRUMENT

Rongeurs

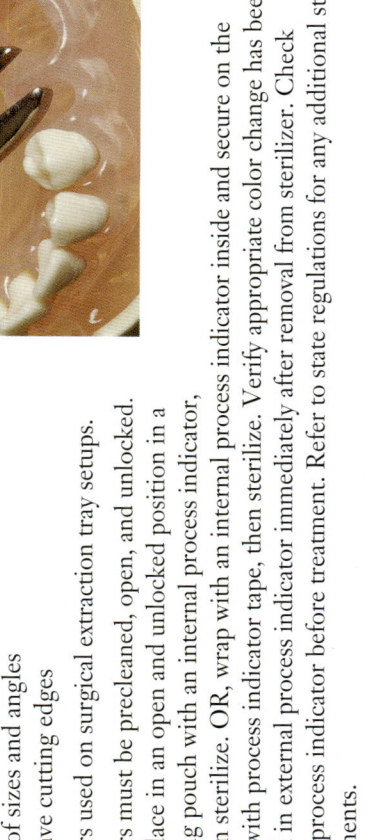

Functions ▶ To trim and remove excess alveolar bone after extraction of teeth

To contour alveolar bone after single or multiple extractions

Characteristics ▶ Variety of sizes and angles

Beaks have cutting edges

Practice Note ▶ Rongeurs used on surgical extraction tray setups.

Sterilization Notes ▶ Rongeurs must be precleaned, open, and unlocked. Then, place in an open and unlocked position in a sterilizing pouch with an internal process indicator, seal, then sterilize. OR, wrap with an internal process indicator inside and secure on the outside with process indicator tape, then sterilize. Verify appropriate color change has been achieved in external process indicator immediately after removal from sterilizer. Check internal process indicator before treatment. Refer to state regulations for any additional state requirements.

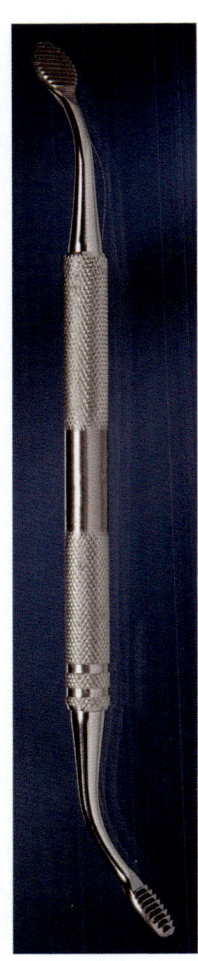

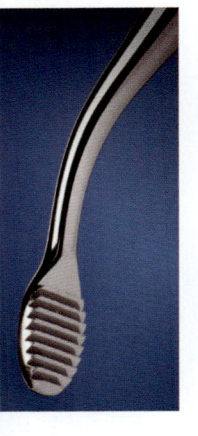

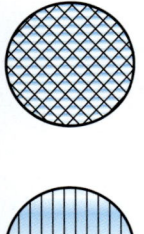

Bone File

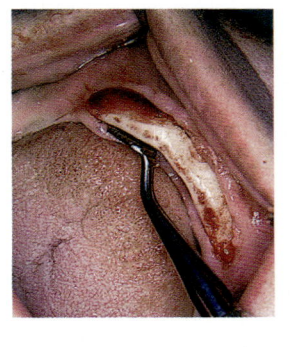

Function ▶ To remove or smooth rough edges of alveolar bone

Characteristics ▶ Used with push-pull motion
Straight-cut or crosscut cutting end
Variety of sizes, angles, and shapes

Practice Note ▶ Bone File is used on surgical extraction tray setups.

Sterilization Notes ▶ Bone File must be precleaned. Then, place in a sterilizing pouch with an internal process indicator, seal, then sterilize. OR, wrap with an internal process indicator inside and secure on the outside with process indicator tape, then sterilize. Verify appropriate color change has been achieved in external process indicator immediately after removal from sterilizer. Check internal process indicator before treatment. Refer to state regulations for any additional state requirements.

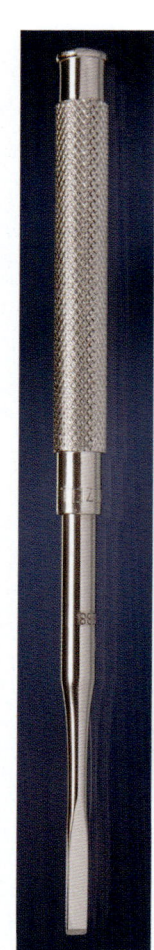

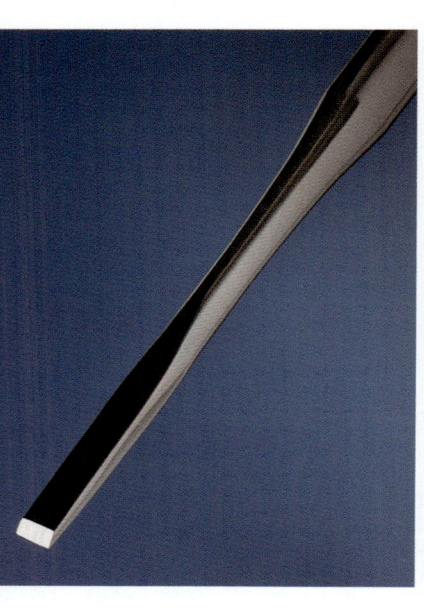

■ INSTRUMENT

Surgical Chisel

Functions ▸ To split or section a tooth for easier removal by tapping on chisel with mallet

To reshape or contour alveolar bone

Characteristics ▸ Single-bevel chisel—For contouring or removing alveolar bone

Bi-bevel chisel—For splitting teeth

Styles—Surgical chisel, bone splitter

Range of sizes available

Practice Note ▸ Surgical Chisel is used on surgical extraction and other types of surgical procedure tray setups.

Sterilization Notes ▸ Surgical Chisel must be precleaned. Then, place in a sterilizing pouch with an internal process indicator, seal, then sterilize. OR, wrap with an internal process indicator inside and secure on the outside with process indicator tape, then sterilize. Verify appropriate color change has been achieved in external process indicator immediately after removal from sterilizer. Check internal process indicator before treatment. Refer to state regulations for any additional state requirements.

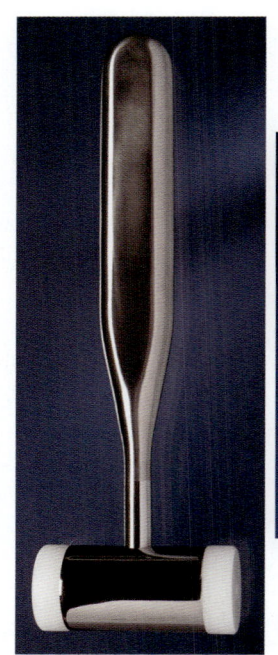
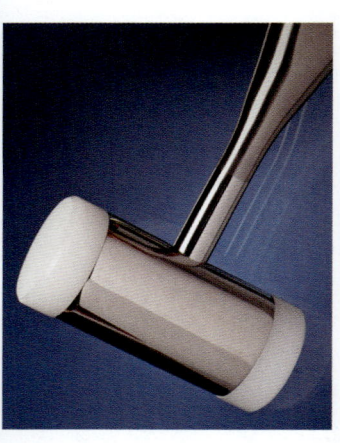

■ INSTRUMENT

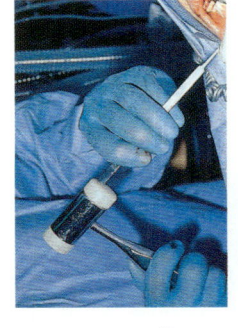

Surgical Mallet

Functions ▶ To use with bone chisel to section tooth for easier removal by tapping on chisel with surgical mallet

To use with bone chisel to reshape or contour alveolar bone

Characteristic ▶ Range of sizes available

Practice Note ▶ Surgical Mallet is used on surgical extraction and other types of surgical procedure tray setups.

Sterilization Notes ▶ Surgical Mallet must be precleaned. Then, place in a sterilizing pouch with an internal process indicator, seal, then sterilize. OR, wrap with an internal process indicator inside and secure on the outside with process indicator tape, then sterilize. Verify appropriate color change has been achieved in external process indicator immediately after removal from sterilizer. Check internal process indicator before treatment. Refer to state regulations for any additional state requirements.

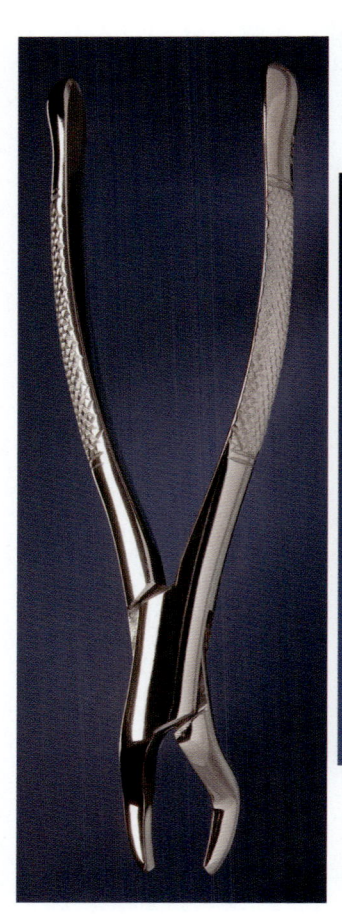
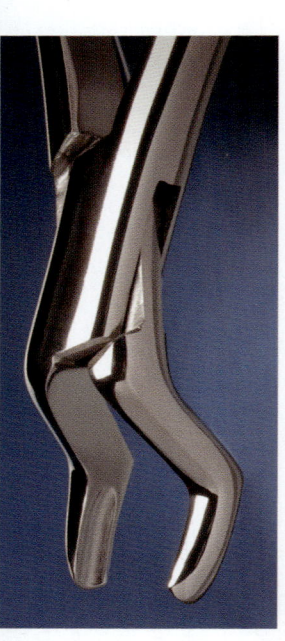

Universal Maxillary Forceps No. 10S

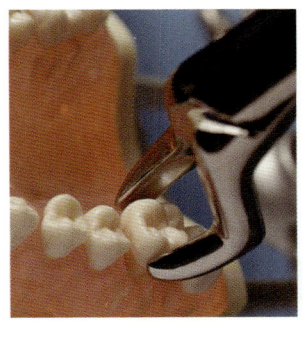

INSTRUMENT

Function ▶ To extract maxillary molars

Characteristic ▶ Straight handle

Practice Note ▶ Universal Maxillary Forceps No. 10S are used on surgical extraction tray setups.

Sterilization Notes ▶ Universal Maxillary Forceps No. 10S must be precleaned, open, and unlocked. Then, place in an open and unlocked position in a sterilizing pouch with an internal process indicator, seal, then sterilize. OR, wrap with an internal process indicator inside and secure on the outside with process indicator tape, then sterilize. Verify appropriate process indicator color change has been achieved in external process indicator immediately after removal from sterilizer. Check internal process indicator before treatment. Refer to state regulations for any additional state requirements.

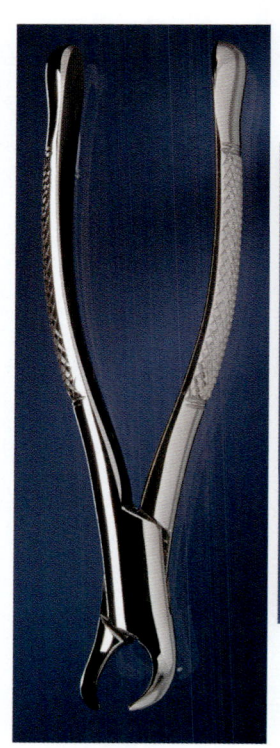
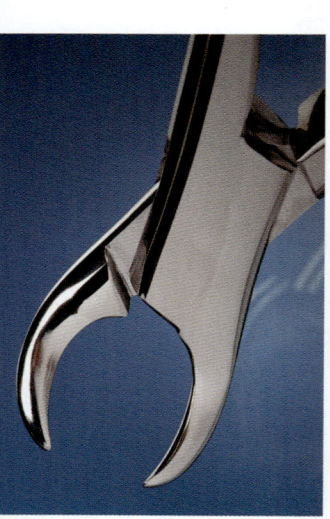

Universal Mandibular Forceps No. 16

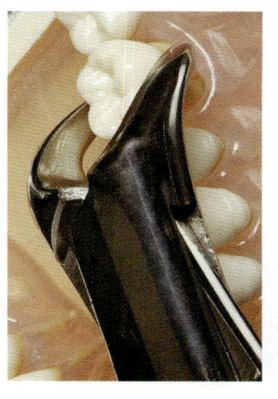

INSTRUMENT

Function ▶ To extract mandibular first and second molars

Characteristics ▶ Straight handles or one curved handle
Referred to as Cowhorn Forceps

Practice Note ▶ Universal Mandibular Forceps No. 16 Cowhorn is used on surgical extraction tray setups.

Sterilization Notes ▶ Universal Mandibular Forceps No. 16 must be precleaned, open, and unlocked. Then, place in an open and unlocked position in a sterilizing pouch with an internal process indicator, seal, then sterilize. OR, wrap with an internal process indicator inside and secure on the outside with process indicator tape, then sterilize. Verify appropriate color change has been achieved in external process indicator immediately after removal from sterilizer. Check internal process indicator before treatment. Refer to state regulations for any additional state requirements.

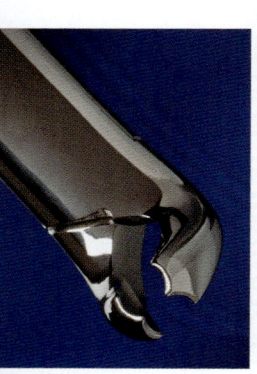

■ INSTRUMENT

Mandibular Forceps No. 17

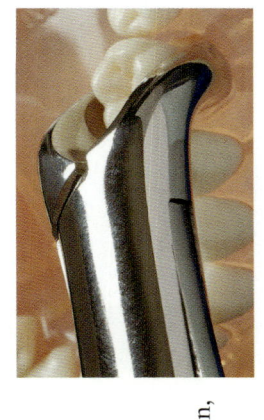

Function ▶ To extract bifurcated mandibular first or second molars

Characteristic ▶ Straight handles

Practice Note ▶ Mandibular Forceps No. 17 are used on surgical extraction tray setups.

Sterilization Notes ▶ Mandibular Forceps No. 17 must be precleaned, open, and unlocked. Then, place in an open and unlocked position in a sterilizing pouch with an internal process indicator, seal, then sterilize. OR, wrap with an internal process indicator inside and secure on the outside with process indicator tape, then sterilize. Verify appropriate color change has been achieved in external process indicator immediately after removal from sterilizer. Check internal process indicator before treatment. Refer to state regulations for any additional state requirements.

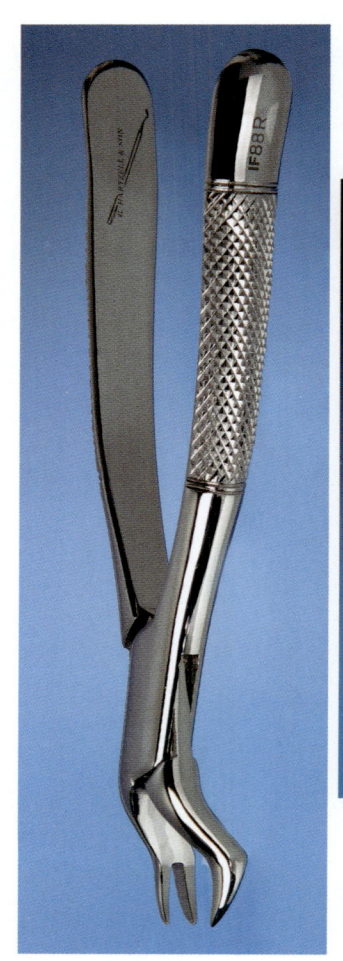
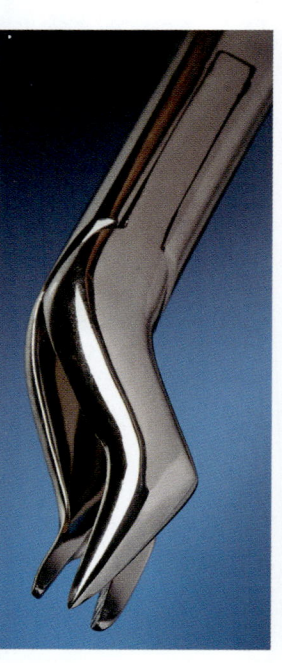

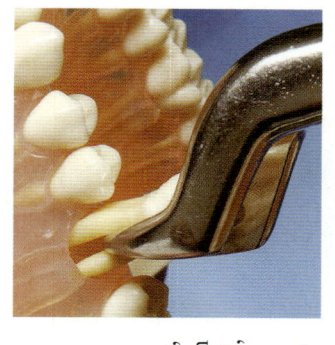

■ **INSTRUMENT**

Maxillary Right Forceps No. 88R

Function ▸ To extract trifurcated maxillary right first or second molars

Characteristic ▸ Right split beak—For engaging lingual root

Practice Note ▸ Maxillary Right Forceps No. 88R are used on surgical extraction tray setups.

Sterilization Notes ▸ Maxillary Right Forceps No. 88R must be precleaned, open, and unlocked. Then, place in an open and unlocked position in a sterilizing pouch with an internal process indicator, seal, then sterilize. OR, wrap with an internal process indicator inside and secure on the outside with process indicator tape, then sterilize. Verify appropriate color change has been achieved in external process indicator immediately after removal from sterilizer. Check internal process indicator before treatment. Refer to state regulations for any additional state requirements.

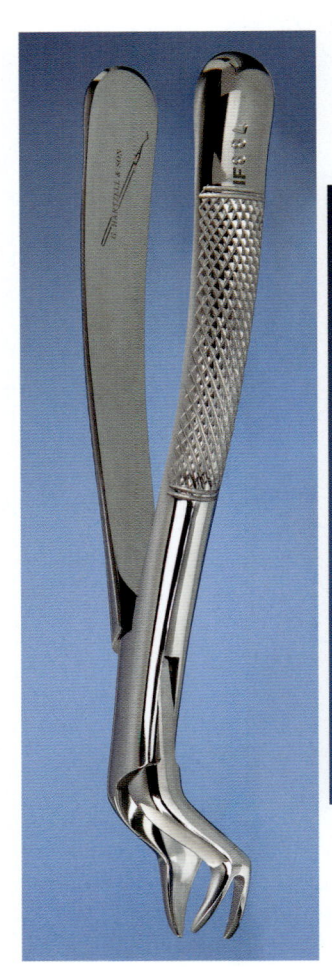
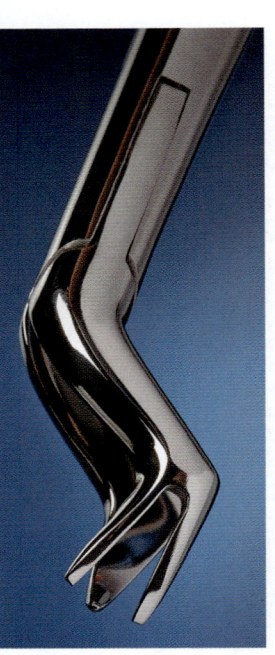

INSTRUMENT

Maxillary Left Forceps No. 88L

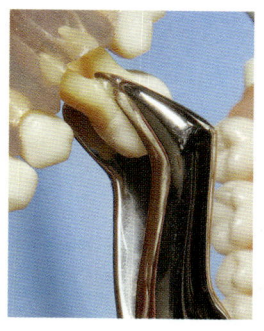

Function ▶ To extract trifurcated maxillary left first or second molars

Characteristic ▶ Left split beak—For engaging lingual root

Practice Note ▶ Maxillary Left Forceps No. 88L are used on surgical extraction tray setups.

Sterilization Notes ▶ Maxillary Left Forceps No. 88L must be precleaned, open, and unlocked. Then, place in an open and unlocked position in a sterilizing pouch with an internal process indicator, seal, then sterilize. OR, wrap with an internal process indicator inside and secure on the outside with process indicator tape, then sterilize. Verify appropriate color change has been achieved in external process indicator immediately after removal from sterilizer. Check internal process indicator before treatment. Refer to state regulations for any additional state requirements.

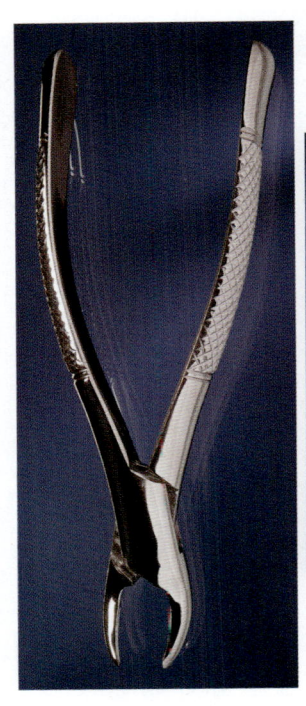
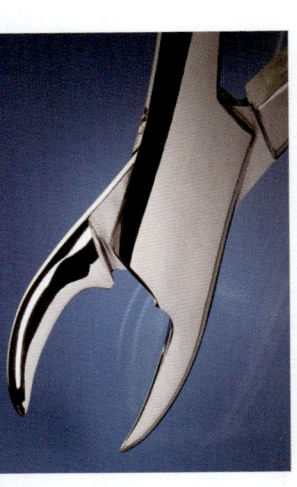

■ INSTRUMENT

Maxillary Universal Forceps—Cryer 150

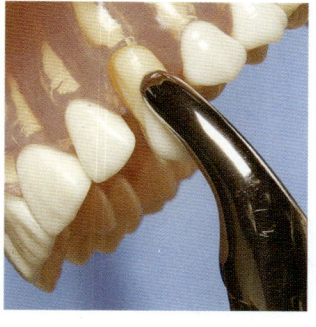

Function ▸ To extract maxillary centrals, laterals, cuspids, premolars, and roots

Characteristics ▸ Straight handles or one curved handle

Practice Note ▸ Maxillary Universal Forceps—Cryer 150 are used on surgical extraction tray setups.

Sterilization Notes ▸ Maxillary Universal Forceps—Cryer 150 must be precleaned, open, and unlocked. Then, place in an open and unlocked position in a sterilizing pouch with an internal process indicator, seal, then sterilize. OR, wrap with an internal process indicator inside and secure on the outside with process indicator tape, then sterilize. Verify appropriate color change has been achieved in external process indicator immediately after removal from sterilizer. Check internal process indicator before treatment. Refer to state regulations for any additional state requirements.

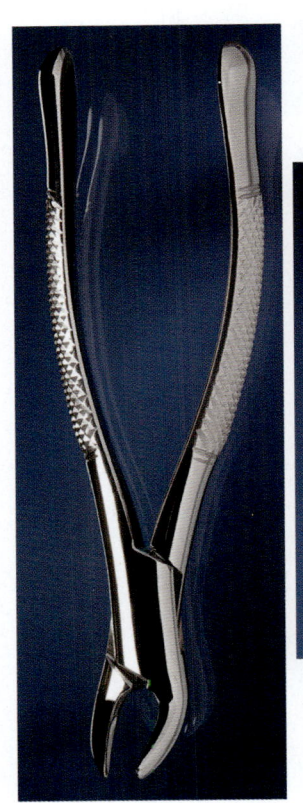

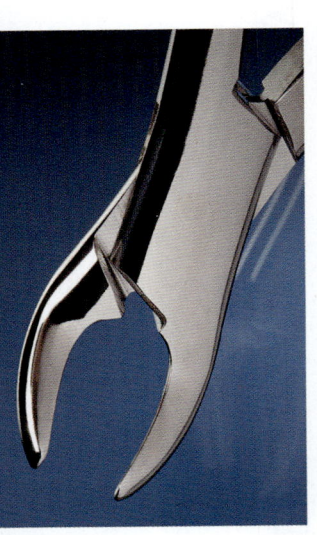

■ INSTRUMENT

Mandibular Universal Forceps—Cryer 151

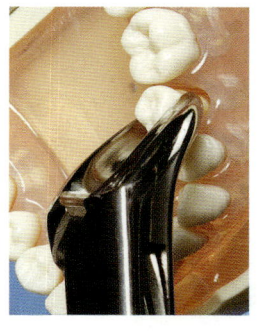

Function ▸ To extract mandibular centrals, laterals, cuspids, premolars, and roots

Characteristics ▸ Straight handles or one curved handle

Practice Note ▸ Mandibular Universal Forceps—Cryer 151 are used on surgical extraction tray setups.

Sterilization Notes ▸ Mandibular Universal Forceps—Cryer 151 must be precleaned, open, and unlocked. Then, place in an open and unlocked position in a sterilizing pouch with an internal process indicator, seal, then sterilize. OR, wrap with an internal process indicator inside and secure on the outside with process indicator tape, then sterilize. Verify appropriate color change has been achieved in external process indicator immediately after removal from sterilizer. Check internal process indicator before treatment. Refer to state regulations for any additional state requirements.

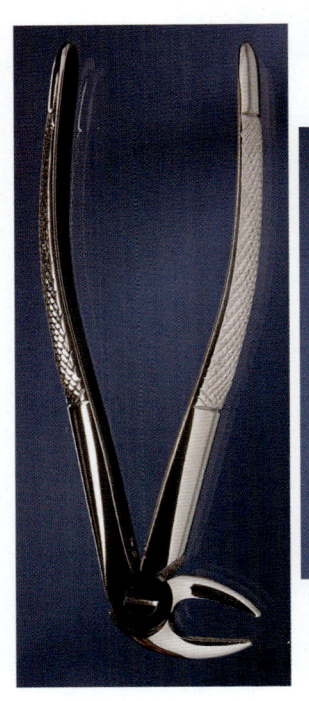
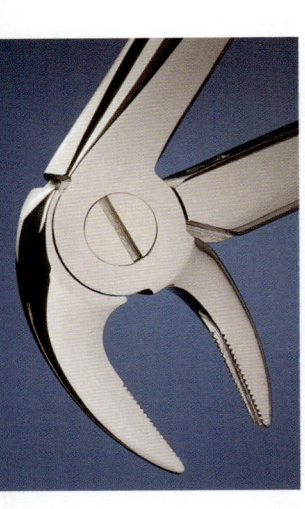

Mandibular Anterior Forceps

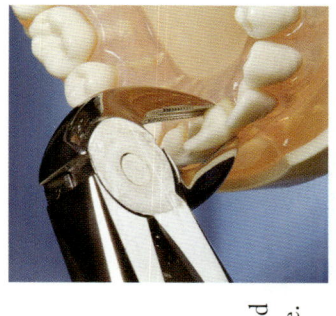

Function ▶ To extract mandibular anterior teeth

Characteristic ▶ Serrated beaks

Practice Note ▶ Mandibular Anterior Forceps are used on surgical extraction tray setups.

Sterilization Notes ▶ Mandibular Anterior Forceps must be precleaned, open, and unlocked. Then, place in an open and unlocked position in a sterilizing pouch with an internal process indicator, seal, then sterilize. OR, wrap with an internal process indicator inside and secure on the outside with process indicator tape, then sterilize. Verify appropriate color change has been achieved in external process indicator immediately after removal from sterilizer. Check internal process indicator before treatment. Refer to state regulations for any additional state requirements.

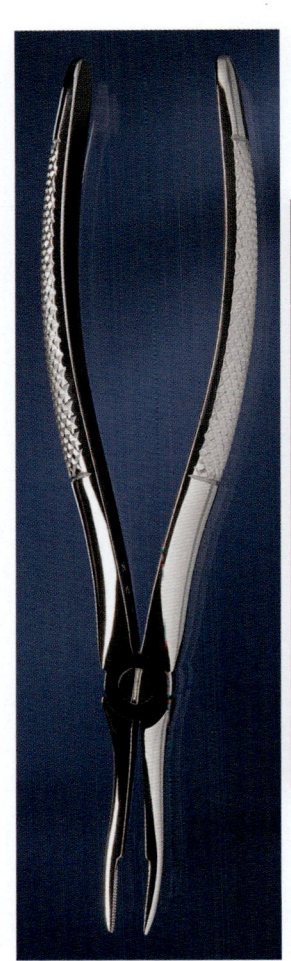

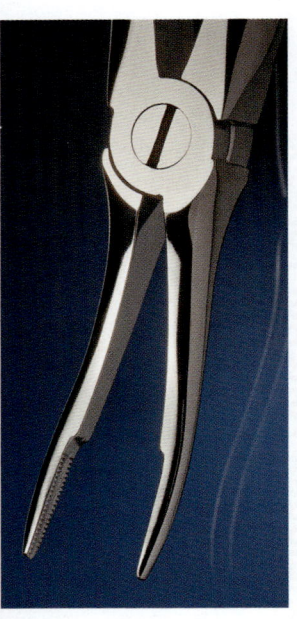

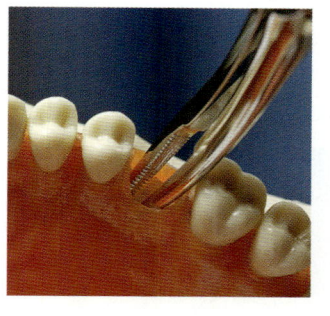

INSTRUMENT ▪ Maxillary Root Forceps

Function ▸ To extract maxillary roots

Characteristics ▸ Narrow, serrated beaks
Straight handles

Practice Note ▸ Maxillary Root Forceps are used on surgical extraction tray setups.

Sterilization Notes ▸ Maxillary Root Forceps must be precleaned, open, and unlocked. Then, place in an open and unlocked position in a sterilizing pouch with an internal process indicator, seal, then sterilize. OR, wrap with an internal process indicator inside and secure on the outside with process indicator tape, then sterilize. Verify appropriate color change has been achieved in external process indicator immediately after removal from sterilizer. Check internal process indicator before treatment. Refer to state regulations for any additional state requirements.

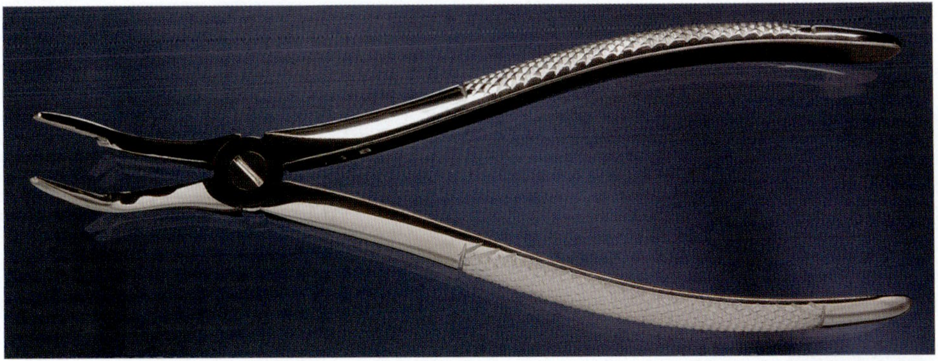

Mandibular Root Forceps

■ INSTRUMENT

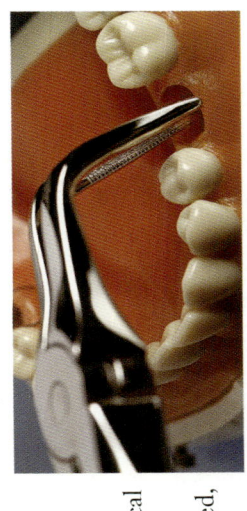

Function ▶ To extract mandibular roots

Characteristics ▶ Narrow, serrated beaks
Straight handles

Practice Note ▶ Mandibular Root Forceps are used on surgical extraction tray setups.

Sterilization Notes ▶ Mandibular Root Forceps must be precleaned, open, and unlocked. Then, place in an open and unlocked position in a sterilizing pouch with an internal process indicator, seal, then sterilize. OR, wrap with an internal process indicator inside and secure on the outside with process indicator tape, then sterilize. Verify appropriate color change has been achieved in external process indicator immediately after removal from sterilizer. Check internal process indicator before treatment. Refer to state regulations for any additional state requirements.

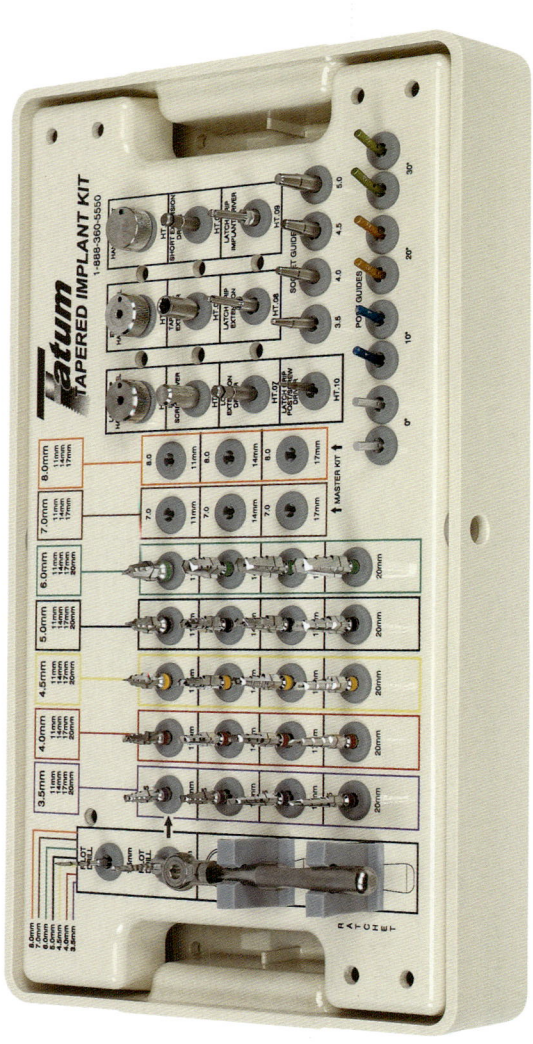

Implant System

Function ▸ To use for implant surgery

Characteristics ▸ Components—Depth drills, thread formers, hand wrench, ratchet, ratchet adapter, hex driver
Many types of implant systems available

Practice Notes ▸ Implant System is used on a surgical tray setup.
Sterile technique must be kept during procedure.

Sterilization Notes ▸ Implant System must be precleaned. Then, place in a sterilizing pouch or wrapped for sterilization. Then each load should have a Biological Indicator also known as Process Integrators (spore testing) and place internally in a pouch or wrapped instrument cassette for all implant devices.

Weekly Spore testing is still recommended. Verify Biological indicator (Process Integrators) before treatment. Refer to state regulations for any additional requirements. Refer to specific sterilization guidelines for implants according to Center for Disease Control and Prevention Guidelines for Infection Control in Dental Health-Care Settings—2003. Recommendations, Category IB. Strongly recommended for implementation and supported by experimental, clinical, or epidemiologic studies and a strong theoretical rationale.

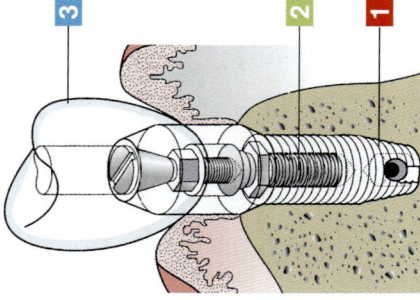

Implant

Function ▶

To use for implant surgery

Characteristics ▶

Endosteal implant—An implant surgically embedded into the bone

Osseointegration—The attachment of healthy bone to a dental implant, also referred to as stably integrated

Two other types of implants—Subperiosteal and transosteal

Components:

1 Implant fixture (titanium) embedded into bone; many styles of implants available

2 Center screw

3 Crown

Practice Notes ▶

Implant is used on a surgical tray setup.

Sterile technique must be kept during procedure.

Sterilization Notes ▶

Implant System must be precleaned. Then, place in a sterilizing pouch or wrapped for sterilization. Then each load should have a Biological Indicator also known as Process Integrators (spore testing) and place internally in a pouch or wrapped instrument cassette for all implant devices. Verify Biological indicator (Process Integrators) before treatment. Refer to specific sterilization Weekly Spore testing is still recommended. Refer to state regulations for any additional requirements. Refer to specific sterilization guidelines for implants according to Center for Disease Control and Prevention Guidelines for Infection Control in Dental Health-Care Settings—2003. Recommendations, Category IB. Strongly recommended for implementation and supported by experimental, clinical, or epidemiologic studies and a strong theoretical rationale.

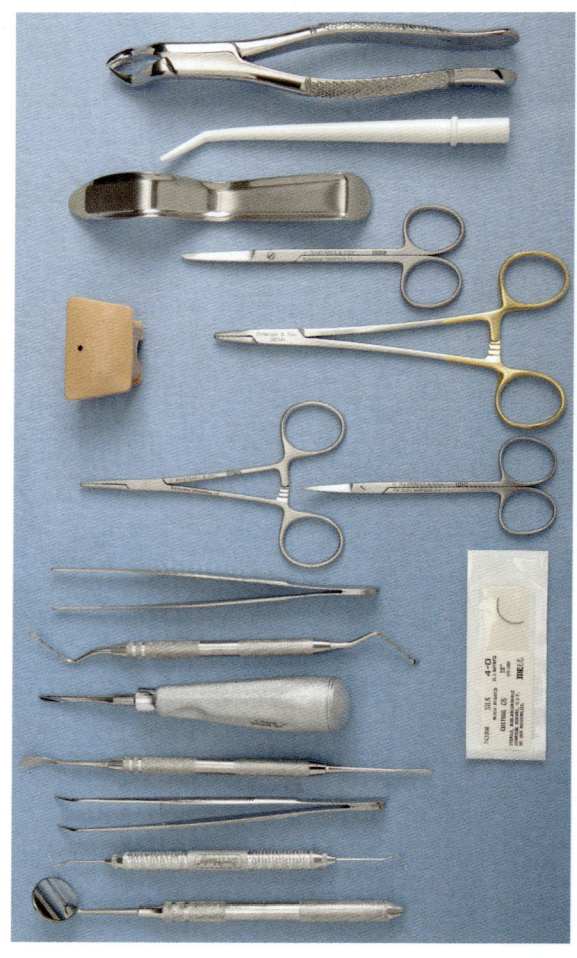

Extraction of Maxillary Right First Molar

TOP ROW (LEFT TO RIGHT)

Mouth mirror, explorer, cotton forceps, periosteal elevator, straight elevator, surgical curette, tissue forceps, hemostat, tissue scissors, mouth prop, needle holder, suture scissors, tongue and cheek retractor (Minnesota), disposable high–volume surgical evacuation tip, and maxillary right forceps No. 88R

BOTTOM ROW

Silk suture with needle in sterile package

Sterilization Notes ▶

Refer to each picture for correct procedure for instrument sterilization or disposal of instrument or material. Refer to Chapter 15 to see additional instruments used in oral surgery extractions. Also refer to other chapters for additional instruments on this tray setup that are not included in this chapter.

For mandibular first or second molar extraction, the tray setup is identical to the tray setup for the extraction of a maxillary right first molar, except that a mandibular right forceps No. 17 is used in place of a maxillary right forceps No. 88R.

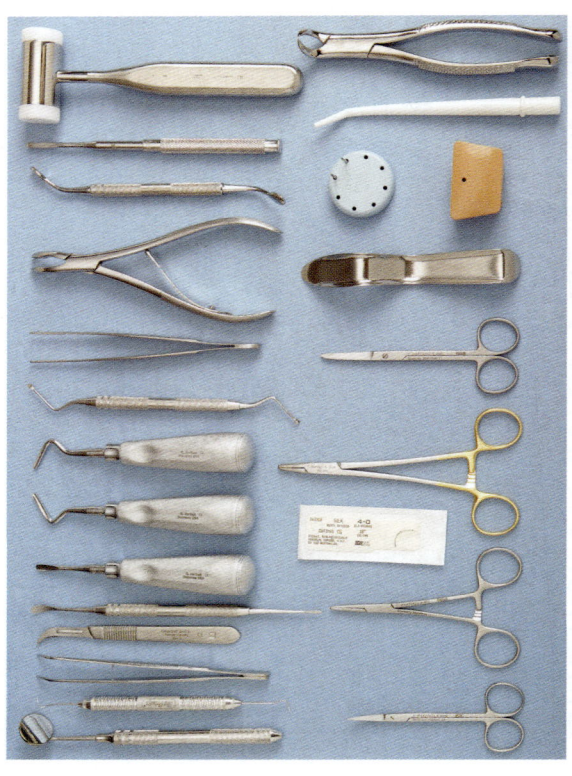

Extraction of Impacted Mandibular Molar

TOP ROW (LEFT TO RIGHT)

Mouth mirror, explorer, cotton forceps (pliers), scalpel #12 with blade, periosteal elevator, straight elevator, right and left root-tip elevators, surgical curette, tissue forceps, rongeurs, bone file, surgical chisel, surgical mallet

BOTTOM ROW (LEFT TO RIGHT)

Tissue scissors, hemostat, silk suture with needle in sterile package, needle holder, suture scissors, tongue and cheek retractor (Minnesota), surgical long-shank burs in bur holder, mouth prop, disposable high-volume surgical evacuation tip, universal mandibular forceps No. 16

Sterilization Notes ▶ Refer to each picture for correct procedure for instrument sterilization or disposal of instrument or material. Refer to Chapter 15 to see additional instruments used in oral surgery extractions. Also refer to other chapters for additional instruments on this tray setup that are not included in this chapter.

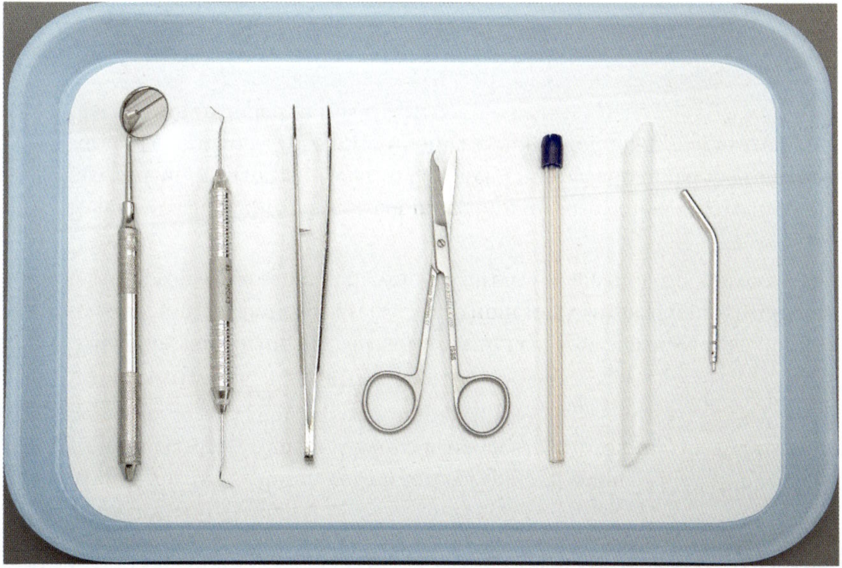

Suture Removal

LEFT TO RIGHT

Mouth mirror, pigtail explorer, cotton forceps (pliers), suture scissors, saliva ejector, high-volume evacuator (HVE) tip, air/water syringe tip

Sterilization Notes ▶ Refer to each picture for correct procedure for instrument sterilization or disposal of instrument or material. Refer to other chapters for instruments on this tray setup.

18

Sterilization and Protective Equipment

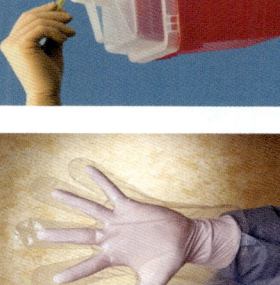

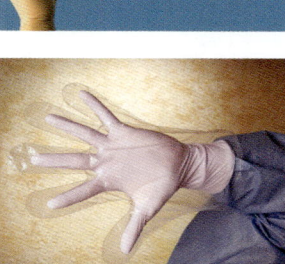

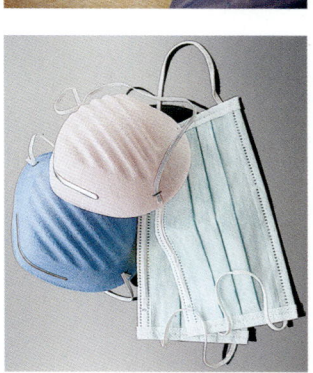

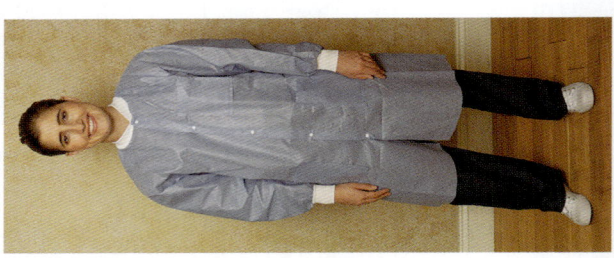

Protective Gown

■ INSTRUMENT	
Function ▶	To protect clothing, surgical scrubs, and skin during patient care and sterilization process to prevent contamination from blood and body substances
Characteristics ▶	Disposable, pictured, or cloth gowns. Cloth gowns must be made of polyester and cotton in accordance with state and federal regulations.
	Cuffed long sleeves
	Closure at neckline
	Moisture resistant (against contamination with liquids)
	Many styles available
Practice Notes ▶	All protective clothing should be removed before leaving the workplace.
	Follow regulations within the state for standard precautions.
Sterilization Notes ▶	Dispose of Protective Gown in garbage at the end of the day. If lab coat becomes visibly soiled during the work day, change to a new lab coat. Cloth lab coats must be laundered each day.

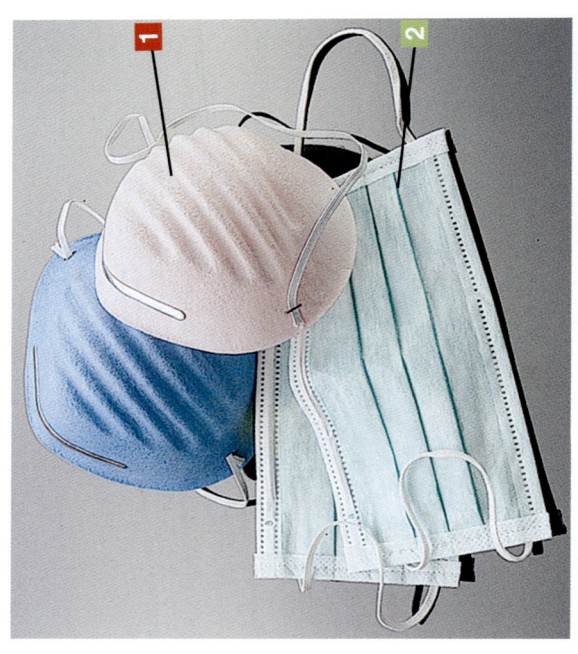

■ INSTRUMENT

Protective Mask

Functions ▶ To protect against chemicals, airborne pathogens, bacteria, and viruses during processing of instruments for sterilization

To protect against airborne pathogens, bacteria, and viruses and against scrap filling material during all phases of patient treatment

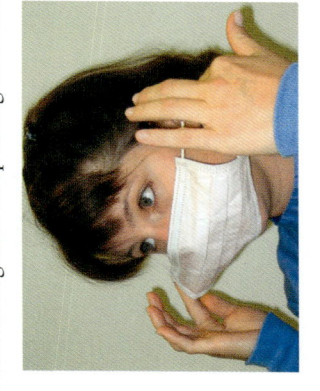

Characteristics ▶ **1** Dome shaped or **2** flat style

Different levels of filtration available

Practice Notes ▶ Protective Mask must cover nose and mouth.

Protective Face Shields available.

Protective Mask must be worn during dental procedures with a patient and during any exposure to dental material that is airborne.

Sterilization Notes ▶ Protective Mask should be disposed of in the garbage. A new mask must be used with each patient.

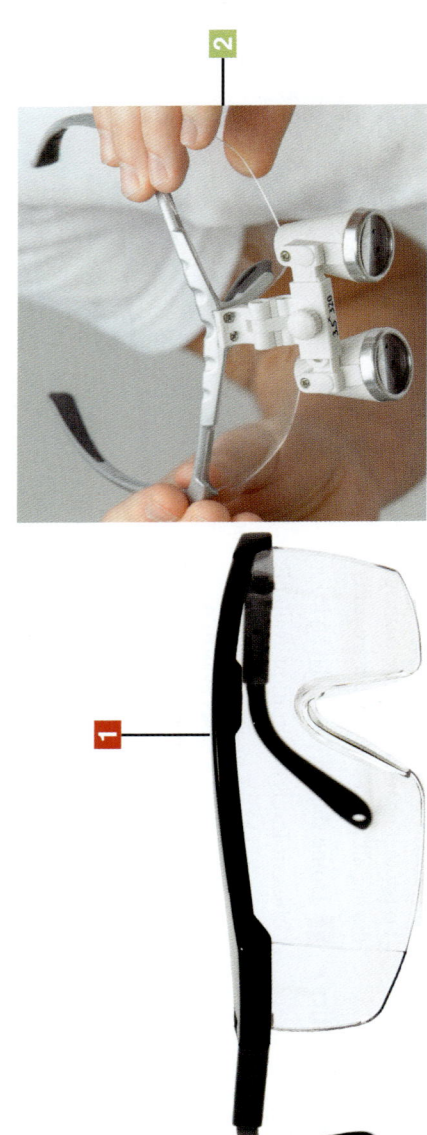

■ INSTRUMENT

Protective Glasses/Loupes

Functions ▸ To protect against chemicals, airborne pathogens, bacteria, and viruses during processing of instruments for sterilization

To protect against airborne pathogens, bacteria, and viruses during patient care and against filling material during restorative and rinsing phases of patient treatment

To enhance (Loupes) depth-of-focus and field-of-view during treatment

Extend to sides, top, and bottom of eyes for complete protection

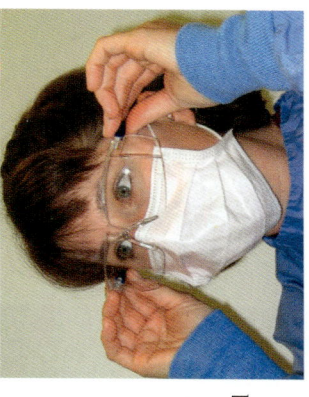

Characteristics ▸

1 Protective Glasses—Variety of styles available; some styles are larger to fit over prescription glasses. Must have side shields.

2 Loupes—Have different levels of magnification; may have a light source attached to the glasses for regular patient treatment, as well as availability to change the light source for sensitive material such as composite restorations.

Practice Notes ▸ Facial shields available for eye protection (mask must be worn)

Protective glasses must be worn during dental procedures with a patient, sterilization, and during any exposure to dental material that is airborne.

Loupes allow a practitioner to maintain a more physiologic posture promoting ergonomically correct chair position during treatment.

Sterilization Notes ▸ Protective glasses/loupes are disinfected between patients according to the manufacturer's recommendation. Refer to state regulations for any additional state requirements.

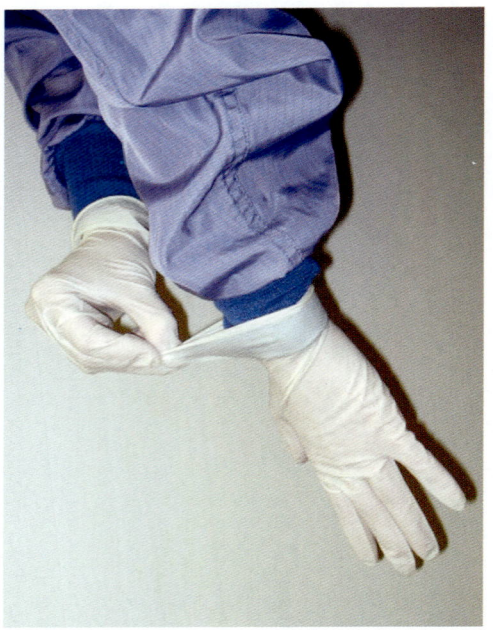

Examination Gloves

Functions ▶

To wear during patient care

To wear as a protective barrier

To wear during treatment room disinfection

Characteristics ▶

Latex (pictured), nitrile, or vinyl—Nonsterile and sterile gloves are available.

Nonsterile gloves worn for most dental procedures; sterile gloves may be worn for surgical procedures.

Examination Gloves should be worn over cuff of protective gown.

Various sizes available

Practice Notes ▶

Examination Gloves are single use only. Wash or sanitize hands before putting on gloves and after removing gloves. Must change if leaving patient care, or use overgloves (refer to pages 590 and 591). Replace worn or torn gloves immediately (along with washing hands or using hand sanitizer [follow state guidelines]). If procedure is long, change gloves every hour. Gloves must go over cuff of lab coat.

Sterilization Notes ▶

Examination Gloves must be disposed of in the garbage.

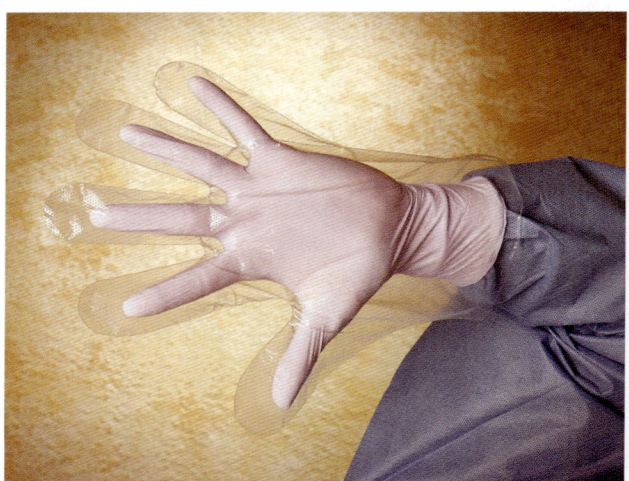

■ INSTRUMENT   Overgloves

Functions ▲ To wear over examination gloves when leaving each treatment area

To wear as a protective barrier over examination gloves as not to cross-contaminate

Characteristics ▲ Lightweight clear gloves

Not to be worn for dental procedures

Various sizes available

Practice Notes ▲ New set of overgloves must be used for each patient. Keep overgloves in an uncontaminated area of the treatment room. Must be careful to not contaminate outside of overgloves when putting on over examination gloves.

Sterilization Notes ▲ Overgloves must be disposed of in the garbage.

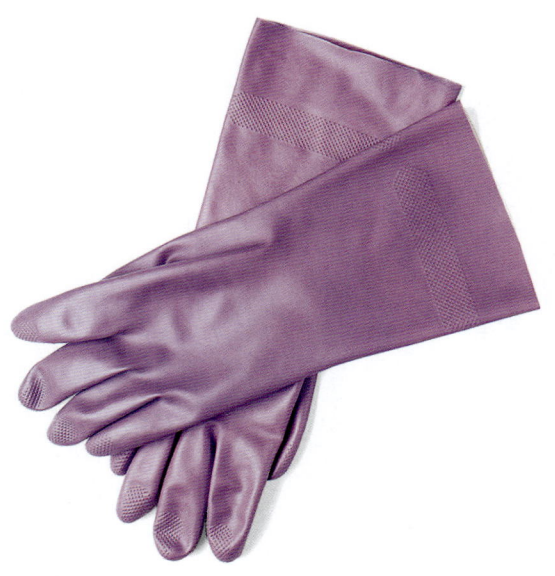

▪ INSTRUMENT

Nitrile Utility Gloves

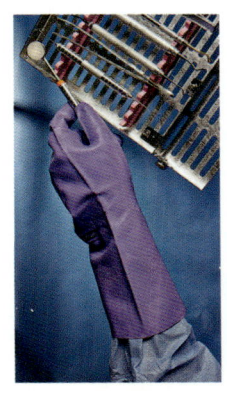

Functions ▸

To protect hands during processing of instruments for
sterilization procedures

To wear for preparation and handling of chemicals

To disinfect operatory

To transport cassettes of tray setups to sterilization
area from treatment area

Characteristics ▸

Chemical resistant

Puncture resistant

Ribbed for nonslip grip

Range of sizes and colors

Refer to state regulations regarding when utility gloves should be worn

Practice Note ▸

Nitrile Utility Gloves should be kept in sterilization area of office.

Sterilization Notes ▸

Nitrile Utility Gloves are disinfected after each use. Sterilize according to the
manufacturer's recommendation and refer to local and state regulations.

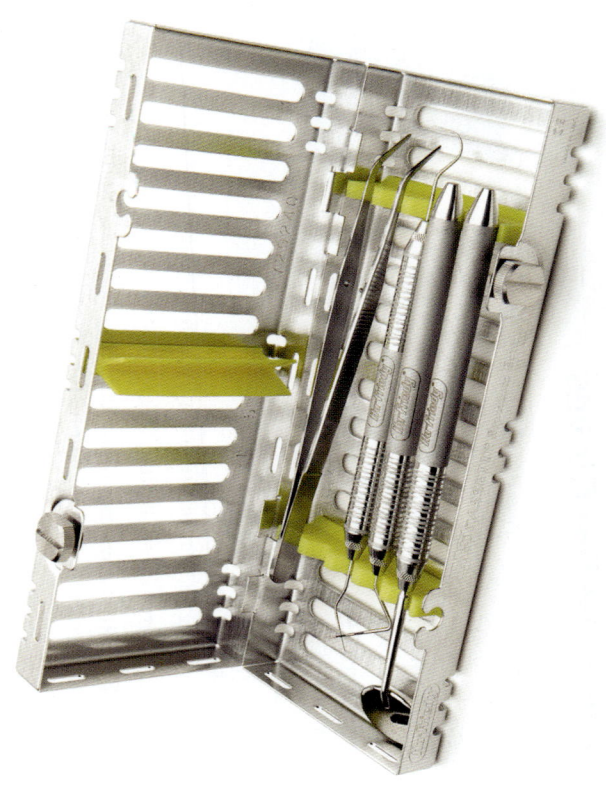

Cassette

Functions ▶ To use for instruments as tray setup

To use for precleaning and sterilization of instruments

Characteristics ▶ Available in metal or resin—different styles of cassettes available

Color coded

Range of sizes

Practice Notes ▶ Instruments in the cassette may be cleaned in an ultrasonic cleaner and then wrapped and sterilized.

Color coding aids in the identification of cassettes and tray setups.

Sterilization Notes ▶ Cassette with instruments must be precleaned. Then, place in a sterilizing pouch with an internal process indicator, seal, then sterilize. OR, wrap with an internal process indicator inside and secure on the outside with process indicator tape, then sterilize. Verify appropriate color change has been achieved in external process indicator immediately after removal from sterilizer. Check internal process indicator before treatment. Refer to state regulations for any additional state requirements.

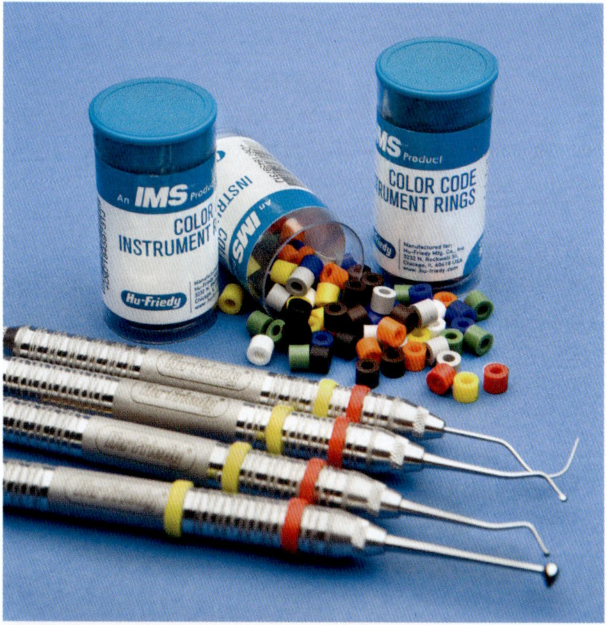
An IMS Product
COLOR CODE
INSTRUMENT RINGS
Hu-Friedy

Color-Coding System for Instruments

■ INSTRUMENT

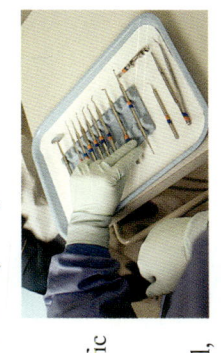

Function ▶ To color code instruments for organization and identification of tray setups

Characteristic ▶ Variety of colors—Color coding coordinates with color cassettes

Practice Note ▶ The Color-Coding System makes it easier to identify specific tray setups and instruments within the tray setup.

Sterilization Notes ▶ Color-Coded Instruments must be precleaned. Then, place in a sterilizing pouch with an internal process indicator, seal, then sterilize. OR, wrap with an internal process indicator inside and secure on the outside with process indicator tape, then sterilize. Verify appropriate color change has been achieved in external process indicator immediately after removal from sterilizer. Check internal process indicator before treatment. Refer to state regulations for any additional state requirements.

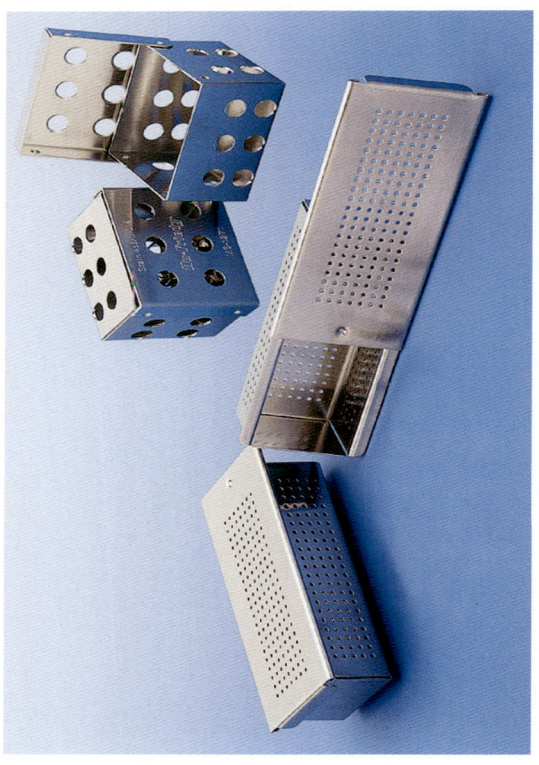

Parts Box for Sterilization

Function ▶ To use for sterilization of small items
Examples: Burs, dental dam clamps

Characteristic ▶ Range of sizes to accommodate sterilization needs

Practice Note ▶ Parts Box helps hold and organize small items for tray setups.

Sterilization Notes ▶ Parts Box must be precleaned. Then, place in a sterilizing pouch with an internal process indicator, seal, then sterilize. OR, wrap with an internal process indicator inside and secure on the outside with process indicator tape, then sterilize. Verify appropriate color change has been achieved in external process indicator immediately after removal from sterilizer. Check internal process indicator before treatment. Refer to state regulations for any additional state requirements.

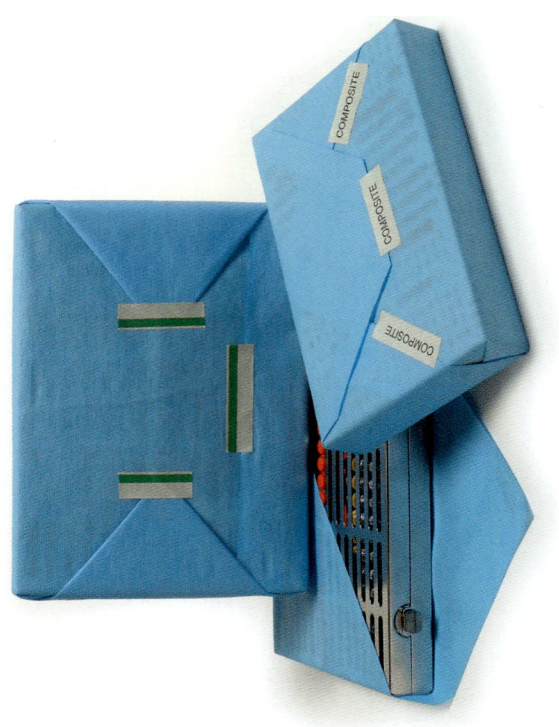

Cassette Wrap

Functions ▶ To use to wrap cassette for sterilization
To store cassette with wrapping after sterilization
To use for tray cover during dental procedure

Characteristic ▶ Range of sizes—To accommodate Cassette

Practice Note ▶ Cassettes should be kept in sterile wrap until the patient is seated. Refer to local and state regulations.

Sterilization Notes ▶ All instruments or cassettes must be precleaned. Then, place in a sterilizing pouch with an internal process indicator, seal, then sterilize. OR, wrap with an internal process indicator inside and secure on the outside with process indicator tape, then sterilize. Verify appropriate color change has been achieved in external process indicator immediately after removal from sterilizer. Check internal process indicator before treatment. Refer to state regulations for any additional state requirements. Indicator tape verifies that the instruments have reached a specific temperature.

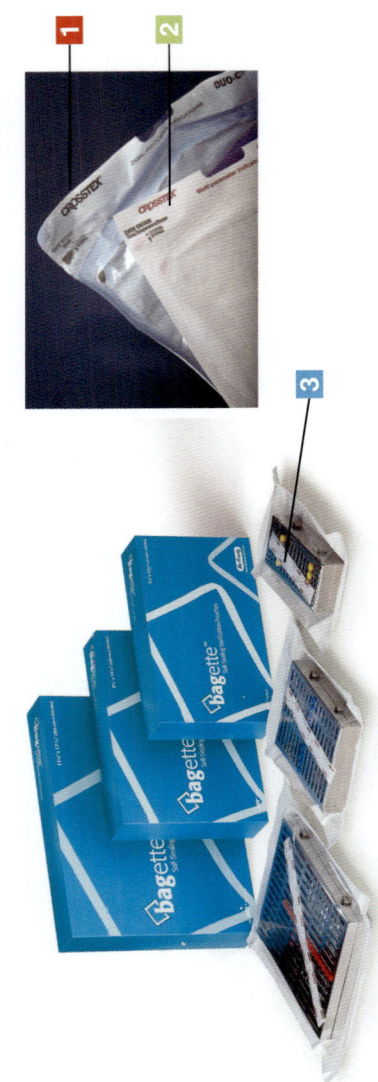

Sterilization Pouches

Function ▸ To be used for sterilization of instruments and cassettes

Characteristic ▸ Pouches have range of sizes to accommodate all sizes of instruments and cassettes.

Available with Self Seal Pouches

Available with indicator strip on pouch

1 Indicator strip changes color after sterilization. Indicator strip verifies that the instruments have reached a specific temperature.

2 Indicator strip color before sterilization

3 Cassette with indicator tape on outside of pouch

Practice Note ▸ Instruments should be kept in the pouches until the patient is seated. Refer to state regulations.

Sterilization Notes ▸ All instruments must be precleaned. Then, place in a sterilizing pouch with an internal process indicator, seal, then sterilize. OR, wrap with an internal process indicator inside and secure on the outside with process indicator tape, then sterilize. Verify appropriate color change has been achieved in external process indicator immediately after removal from sterilizer. Check internal process indicator before treatment. Refer to state regulations for any additional state requirements.

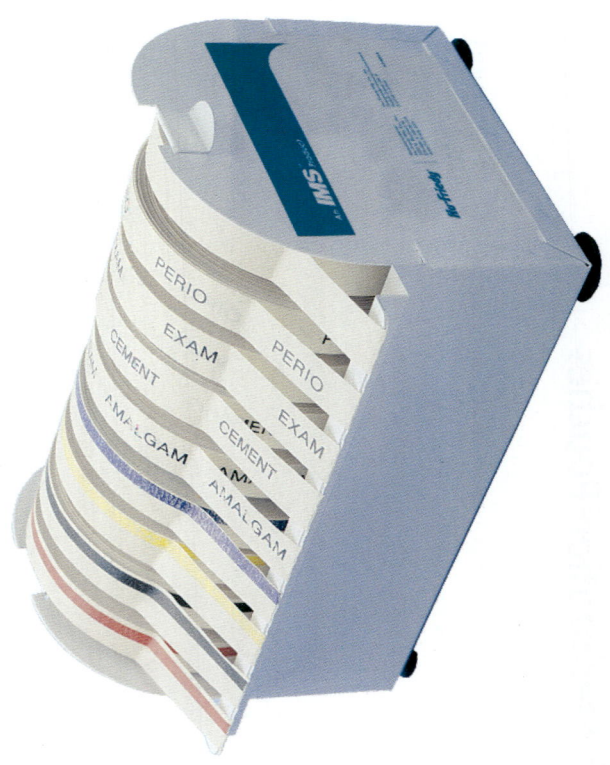

Indicator Tape and Dispensing Unit

Functions ▶

To secure wrap on outside of cassette

To use outside cassettes or sterilization pouches to indicate exposure of instruments to a specific temperature—Color will change on the tape.

Characteristics ▶

Available in preprinted tray setup procedures—as shown in picture.

Available with color coding

Available blank for labeling tape with procedure and/or instrument content

Practice Note ▶

Instruments should be kept in the pouches until the patient is seated. Refer to state regulations.

Sterilization Notes ▶

When Indicator Tape is placed outside and/or inside a cassette, the strip changes color with exposure to a specific temperature of the sterilization process; they do not determine the actual sterilization. Refer to sterilization monitoring. If the indicator tape does not change color, the pouch or wrap must be resterilized.

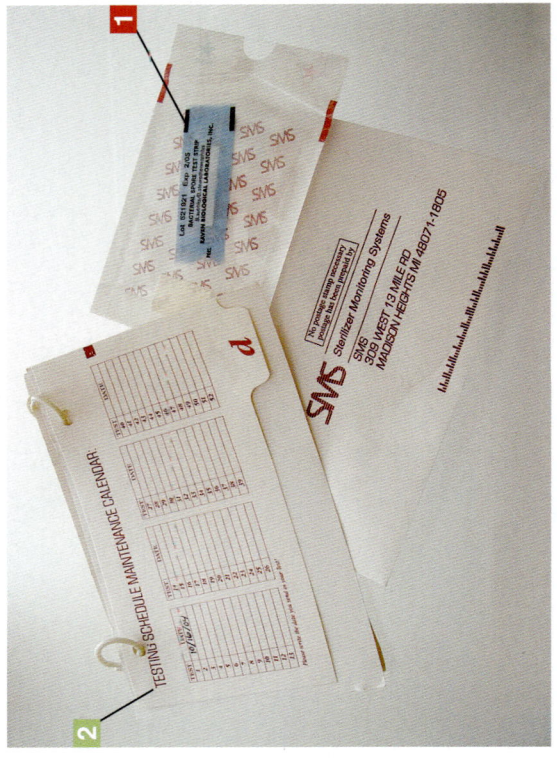

Biological Monitors for Sterilizers

■ INSTRUMENT

Function ▶ To confirm efficacy of sterilization, documentation of results is recorded in office sterilization log.

Biological Monitors, Spore Testing, measures Time, Temperature and Pressure to verify proper sterilization.

Characteristic ▶ Many systems available

Practice Note ▶ **1** Biological Monitor Testing device is placed in the sterilizer for one cycle of instruments. It is then mailed to the manufacturer, which mails back the findings.

2 The results are logged in the office sterilization records.

Biological Indicators also known as Process Integrators. They are placed internally in a pouch or wrapped instrument cassette.

Weekly Spore testing is still recommended.

A Process Integrator should be included for sterilization for all implant devices.

Sterilization Notes ▶ The Centers for Disease Control and Prevention, the American Dental Association, and the Office Safety and Asepsis Procedures Research Foundation recommend at least weekly testing of each sterilizer in the office. Refer to local and state requirements. Requirements may be different for each state.

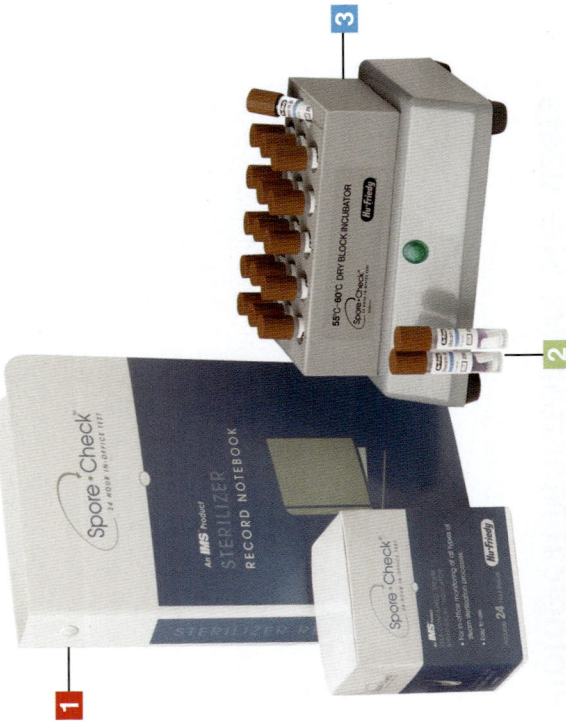

Sterilization Spore Check—In Office

INSTRUMENT

Function ▶ To monitor and confirm the effectiveness of steam sterilizers

Characteristics ▶

1. Record Notebook
2. Self-contained biological indicator
3. Dry block incubator

Practice Note ▶ A vial with the solution is marked and placed in a sterilization pouch, and the sterilization cycle is processed. After the cycle is complete, follow the directions; then place vial in incubator. Results will occur in 24 hours.

Record results.

Biological Indicators also known as Process Integrators. They are placed internally in a pouch or wrapped instrument cassette.

Weekly Spore testing is still recommended.

A Process Integrator should be included for sterilization for all implant devices.

Sterilization Notes ▶ All sterilizers should be checked for effectiveness every week. Every load of implants should be monitored for effectiveness when possible with each implant before each implant procedure.

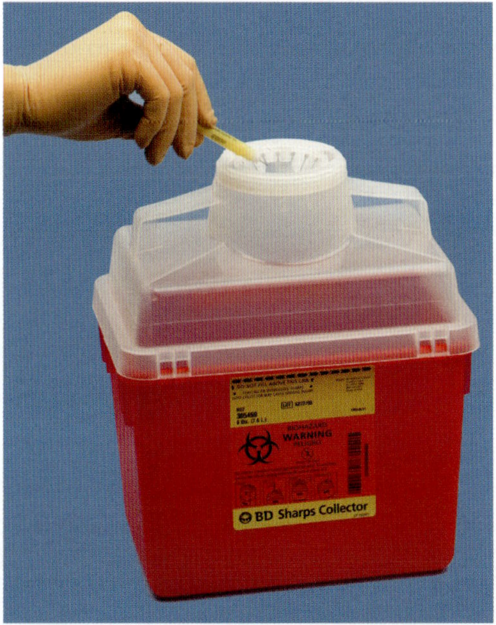
WARNING
BD Sharps Collector

Sharps Container

Function ▶ To serve as storage receptacle for used needles, old burs, scalpel blades, orthodontic wires, endodontic files, and all other disposable sharp items used during dental procedures

Characteristics ▶ Must be puncture resistant
Must be labeled "Biohazard"
Must have a reclosable top

Practice Note ▶ Sharps containers must be disposed of according to local, state, and federal regulations and by an Environmental Protection Agency regulatory disposal company. Required paperwork must be kept according to state and federal regulations.

Sterilization Notes ▶ Refer to state and local regulations on the type of gloves to use, utility gloves or patient gloves, to handle sharps that are disposed in the Sharps Container.
Refer to state and local regulations on where Sharps Container should be placed in the dental office.

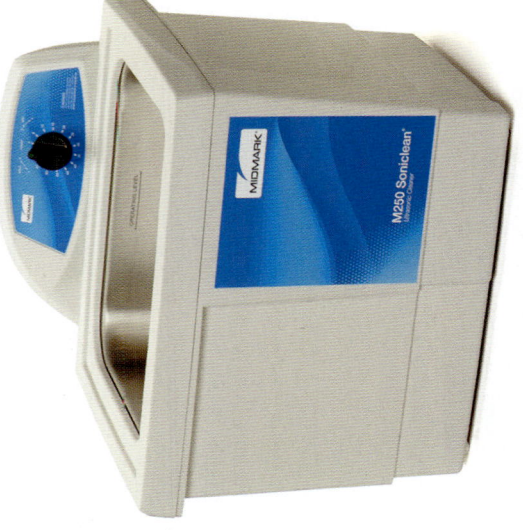

Ultrasonic Cleaning Unit

INSTRUMENT

Function ▶ To remove debris and bioburden from instruments

Characteristic ▶ Reduces risk of exposure to pathogens during the cleaning stage of the sterilization process

Practice Notes ▶ Tank is filled with antimicrobial or general all-purpose solution specially designed for the ultrasonic unit. Fill and drain solution daily.

Debris is removed by mechanical means; sound waves create tiny bubbles that cause inward collapse (implosion) and removal of material. Lid must be closed during operation of unit. Available in some units are racks for cassettes.

Sterilization Notes ▶ After cleaning the instruments in the ultrasonic cleaning unit, instruments must be precleaned. Then, place in a sterilizing pouch with an internal process indicator, seal, then sterilize. OR, wrap with an internal process indicator inside and secure on the outside with process indicator tape, then sterilize. Verify appropriate color change has been achieved in external process indicator immediately after removal from sterilizer. Check internal process indicator before treatment. Refer to state regulations for any additional state requirements.

For precleaning instruments *Guidelines for Infection Control in Dental Health-Care Settings—2003* states "that the use of automated cleaning equipment such as ultrasonic cleaner or washer-disinfector is safer than hand scrubbing instruments prior to continuing the sterilization process even though hand washing is acceptable."

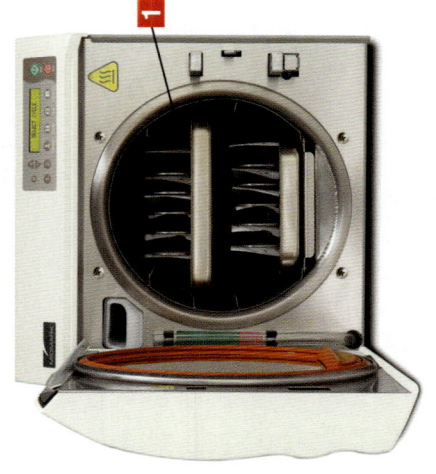

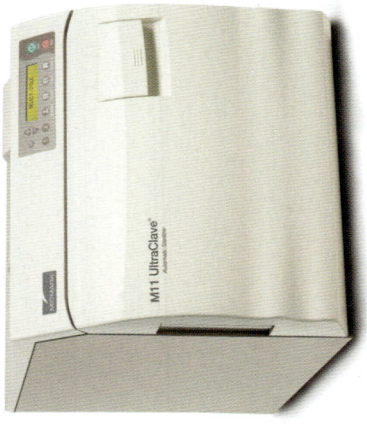

INSTRUMENT Sterilizer—Autoclave (Saturated Steam)

Function ▶ To kill all microbes, viruses, bacteria, and fungi, thereby sterilizing instruments

Characteristics ▶ Uses steam under pressure—15 pounds per square inch (psi) at 250°F for 20 minutes

1 Shelves and racks are available for cassettes

Various styles and manufacturers

Range of sizes

Practice Notes ▶ Refer to federal, state, and manufacturer's sterilization techniques as well as manufacturer's maintenance requirements.

Sterilization Notes ▶ The Centers for Disease Control and Prevention, the American Dental Association, and the Office Safety and Asepsis Procedures Research Foundation recommend at least weekly testing of Sterilizers. Local and state requirements may be different. Refer to pages 606 and 607 for Biological Monitors for Sterilization.

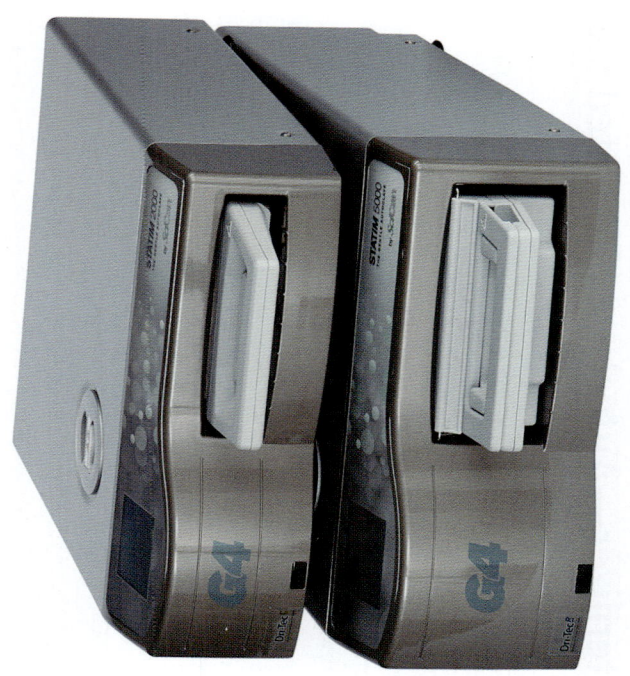

Statim G4 Cassette Autoclave

INSTRUMENT

Functions ▲

To kill all microbes, viruses, bacteria, and fungi
To sterilize instruments and handpieces

Characteristics ▲

Statim 2000 G4 cycle times: 6 minutes unwrapped, 14 minutes wrapped
Statim 5000 G4 cycle times: 9 minutes unwrapped, 17.5 minutes wrapped
Uses fresh steam–distilled water with every cycle
Uses Dri-Tec drying system for fast dry loads
Readout Screen available for each cycle

Practice Note ▲

Refer to federal, state, and manufacturer's sterilization techniques as well as manufacturer's maintenance requirements.

Sterilization Notes ▲

The Centers for Disease Control and Prevention, the American Dental Association, and the Office Safety and Asepsis Procedures Research Foundation recommend at least weekly testing of sterilizers. Local and state requirements may be different. Refer to pages 606 and 607 for Biological Monitors for Sterilization.

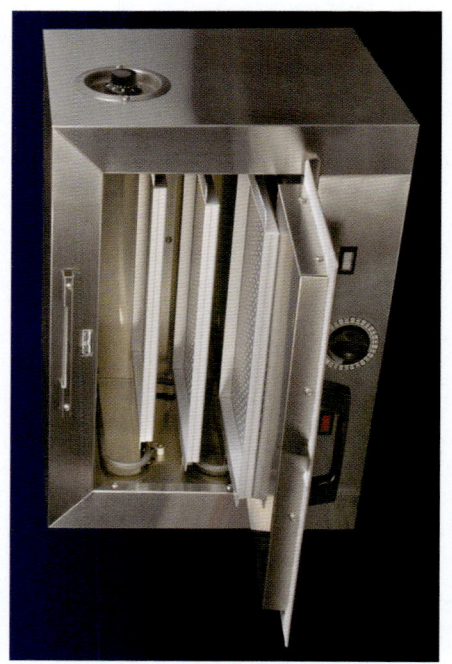

Sterilizer—Dry Heat (Static Air)

INSTRUMENT

Function ▶ To kill all microbes, viruses, bacteria, and fungi, thereby sterilizing instruments

Characteristics ▶ Oven-type sterilizer

340°F for 60 to 120 minutes, wrapped instruments

Shelves available for cassettes

Various styles and manufacturers

Range of sizes

Practice Notes ▶ Packaging and wrapped material must be able to withstand high temperatures.

Door cannot be opened during sterilization cycle.

Items cannot be layered or stacked but should be placed on their edges.

Sterilization Notes ▶ The Centers for Disease Control and Prevention, the American Dental Association, and the Office Safety and Asepsis Procedures Research Foundation recommend at least weekly testing of Sterilizers. Local and state requirements may be different. Refer to pages 606 and 607 for Biological Monitors for Sterilization.

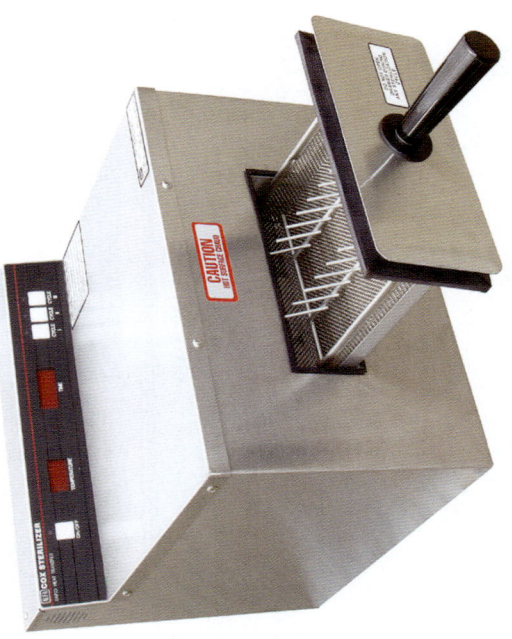

Sterilizer—Dry Heat (Rapid Heat Transfer)

Function ▶ To kill all microbes, viruses, bacteria, and fungi, thereby sterilizing instruments

Characteristics ▶ Forced air–type sterilizer

375°F for 12 minutes, wrapped instruments

375°F for 6 minutes, unwrapped instruments

Instruments placed in preheated chamber

Various styles and manufacturers

Range of sizes

Practice Notes ▶ Packaging and wrapped material must be able to withstand high temperatures.

Door cannot be opened during sterilization cycle.

Sterilization Notes ▶ The Centers for Disease Control and Prevention, the American Dental Association, and the Office Safety and Asepsis Procedures Research Foundation recommend at least weekly testing of Sterilizers. Local and state requirements may be different. Refer to pages 606 and 607 for Biological Monitors for Sterilization.

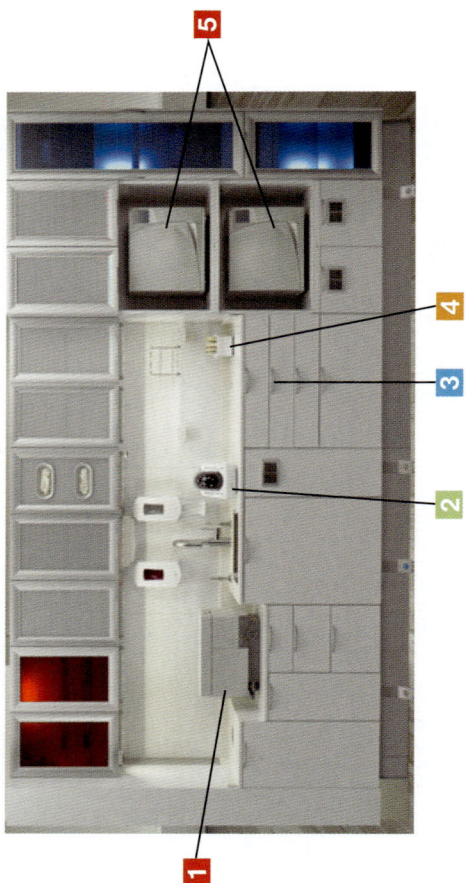

Sterilization Center

Function ▶ To process instruments for precleaning and sterilization

Characteristics ▶ Main components of sterilization center:

1 Ultrasonic Cleaning Unit – Preclean all Instruments
2 Handpiece Maintenance System – Refer to Chapter 5 – Page 109
3 Drawers for sterilization pouches and cassette wraps
4 Indicator tape with dispensing unit
5 Sterilizers

Practice Notes ▶ Different designs of sterilization centers available to accommodate each dental office

Sterilization Notes ▶ Nitrile Utility Gloves and appropriate PPE (mask, protective eyewear and gown) should be worn during processing of instruments for sterilization procedures. All instruments must be precleaned, open and unlocked, if applicable. Place in an open and unlocked position. Then, place in a sterilizing pouch with an internal process indicator, seal, then sterilize. OR, wrap with an internal process indicator inside and secure on the outside with process indicator tape, then sterilize. Verify appropriate color change has been achieved in external process indicator immediately after removal from sterilizer. Check internal process indicator before treatment. Refer to state regulations for any additional state requirements. Follow standard precautions and cross-contamination protocol.

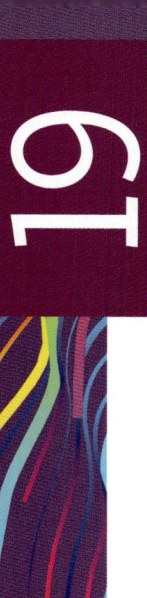

19

Dental Materials Equipment

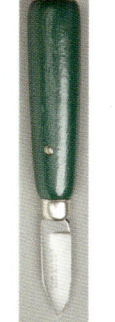

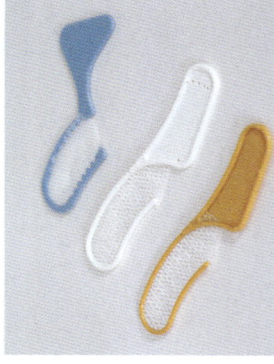

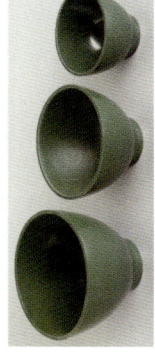

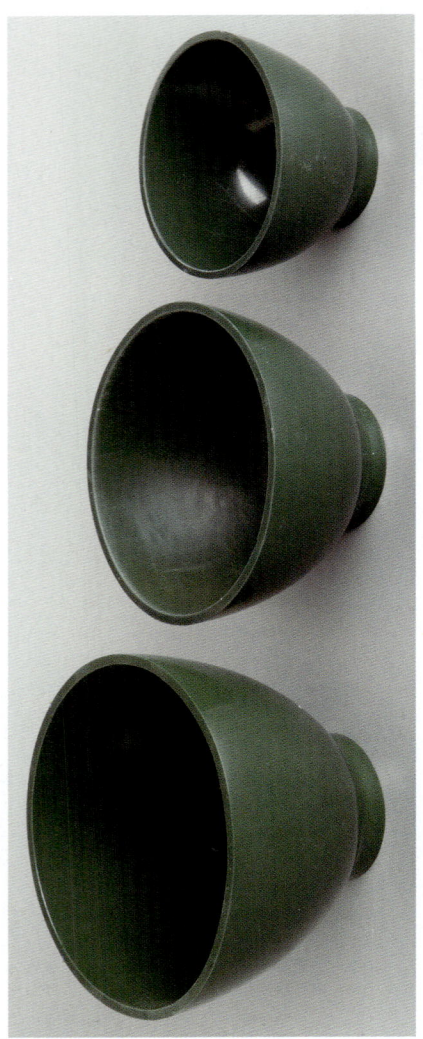

INSTRUMENT

Flexible Rubber Bowl

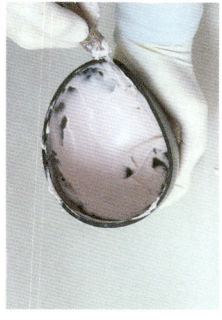

Functions ▶ To mix material, usually a powder and a liquid

To mix impression material and irreversible hydrocolloid, alginate, for study models, opposing models, bleaching trays, night guards, mouth guards, orthodontic appliances, or custom trays for removable appliances

To mix laboratory plaster, stone, and die stone for models

Characteristic ▶ Bowl is flexible to manipulate material.

Different size bowls to accommodate different amounts of material being mixed.

Practice Note ▶ Flexible Rubber Bowl is used with the alginate spatula.

Sterilization Notes ▶ Preclean and disinfect Flexible Rubber Bowl before and after each use according to the manufacturer's recommendation.

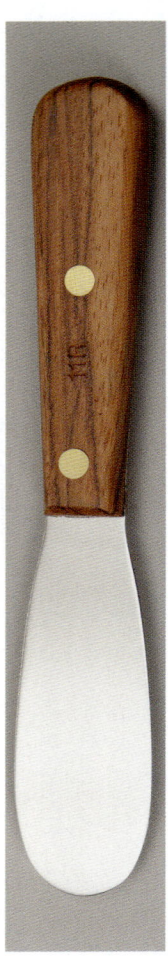

Flexible Alginate (Irreversible Hydrocolloid) Spatula

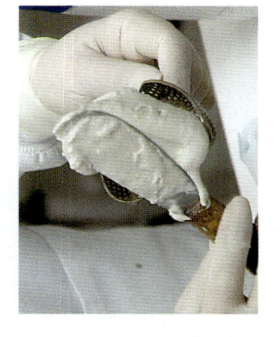

Functions ▶

To mix powder and a liquid in a flexible bowl

To mix impression material such as irreversible hydrocolloid, alginate

To load material into tray

To mix laboratory plaster, stone, and die stone for models

Characteristic ▶

Spatula is flexible to manipulate material.

Practice Note ▶

Flexible Alginate Spatula is used with the flexible rubber bowl.

Sterilization Notes ▶

Preclean and disinfect Flexible Alginate Spatula before and after each use according to manufacturer's recommendation. If contaminated, preclean. Then, place in a sterilizing pouch with an internal process indicator, seal, then sterilize. OR, wrap with an internal process indicator inside and secure on the outside with process indicator tape, then sterilize. Verify appropriate color change has been achieved in external process indicator immediately after removal from sterilizer. Check internal process indicator before treatment. Refer to state regulations for any additional state requirements.

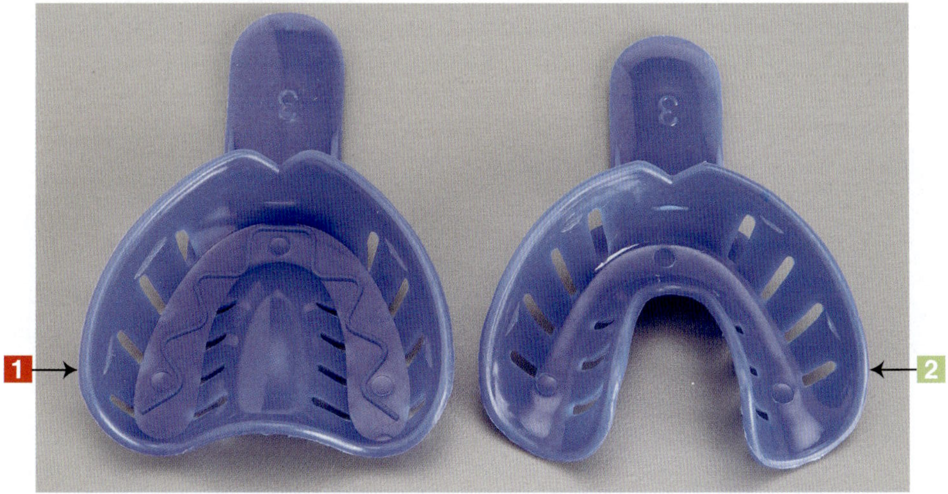
1
2
3
3

Disposable Plastic Perforated Full Arch Impression Trays

■ INSTRUMENT

Function ▶ To use for taking impressions with many types of impression material
Example: Irreversible hydrocolloid (alginate), crown, and bridge impression material

Characteristics ▶
1 Maxillary perforated tray
2 Mandibular perforated tray

Perforated trays allow material to push through the tray, creating a mechanical lock that keeps the material in place.
Range of sizes

Practice Notes ▶ Disposable Plastic Perforated trays are used for many types of dental procedures involving taking impressions.
Impressions must be rinsed then disinfected before pouring up impressions.

Sterilization Notes ▶ Disposable Plastic Perforated Full Arch Impression Trays should be disposed of in the garbage. Single use only.

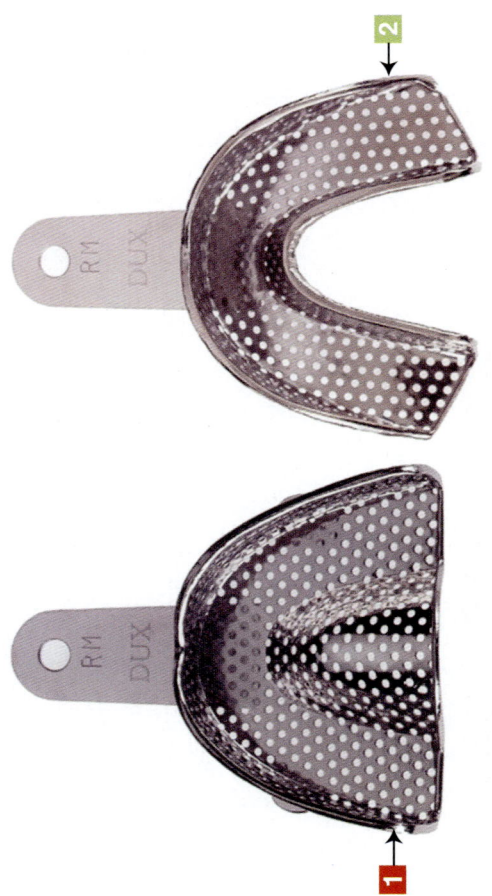

Metal Perforated Full Arch Impression Trays

Function ▶ To use for taking impressions with many types of impression material.
Example: Irreversible hydrocolloid (alginate), crown, and bridge impression material

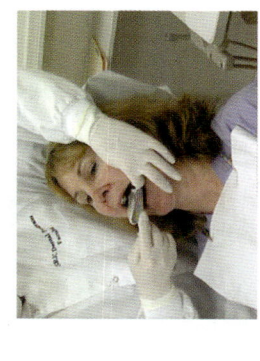

Characteristics ▶ **1** Maxillary Metal Perforated Tray
2 Mandibular Metal Perforated Tray

Perforated trays allow material to push through the tray, creating a mechanical lock that keeps the material in place. Range of sizes

Practice Notes ▶ Metal Perforated Full Arch Impression Trays are used for many types of dental procedures involving taking impressions.

Impression trays must be rinsed then disinfected before pouring up impressions.

Sterilization Notes ▶ Metal Perforated Full Arch Impression Trays must be precleaned. Then, place in a sterilizing pouch with an internal process indicator, seal, then sterilize. OR, wrap with an internal process indicator inside and secure on the outside with process indicator tape, then sterilize. Verify appropriate color change has been achieved in external process indicator immediately after removal from sterilizer. Check internal process indicator before treatment. Refer to state regulations for any additional state requirements.

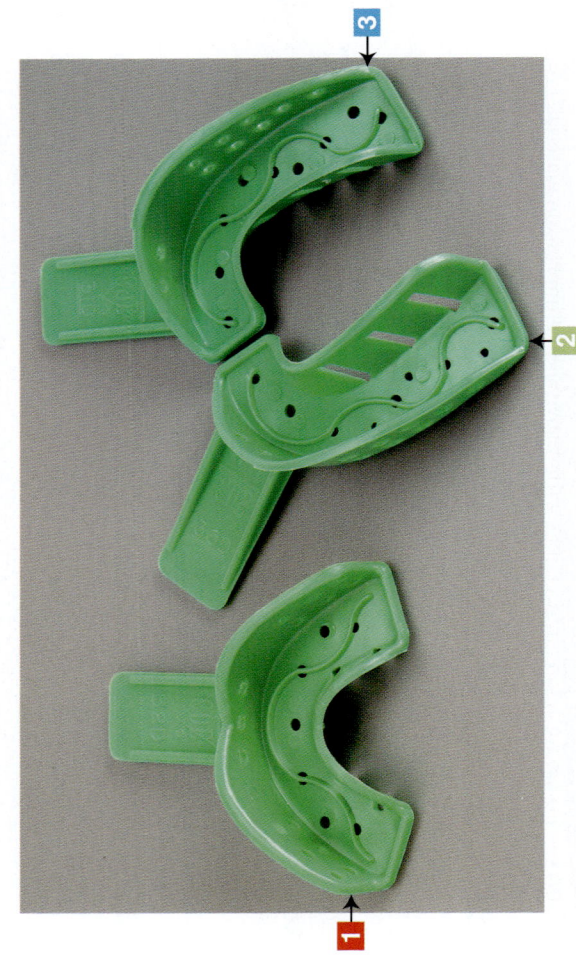

■ INSTRUMENT

Disposable Plastic Perforated Quadrant and Anterior Impression Trays

Functions ▸
To use for taking impressions with many types of impression material
To use for taking a quadrant or anterior portion of the mouth

Characteristics ▸
1 Section tray for anterior maxillary or mandibular perforated tray
2 Maxillary left or mandibular right perforated tray
3 Maxillary right or mandibular left perforated tray

Perforated trays allow material to push through the tray, creating a mechanical lock that keeps the material in place.
Range of sizes
Metal quadrant and anterior trays also available. Refer to sterilization notes below.

Practice Notes ▸
Disposable Plastic Perforated Quadrant and Anterior Impression Trays are used for many types of dental procedures involving taking impressions.
Impressions must be rinsed then disinfected before pouring up impressions.

Sterilization Notes ▸
Disposable Plastic Perforated Quadrant and Anterior Impression Trays should be disposed of in the garbage. Single use only. Metal Trays must follow sterilization procedures.

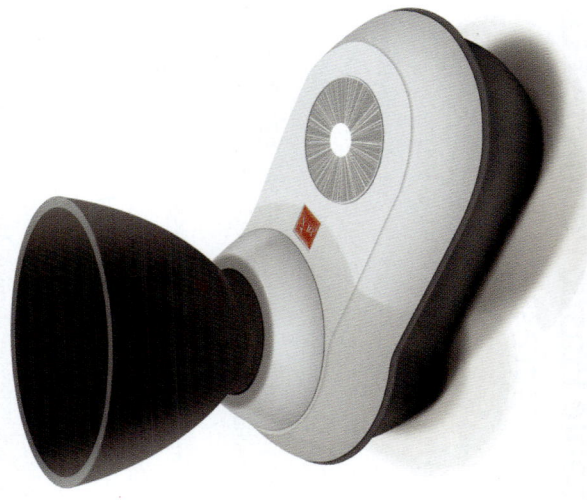

Alginator

■ **INSTRUMENT**

Function ▶ To mix alginate, irreversible hydrocolloid automatically

Characteristics ▶ Flexible bowl attaches to alginator

Low and high buttons allow bowl to rotate, mixing the alginate and water together.

Spatula pressing the material against the bowl along with the rotation of the bowl results in the material being a smooth and bubble-free consistency.

Practice Notes ▶ Alginator is used for many dental procedures involving taking an alginate impression.

Impressions must be cleaned and disinfected before pouring up impressions.

Sterilization Notes ▶ Alginator must be precleaned, sprayed with a disinfectant to wipe clean the surface, then, sprayed a second time to disinfect according the manufacturers guidelines with an approved TB/hospital wipe or spray. The Flexible Alginate Bowl must be precleaned thoroughly after removing alginate from the bowl; then, sprayed a second time to disinfect with an approved TB/hospital wipe or spray. Switch on the unit when wiping the bowl to assure thorough coverage. Refer to state regulations for any additional state requirements.

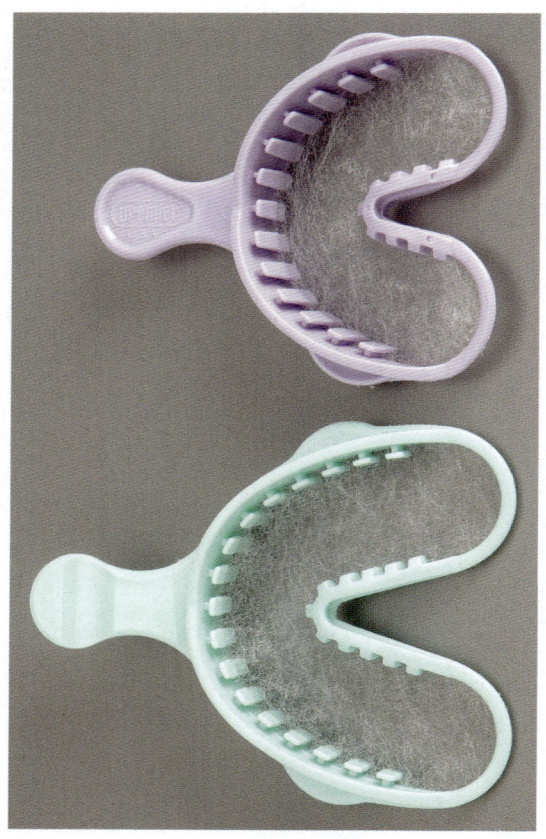

Triple Tray (Disposable)

■ INSTRUMENT

Functions ▸ To use for taking final impressions for crown and bridge restorations, opposing teeth, and bite registration with one impression

To use in the mouth, taking maxillary and mandibular simultaneously

To use with many types of impression material

Characteristics ▸ Trays have a ledge on the side to hold sufficient amount of material for the impression.

Trays have mesh-type material in the middle of the tray to hold material in place.

Trays available:

- Quadrant used for maxillary right/left or mandibular right/left
- Maxillary left or mandibular right perforated tray
- Anterior maxillary or mandibular perforated tray

Practice Note ▸ Triple Trays are used for many types of dental procedures.

Impressions must be rinsed then disinfected before pouring up impressions.

Sterilization Notes ▸ Triple Trays should be disposed of in the garbage. Single use only.

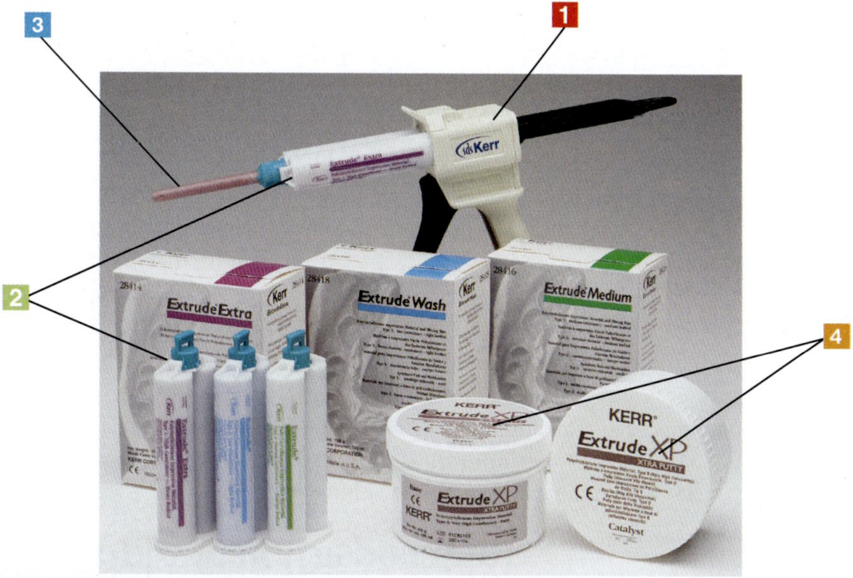
1
2
3
4
sds Kerr
Extrude Extra
Extrude Wash
Extrude Medium
28414
28418
28416
KERR
Extrude XP
XTRA PUTTY
Catalyst
Base

Mixing Gun for Dental Impression Material

Functions ▶

To mix polyvinylsiloxane, polysulfide, and polyether material for final impression

To mix base and catalyst for impression tray

To mix wash material for the syringe

To mix material for bite registration and temporary crowns

Characteristics ▶

1 Mixing gun
2 Material used in gun
3 Mixing rod attached to mix material

Manufacturers have different-style guns to accommodate their material.

4 A different technique for the tray material is to mix a putty material that is a base and a catalyst.

Practice Notes ▶

A tube with the base and catalyst is inserted into the mixing gun with a mixing rod attached. Pressure is placed on the trigger of the gun, and the material extrudes from the tubes into the mixing rod and onto the impression tray or into the tube of the syringe.

Tray material and wash (syringe) material are different.

Sterilization Notes ▶

Use overgloves to handle Mixing Gun or preclean and disinfect after each use according to the manufacturer's recommendation. Mixing rod tips should be disposed of in the garbage. Single use only.

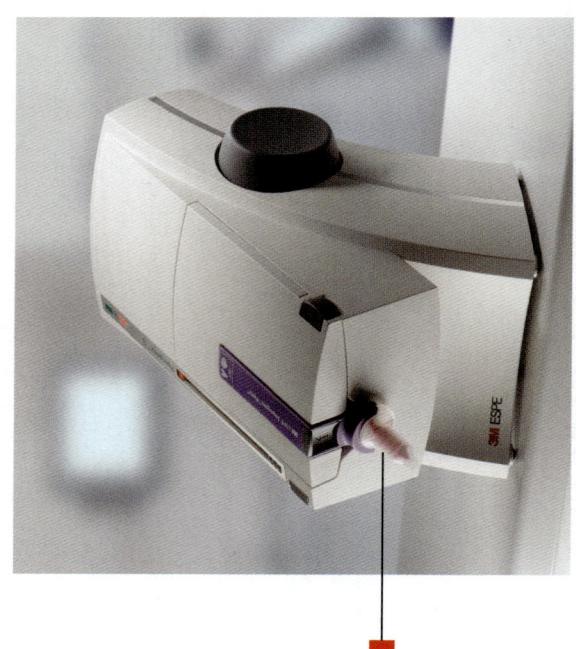

■ INSTRUMENT

Automixer

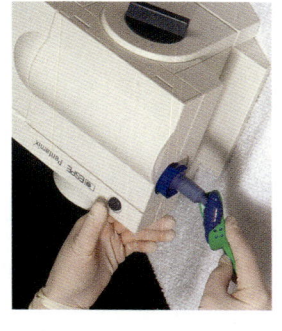

Functions ▶
To automatically mix impression material
To mix base and catalyst for polyvinylsiloxane and polyether material
To place material after dispensing from automixer into impression trays for final impressions

Characteristics ▶
Different styles of automixers available
1 Must attach mixing tips

Practice Notes ▶
A wash material (delivered from a syringe) is placed on the prepared tooth by the operator before the tray with the impression material is placed in the patient's mouth. Polyvinylsiloxane can also be mixed manually.

Sterilization Notes ▶
Use overgloves to handle Automixer or preclean and disinfect after each use according to the manufacturer's recommendation. Mixing rod tips should be disposed of in the garbage. Single use only.

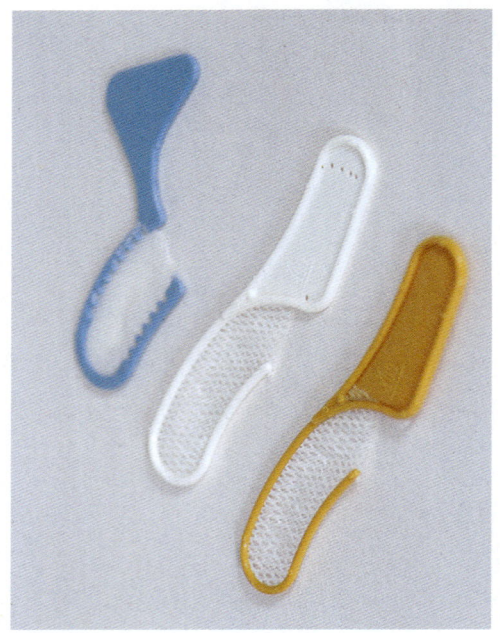

■ INSTRUMENT ▪ Bite Registration Tray

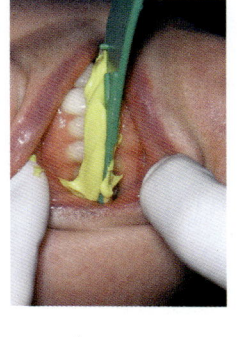

Functions ▶ To use for taking bite registration for crown and bridge procedures
To use in the mouth, taking maxillary and mandibular simultaneously
To use with many types of bite registration material

Characteristics ▶ Trays have mesh-type material in the middle of the tray to hold material in place.
Range of sizes
Trays can be used in right or left quadrant.
Anterior section bite registration tray is also available.

Practice Notes ▶ Bite Registration Trays are used with crown and bridge tray setup.
Mixing guns may be used to mix material.
Bite Registration Trays should be rinsed then disinfected before sending to laboratory.

Sterilization Notes ▶ Bite Registration Trays should be disposed of in the garbage.
Single use only.

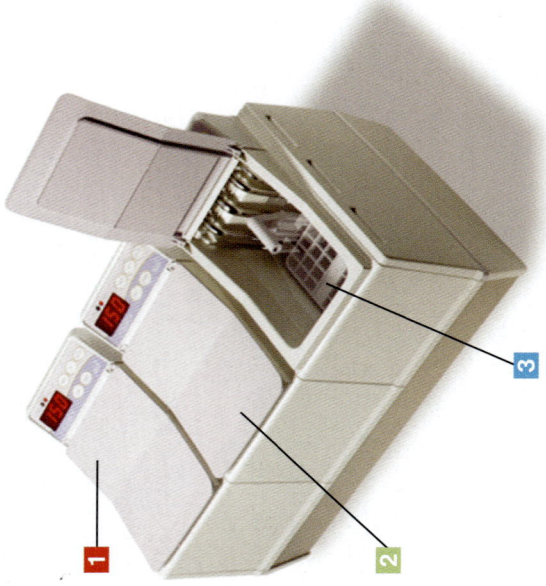

Reversible Hydrocolloid Unit

Function ▶ To boil reversible hydrocolloid, store, and temper material for final impressions

Characteristics ▶ Hydrocolloid unit has three baths:

1 Liquefying the semisolid material at 212°F (100°C)

2 Storage bath that cools the material and keeps it ready for impressions at 150°F (65.5°C)

3 Tempering bath holds the filled impression tray for 5 minutes before it is placed in the patient's mouth at 110°F (44°C).

Tubes of the material are for the impression tray.

Small cylinders are for the wash material and are used in syringes for operator to place around tooth before impression is taken.

Practice Note ▶ Reversible hydrocolloid water-cooled impression trays need to be used for this type of impression material.

Sterilization Notes ▶ Preclean and disinfect Reversible Hydrocolloid Unit, if contaminated, before and after each use according to the manufacturer's recommendation.

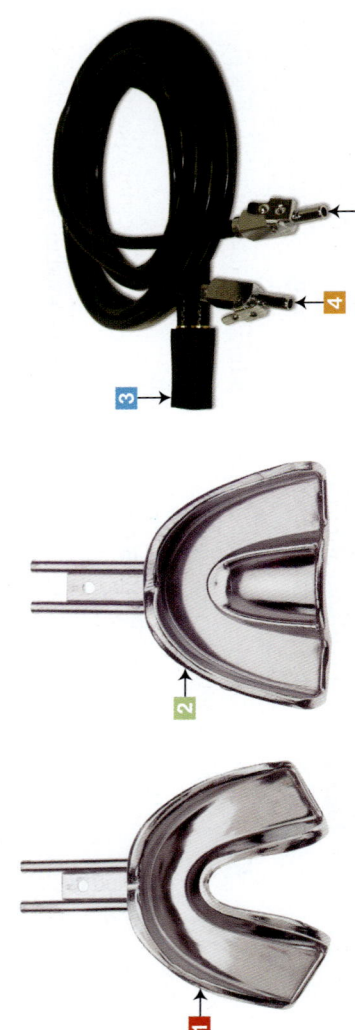

Reversible Hydrocolloid Water-Cooled Impression Trays and Hose

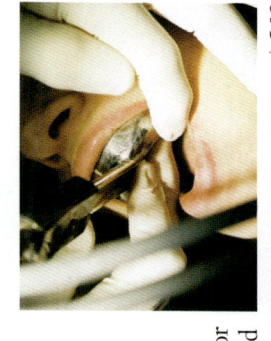

Function ▶ To take impression with reversible hydrocolloid

Characteristics ▶

1 Mandibular water-cooled tray

2 Maxillary water-cooled tray

3 Attaches to tray

4 Attaches to water source on dental unit

5 Attaches to vacuum system of dental unit

A hose attaches to the tray on one end; the other end attaches to a water source and a vacuum for the water.

The water runs inside the tray, which cools and sets the material once in the patient's mouth.

Practice Note ▶ Important to connect all parts of the hose before turning on the water source

Impression must be rinsed then disinfected before sending to lab

Sterilization Notes ▶ Irreversible Hydrocolloid Water-Cooled Impression Trays must be precleaned. Then, place in a sterilizing pouch with an internal process indicator, seal, then sterilize. OR, wrap with an internal process indicator inside and secure on the outside with process indicator tape, then sterilize. Verify appropriate color change has been achieved in external process indicator immediately after removal from sterilizer. Check internal process indicator before treatment. Refer to state regulations for any additional state requirements. Hose must be precleaned and disinfected according to the manufacturer's recommendation.

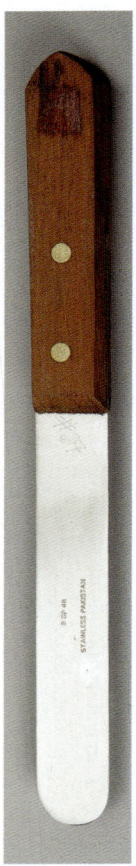

INSTRUMENT

Laboratory Spatula

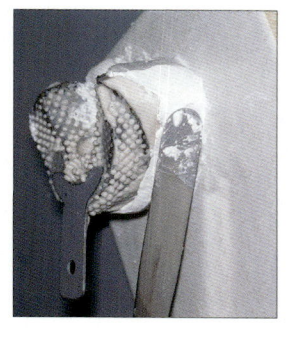

Functions ▶ To mix powder and a liquid in a flexible bowl

To mix and shape laboratory plaster, stone, and die stone for models

Characteristics ▶ Spatula straight to help manipulate material

Range of sizes

Practice Note ▶ Laboratory Spatula is used with vibrator to mix material.

Sterilization Notes ▶ Preclean and disinfect Laboratory Spatula, if contaminated, after each use according to the manufacturer's recommendation. Refer to state regulations for any additional state requirements.

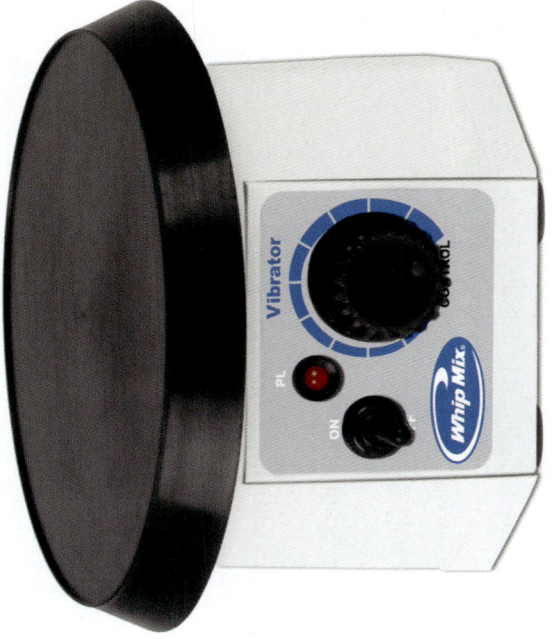

Vibrator for Laboratory

Function ▶ To vibrate material in mixing bowl to remove air bubbles from mixing plaster, stone, or die stone

Characteristics ▶ Use vibrator after manually mixing the plaster or stone.

Use vibrator while adding plaster or stone to impression to eliminate air bubbles in impression.

Practice Note ▶ Place plastic cover on vibrator work surface to keep vibrator free from material.

Sterilization Notes ▶ Preclean and disinfect vibrator, if contaminated, according to the manufacturer's recommendation.

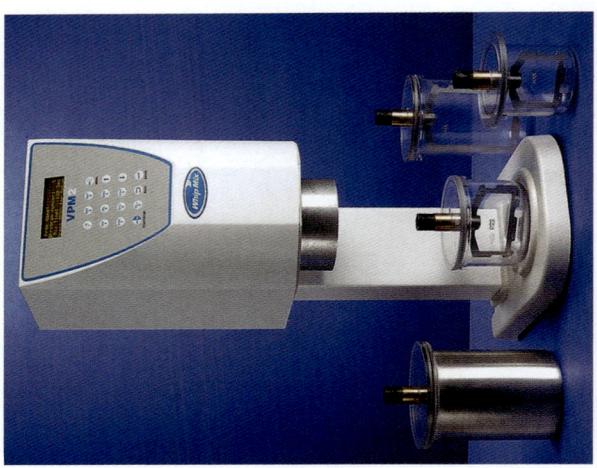

Vacuum Mixing Unit

Functions ▶
To vacuum mix all types of gypsums, plasters, and investment materials
To program digitally type of material being mixed
To remove excessive air from material while mixing

Characteristics ▶
Vacuum Mixing Unit uses blades to mix material and vacuum air bubbles
Bowl with blades attaches to unit and mixes material automatically
Vacuum system within the unit removes excess air for smoother material consistency

Practice Note ▶
Vacuum Mixer is used in dental office labs and dental laboratories for better consistency of material for models and investment material for cast crowns.

Sterilization Notes ▶
Preclean and disinfect Vacuum Mixing Unit and Mixing Bowls, if contaminated, according to manufacturer's recommendation.

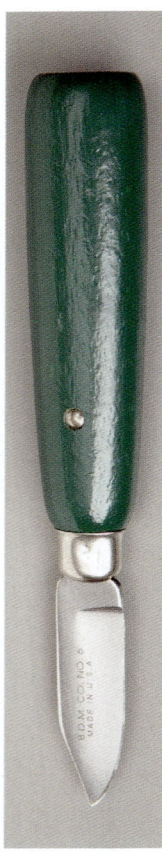

▪ INSTRUMENT | Laboratory Knife

Functions ▶

To use for separating impressions from model(s)

To use for hand-trimming models

To use on any type of appliance for hand trimming

Characteristics ▶

Range of sizes

Usually has green wooden handle—Referred to as Green Handle Lab Knife

Practice Note ▶

Laboratory Knife is used in dental office setting and dental laboratories.

Sterilization Notes ▶

Preclean and disinfect Laboratory Knife. If contaminated then preclean. Then, place in a sterilizing pouch with an internal process indicator, seal, then sterilize. OR, wrap with an internal process indicator inside and secure on the outside with process indicator tape, then sterilize. Verify appropriate color change has been achieved in external process indicator immediately after removal from sterilizer. Check internal process indicator before treatment. Refer to state regulations for any additional state requirements.

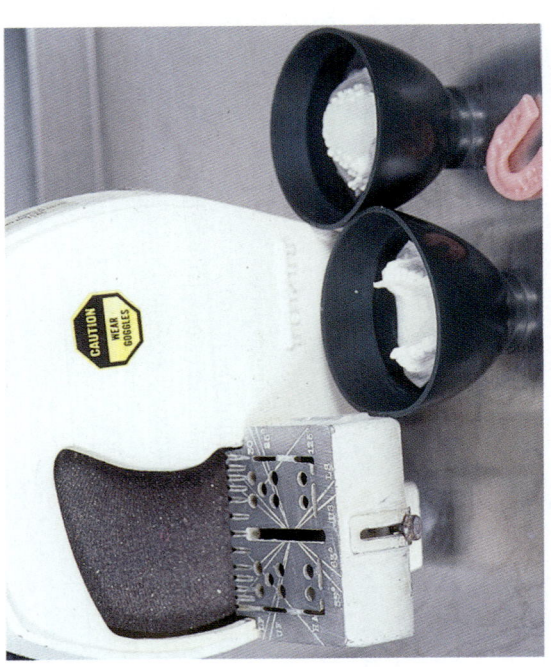

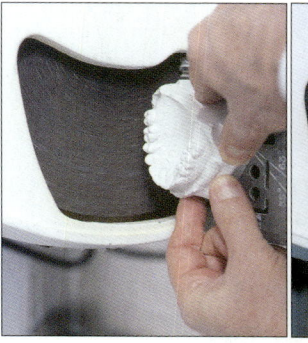 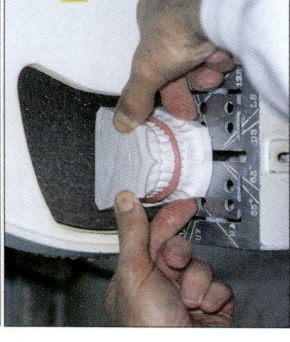

Model Trimmer

Function ▶ To trim plaster, stone, or die stone models

Characteristics ▶ Trimmer has an abrasive grinding wheel to grind excess plaster, stone, and die stone from the models.

Water runs next to the grinding wheel to reduce heat, reduce the dust created by grinding, and keep the wheel clean.

Practice Notes ▶ Diagnostic models, orthodontic models, and crown and bridge models are all trimmed differently.

Glasses and mask should be worn while trimming models.

Unit should have splash guards.

Soaking the base of the models in water helps soften the material for grinding.

Be careful not to submerge teeth on the model.

Sterilization Notes ▶ Preclean and disinfect Model Trimmer, if contaminated, according to the manufacturer's recommendation.

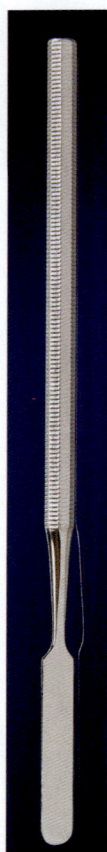

Flexible Mixing Spatula

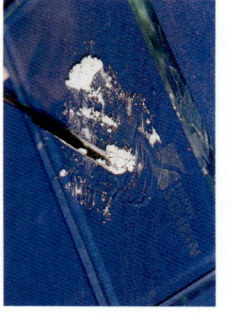

Function ▶ To mix dental materials

Characteristics ▶ Flexible metal spatula allows for proper manipulation of material. Range of sizes

Practice Note ▶ Flexible Mixing Spatula is used on most restorative, endodontic, orthodontic, and periodontic tray setups.

Sterilization Notes ▶ Flexible Mixing Spatula must be precleaned. Then, place in a sterilizing pouch with an internal process indicator, seal, then sterilize. OR, wrap with an internal process indicator inside and secure on the outside with process indicator tape, then sterilize. Verify appropriate color change has been achieved in external process indicator immediately after removal from sterilizer. Check internal process indicator before treatment. Refer to state regulations for any additional state requirements.

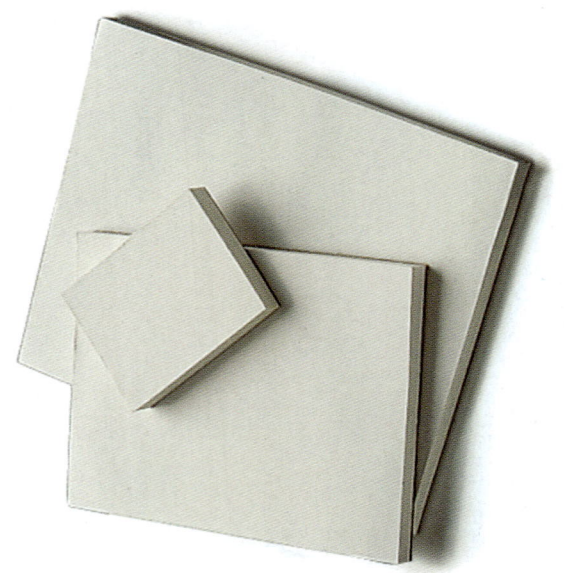

Paper Mixing Pads

Function ▸ To mix all types of dental materials

Characteristics ▸ Each paper on the pad is coated so material will not seep through the paper.
Many types and sizes available

Practice Note ▸ Many materials have special paper pads that must be used when mixing certain materials.

Sterilization Notes ▸ Remove one paper at a time to mix each material and not contaminate the entire mixing pad.
Entire pad should not be used to mix unless overgloves are used.

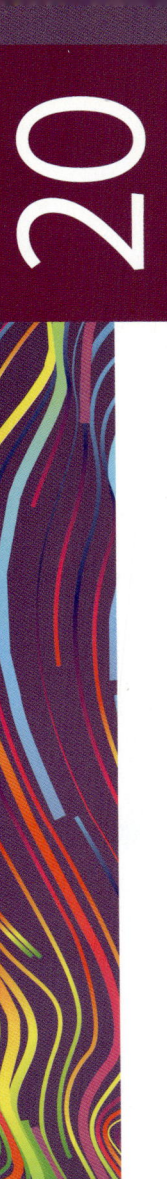

20

Dental Imaging and Diagnostic Equipment

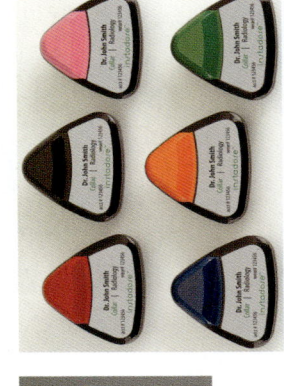

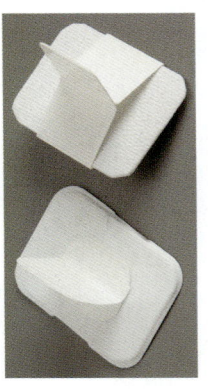

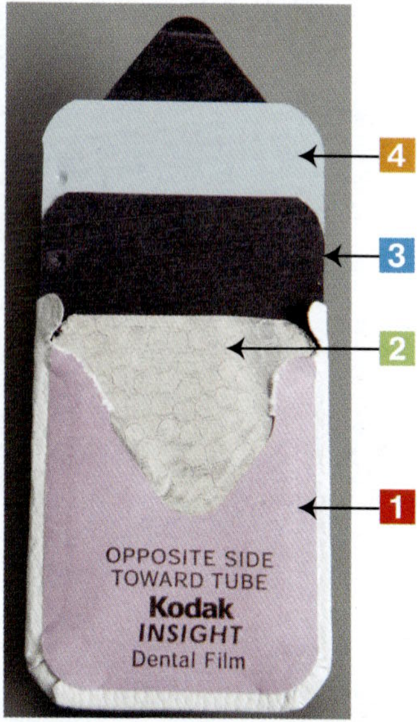

4
3
2
1
OPPOSITE SIDE
TOWARD TUBE
Kodak
INSIGHT
Dental Film

Intraoral Dental Film

Function ▶ To capture the image of teeth in the radiographic process

Characteristics ▶
1. Outside covering of film—Soft plastic or paper (both waterproof)
2. Sheet of lead foil to stop the radiation from extending beyond the film
3. Black paper to protect the film from light penetration
4. Film—Single or double film

Film speed indicated on each packet—Set by American National Standards Institute (ANSI)

Film speed A through F—D, E, F used intraorally

Faster speed of the film reduces the amount of radiation exposure; F speed is faster than D speed.

Film speed determines amount of radiation needed to produce a quality radiograph—Settings are on x-ray unit.

Practice Note ▶ Intraoral Dental X-ray Film is used in all phases of dentistry.

Sterilization Notes ▶ Follow standard precautions and cross-contamination protocol when exposing and processing film for developing. Outer packet and black paper may be disposed of in the garbage. Correct disposal of lead foil must be checked within your state. In some states, lead foil is considered a hazardous waste and must be collected and disposed of properly. For proper recycling protocol, refer to Department of Environmental Health regulations in the state where you practice.

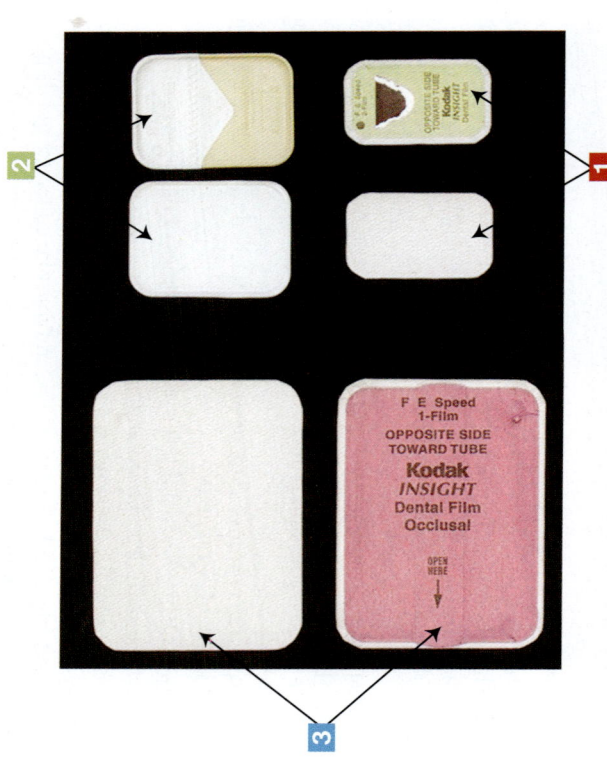

▪ INSTRUMENT

Intraoral Dental Film—Various Sizes

Functions ▸ To project an image of the patient's teeth through radiographic film
To use for intraoral and extraoral projections

Characteristics ▸ Commonly taken radiographs—Front and back view
Size #0—Taken on children under 3 (not pictured)

1 Size #1—Used for Anterior periapical image (narrow view)

2 Size #2—Used for Periapical and bite-wing image

Size #3—Used for extended bitewing projections (not pictured)

3 Size #4—Used for occlusal projections; taken to view maxillary and mandibular teeth: commonly taken on children

Practice Notes ▸ Smooth side of the film (the raised-dot side—convex) faces the x-ray tube or position-indicating device (PID). Raised dot should be toward the occlusal or incisal.

Sterilization Notes ▸ Follow standard precautions and cross-contamination protocol when exposing and processing film for developing. Outer packet and black paper may be disposed of in the garbage. Correct disposal of lead foil must be checked within your state. In some states, lead foil is considered a hazardous waste and must be collected and disposed of properly. For proper recycling protocol, refer to Department of Environmental Health regulations in the state where you practice. Refer to state regulations for any additional state requirements.

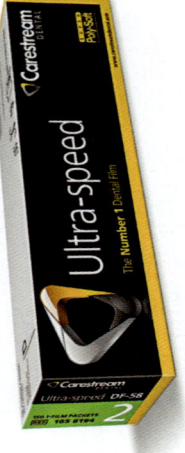

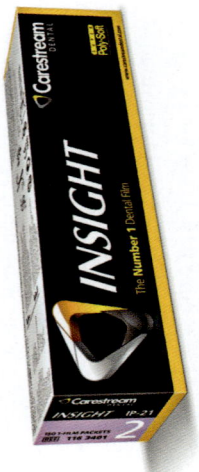

Package of Dental Film

Function ▶ To package intraoral dental film

Characteristics ▶ Box labeled:
- Type of film
- Film speed
- Number of films in individual film packet
- Number of film packets in the box
- Expiration date of film

Film packets—Single or double film

Practice Notes ▶ Each film has an identification dot (raised bump). Concave on one side and convex on the other. Convex/bump faces toward the teeth when placing the x-ray.

Film storage is important to the integrity of the film. Refer to package instructions for storage recommendations.

Sterilization Notes ▶ Follow standard precautions and cross-contamination protocol when processing film for developing. Outer packet and black paper may be disposed of in the garbage. Correct disposal of lead foil must be checked within your state. In some states, lead foil is considered a hazardous waste and must be collected and disposed of properly. For proper recycling protocol, refer to Department of Environmental Health regulations in the state where you practice.

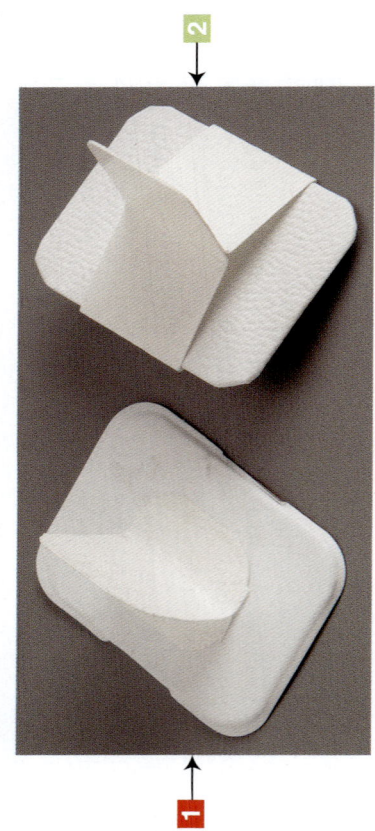

■INSTRUMENT

Bite-Wing Tabs

Function ▸ To take a bite-wing radiograph projection

Characteristics ▸
1 Stick-on tab
2 Slip-on tab

Tab or wing is placed on the occlusal, and patient bites on the tab to secure the film.

Practice Notes ▸ Slip-on tabs are available in different sizes to accommodate different-sized film.

Size #2 film is used for adult bite-wing radiograph.

Bite-wing radiographs are mainly used for diagnosing caries on proximal surfaces (mesial and distal) of the posterior teeth.

Four bite-wings are usually taken on adult dentition—One premolar and one molar projection on each side of the mouth.

Sterilization Notes ▸ Follow standard precautions and cross-contamination protocol when exposing and processing film. Outer packet, black paper, and Bite-Wing Tabs may be disposed of in the garbage. Correct disposal of lead foil must be checked within your state. In some states, lead foil is considered a hazardous waste and must be collected and disposed of properly. For proper recycling protocol, refer to Department of Environmental Health regulations in the state where you practice.

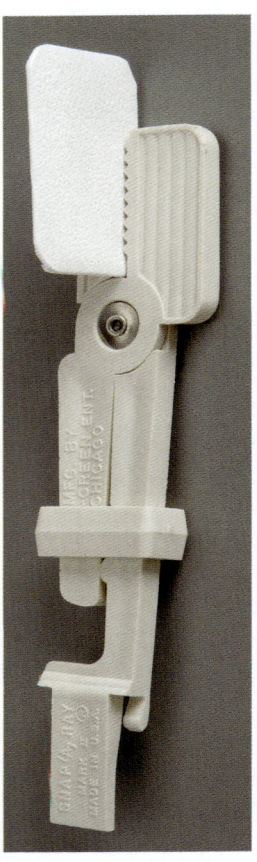

Film Holder—Periapical (EeZee-Grip)

Function ▶ To position and hold the film in patient's mouth for periapical images

Characteristics ▶ Double ended:
- One end holds film for posterior teeth projection, as shown.
- Opposite end holds film for anterior teeth projection.

Practice Notes ▶ Size #2 film used for posterior periapical image

Size #1 or #2 used for anterior periapical image

Periapical images used for viewing the coronal part of the tooth, root, apex, and surrounding bone and tissue

EeZee-Grip formerly called Snap-a-ray

Sterilization Notes ▶ EeZee-Grip Film Holder must be precleaned. Then, place in a sterilizing pouch with an internal process indicator, seal, then sterilize. OR, wrap with an internal process indicator inside and secure on the outside with process indicator tape, then sterilize. Verify appropriate color change has been achieved in external process indicator immediately after removal from sterilizer. Check internal process indicator before treatment. Refer to state regulations for any additional state requirements.

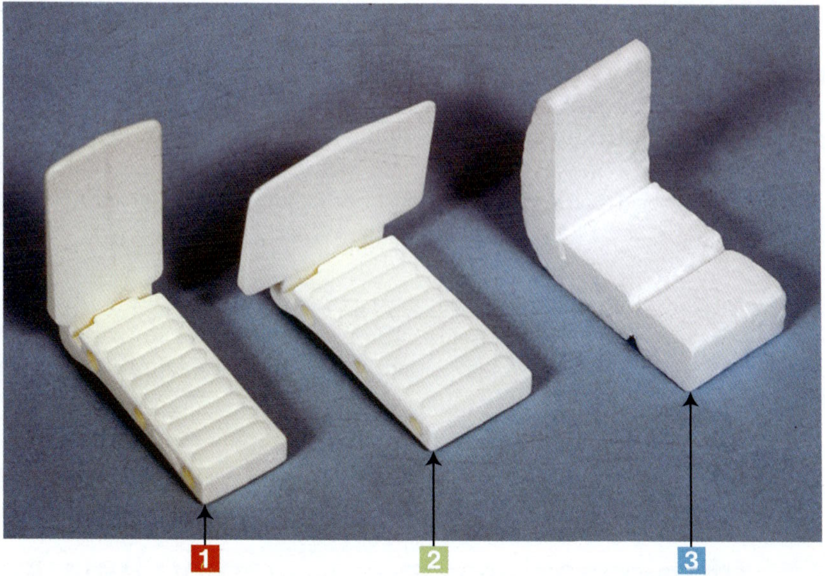
1
2
3

Film Holders—Periapical

INSTRUMENT

Functions ▶ To position and hold a film in patient's mouth for periapical image
To allow patient to bite on holder to keep film in place while positioning the position-indicating device (PID) and exposing the film

Characteristics ▶
1 Holds film for anterior teeth projection—Plastic that can be sterilized
2 Holds film for posterior teeth projection—Plastic that can be sterilized
3 Holds film for anterior and posterior projection—Disposable Styrofoam (one time use)

Slot holds film in place

Practice Note ▶ Periapical images are used for viewing the coronal part of the tooth, root, apex, and surrounding bone and tissue.

Sterilization Notes ▶ Plastic Film Holders must be precleaned. Then, place in a sterilizing pouch with an internal process indicator, seal, then sterilize. OR, wrap with an internal process indicator inside and secure on the outside with process indicator tape, then sterilize. Verify appropriate color change has been achieved in external process indicator immediately after removal from sterilizer. Check internal process indicator before treatment. Refer to state regulations for any additional state requirements. Disposable Styrofoam holder may be disposed of in garbage.

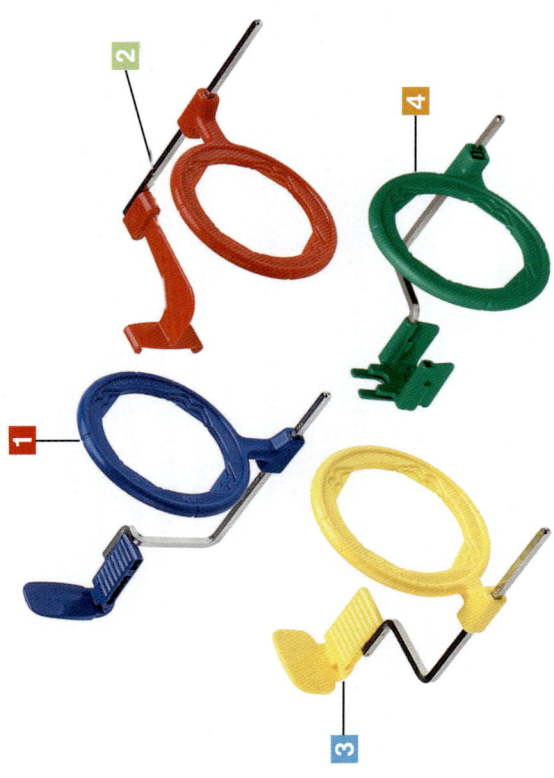

■ INSTRUMENT

Film Holders—XCP

Functions ▸ To position and hold a film in patient's mouth for periapical and bite-wing images using parallel technique

To allow patient to bite on holder to keep film in place while positioning the position-indicating device (PID) and exposing the film

Characteristics ▸
1 Blue—Anterior teeth projection
2 Red—Bite-wing projection
3 Yellow—Posterior teeth projection
4 Green—Projections for endodontic procedures

Slot holds film in place.

Practice Notes ▸ XCP uses the parallel technique for exposing radiation to the film.
PID is parallel with the ring on the XCP.

Sterilization Notes ▸ Film Holders must be disassembled and precleaned. Then, place in a sterilizing pouch with an internal process indicator, seal, then sterilize. OR, wrap with an internal process indicator inside and secure on the outside with process indicator tape, then sterilize. Verify appropriate color change has been achieved in external process indicator immediately after removal from sterilizer. Check internal process indicator before treatment. Refer to state regulations for any additional state requirements.

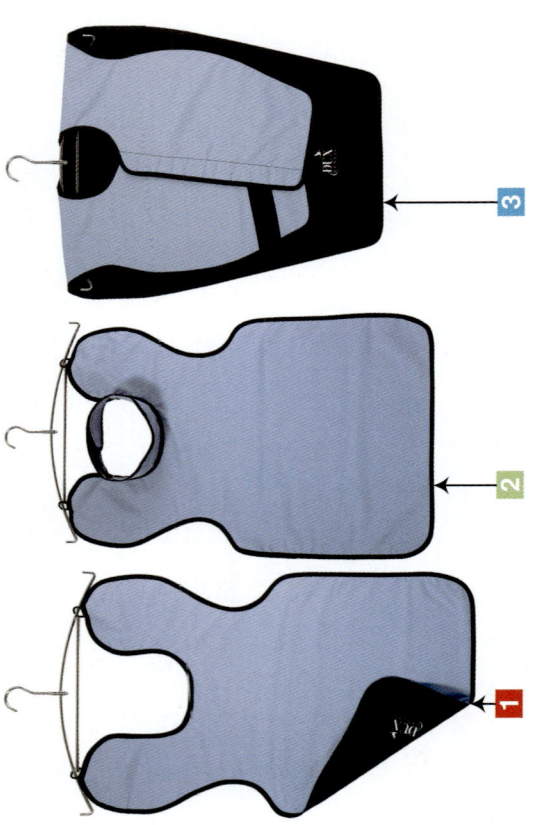

■ INSTRUMENT

Lead Aprons

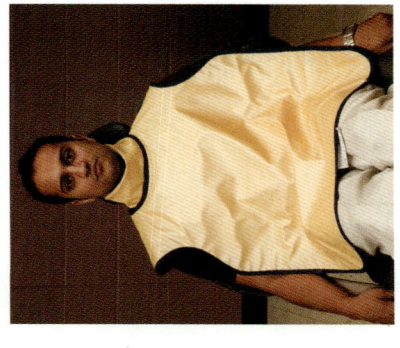

Function ▶ To place on patient for protection against scattered radiation during exposure of x-ray film

Characteristics ▶

1 Lead apron

2 Lead apron with collar to protect thyroid area

3 Lead apron poncho for front and back protection

Practice Notes ▶ Lead Apron must be used when exposing patient to dental x-rays.

Lead aprons should not be folded.

Sterilization Notes ▶ Preclean and disinfect Lead Apron according to the manufacturer's recommendation.

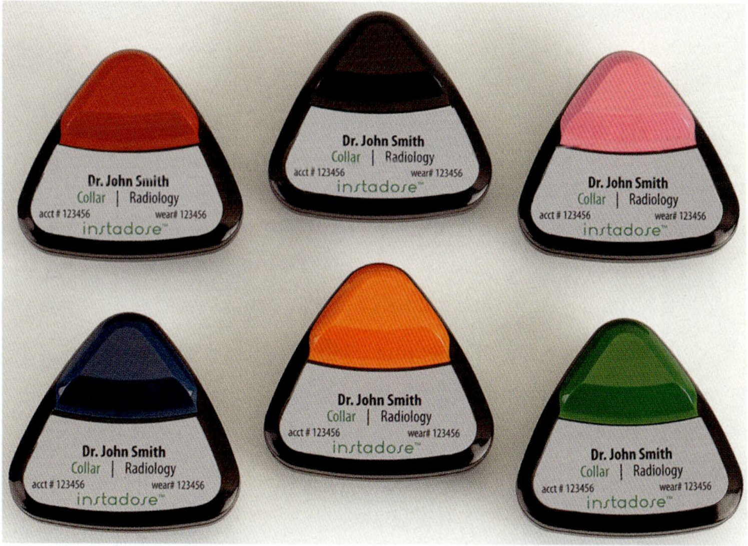
Dr. John Smith
Collar | Radiology
acct # 123456 wear# 123456
instadose™
Dr. John Smith
Collar | Radiology
acct # 123456 wear# 123456
instadose™
Dr. John Smith
Collar | Radiology
acct # 123456 wear# 123456
instadose™
Dr. John Smith
Collar | Radiology
acct # 123456 wear# 123456
instadose™
Dr. John Smith
Collar | Radiology
acct # 123456 wear# 123456
instadose™
Dr. John Smith
Collar | Radiology
acct # 123456 wear# 123456
instadose™

Radiation Monitoring Device

Functions ▶

To place on operator's protective clothing while employee is working in a dental office or radiography lab

To use as a Direct Ion Storage (DIS) dosimeter constructed with non-volatile analog memory cells surround by gas-filled ion chambers

To measure the ionizing radiation exposure dose incident on the dosimeter by calculating the amount of proportional change in the voltage across the memory cells

Characteristics ▶

Each badge includes employee's name, wear and account number, and the radiation monitoring device (dosimeter).

Radiography monitoring device should be worn for traditional and digital projections.

Practice Notes ▶

At the end of a reporting period, or anytime the user wants to check the dose reading on-demand, the dosimeter radiation exposure report can be read instantly and automatically via a mobile device app, localized reader, or computer. The user can also set up high-dose notification alerts or configure badge reassignments online.

Sterilization Notes ▶

If contaminated, disinfect Radiation Monitoring Device according to the manufacturer's recommendation. Refer to state regulations for any additional state requirements.

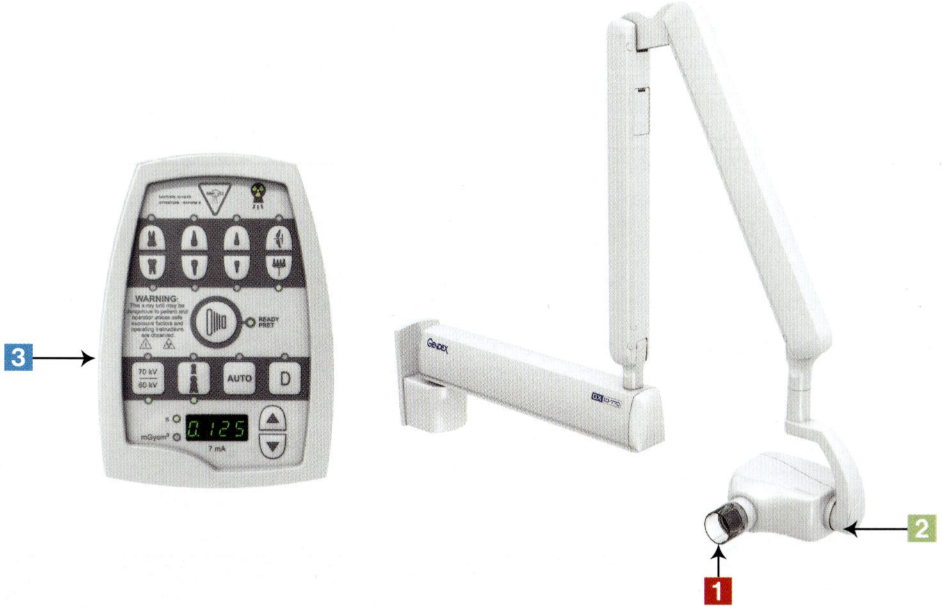
3
WARNING:
READY
PRET
70 kV
80 kV
AUTO
D
0.125
7 mA
mGycm²
GENDEX
GX 770
1
2

INSTRUMENT

Dental Imaging Unit

Function ▶ To expose film with radiation that is generated in the imaging unit

Characteristics ▶
1 Position-indicating device (PID)
2 Tube head
3 Imaging Unit

Round or rectangular PIDs available

Practice Note ▶ Control panel for the imaging unit and button to expose the film are outside patient's treatment room. On some machines, you may adjust the exposure time the x-ray is exposed. Other machines adjust the exposure time, kilovoltage peak (kVp), and milliamperage (mA).

Sterilization Notes ▶ Follow standard precautions and cross-contamination protocol when exposing and processing film. Barriers should be used on x-ray tube head, PID, and panel where x-ray button is pushed. Follow manufacturer's recommendation for precleaning and disinfection of the Dental Imaging Unit. Refer to state regulations for any additional state requirements.

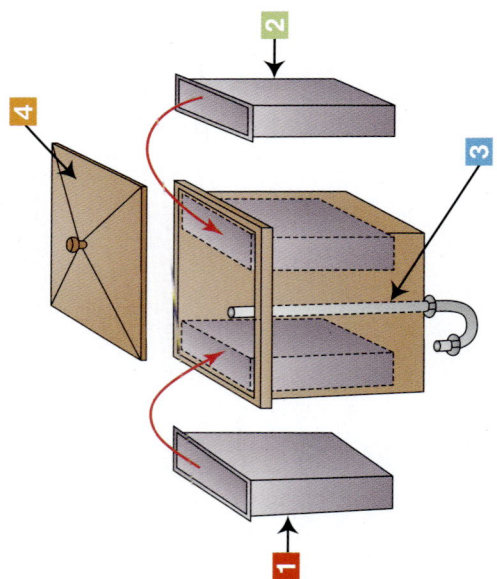

■ INSTRUMENT

Manual Developing Unit

Functions ▶ To manually develop exposed dental radiographic films taken on patients
To develop, rinse, fix, and wash dental radiographic films
To develop dental radiographic films in a darkroom with only a safelight

Characteristics ▶ Tank insert for the developing and fixing solution
1 Developer in left tank; **2** Fixer in right tank
3 Water bath and rinsing tank with constant running water in tank
4 Cover for unit

Practice Note ▶ Developing time depends on the temperature of the running water. The water will determine the temperature of the developer and fixer solutions. A table with the temperature denotes the time to develop and fix. Fixer time is double the developing time. The wash time is 20 minutes after the film has been fixed.

Sterilization Notes ▶ Follow standard precautions and cross-contamination protocol when processing film. For proper recycling protocol for solutions, refer to Department of Environmental Health regulations in the state where you practice. Follow local and state regulations in disposal of developer and fixer solution.

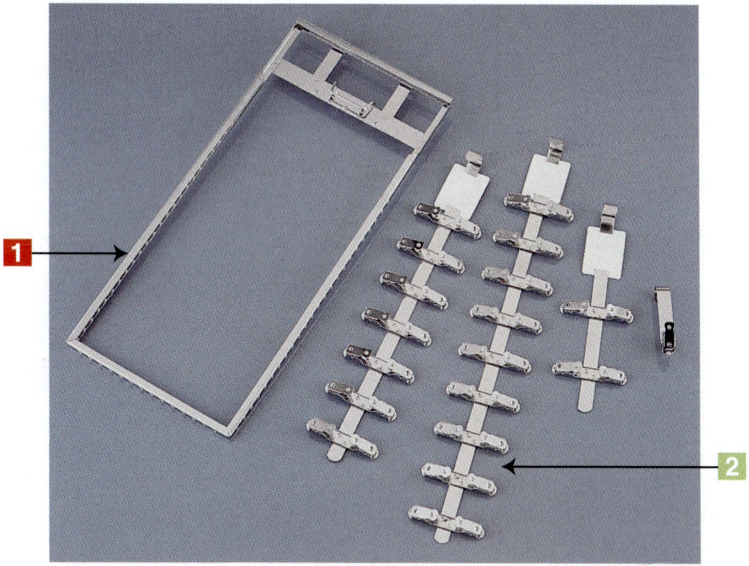
1
2

Film Rack

Functions ▶ To place undeveloped film on the rack in the darkroom with only the safelight before putting rack in the developer

To place film on rack without touching each other

Characteristic ▶ 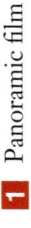 **1** Panoramic film rack

2 Individual single film racks

Various sizes of racks available

Practice Note ▶ Keep all films on rack through the entire process: develop, rinse, fix, wash, and dry.

Sterilization Notes ▶ Follow standard precautions and cross-contamination protocol when processing film. Outer packet and black paper may be disposed of in the garbage. Correct disposal of lead foil must be checked within your state. In some states, lead foil is considered a hazardous waste and must be collected and disposed of properly. For proper recycling protocol, refer to Department of Environmental Health regulations in the state where you practice. Disinfect racks according to manufacturer's recommendation. Refer to state regulations for any additional state requirements.

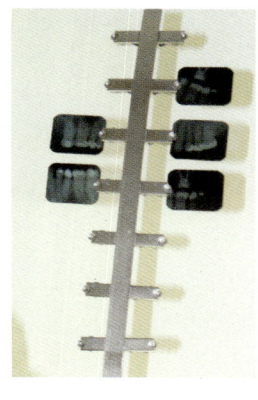

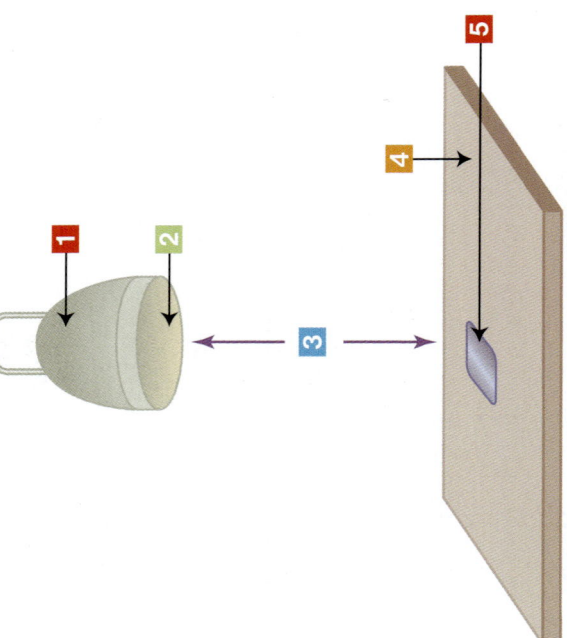

■ INSTRUMENT

Safelight

Function ▶ To provide enough illumination in the darkroom to process films safely without exposing or damaging the film

Characteristics ▶
1 Safelight
2 Safelight filter
3 Minimum distance (at least 4 feet) from safelight to undeveloped x-ray
4 Working area
5 Undeveloped and unwrapped film

Practice Note ▶ Unwrapped film left too close to the safelight or exposed for more than 2 to 3 minutes will appear fogged.

Sterilization Notes ▶ Follow standard precautions and cross-contamination protocol when processing film. Preclean and disinfect area if contaminated.

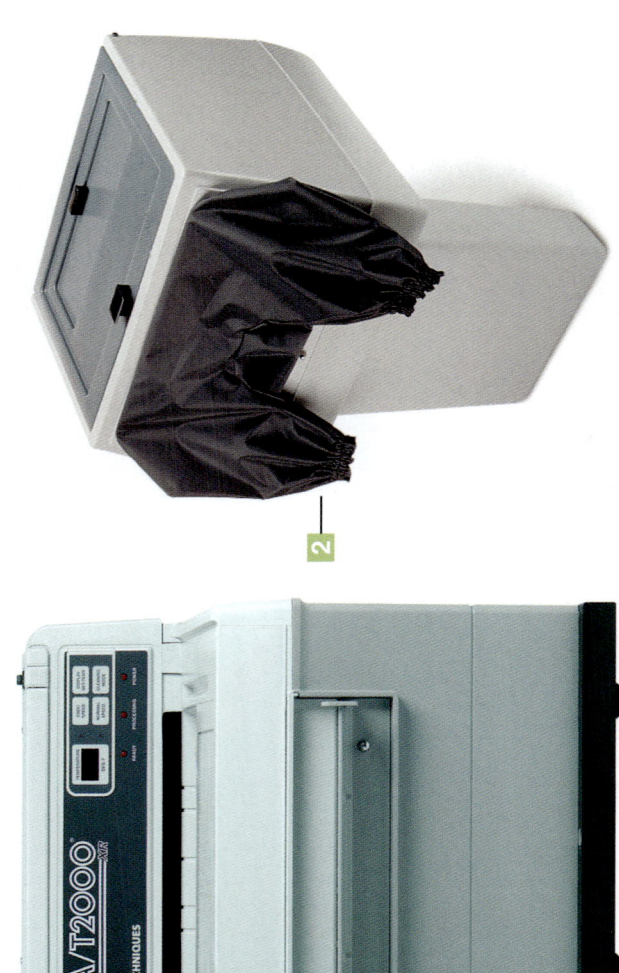

Automatic Film Processor

Functions ▶ To automatically develop radiographs in darkroom
To develop dental film

Characteristics ▶
1 Automatic processor
2 Front loader—Hands go into a dark area to unwrap film. View area from top. Darkroom not needed.

Various types of processors available

Practice Note ▶ Dentist is able to diagnose radiographs once film is dry, which is a great advantage of the automatic processor.

Sterilization Notes ▶ Follow standard precautions and cross-contamination protocol when processing film. Outer packet and black paper may be disposed of in the garbage. Correct disposal of lead foil must be checked within your state. In some states, lead foil is considered a hazardous waste and must be collected and disposed of properly. For proper recycling protocol, refer to Department of Environmental Health regulations in the state where you practice. Follow local and state regulations in disposal of developer and fixer solution. Refer to state regulations for any additional state requirements.

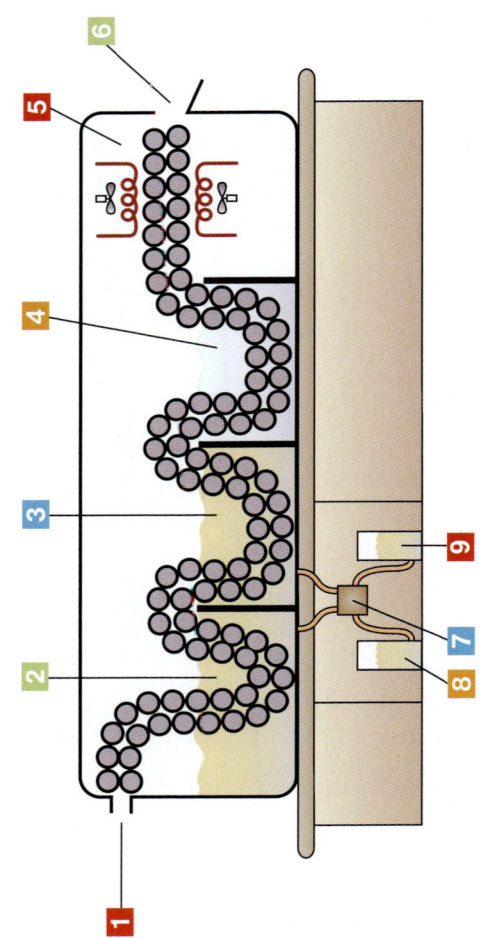

Parts of Automatic Film Processor

■ INSTRUMENT

Functions ▸ To automatically develop radiographic film
To place film in processor to develop, fix, wash, dry; film then ready to mount

Characteristics ▸
1 Slot to feed film
2 Roller transporter in developer tank
3 Roller transporter in fixer tank
4 Roller transporter in water tank
5 Roller transporter in drying compartment
6 Film releases from rollers onto recovery slot
7 Pump to replenish developer and fixer
8 Replenishing solution for developer and **9** Replenishing solution for fixer

Practice Note ▸ Developer and fixer solutions for the automatic processor are different from those for manual processing.

Sterilization Notes ▸ Follow standard precautions and cross-contamination protocol when processing film. Outer packet and black paper may be disposed of in the garbage. Correct disposal of lead foil must be checked within your state. In some states, lead foil is considered a hazardous waste and must be collected and disposed of properly. For proper recycling protocol for solutions, refer to Department of Environmental Health regulations in the state where you practice. Follow local and state regulations in disposal of developer and fixer solution. Refer to state regulations for any additional state requirements.

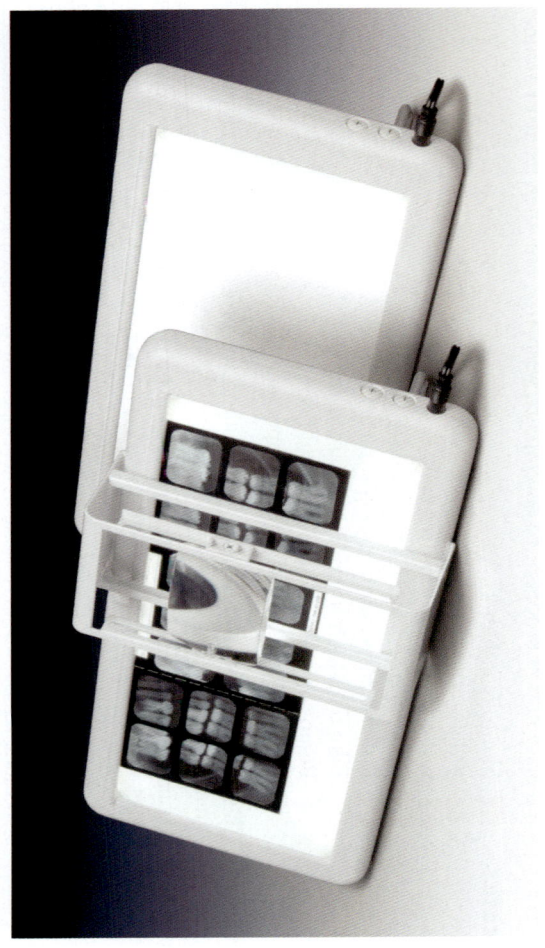

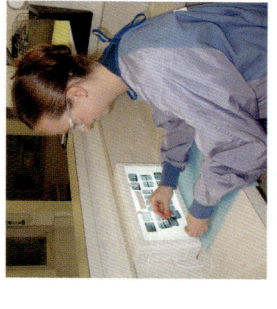

■ INSTRUMENT

View Luminator

Function ▶ To view traditional radiographs for diagnosis

Characteristics ▶ Various sizes and styles of view luminators

Also referred to as view box

Practice Note ▶ View boxes are located in each patient treatment room.

Sterilization Notes ▶ If contaminated, preclean and disinfect View Luminator according to the manufacturer's recommendation.

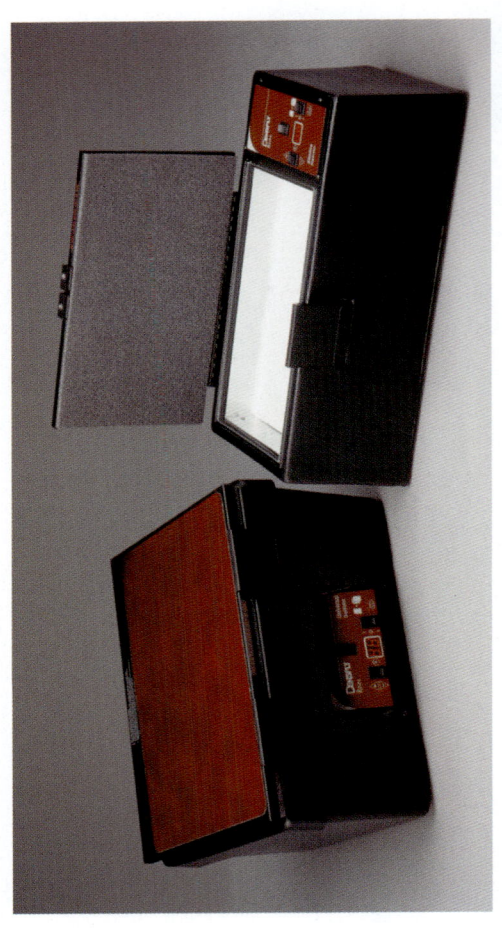

■ INSTRUMENT

Film Duplicator

Function ▶ To duplicate dental radiographic film

Characteristics ▶ Produces white light to expose film

Various sizes and styles available

Practice Notes ▶ All phases of dentistry use film duplicators. Some dental offices use double-pack dental radiographic film instead of duplicating the film.

Electronic devices are available for duplicating dental radiographs.

Duplicated images are sent to insurance companies or referring specialists. If using double-packet dental radiographic film or digital radiography, duplication is not necessary.

Most offices send patient images through the Internet. Internet communication with patient information must be encrypted for Privacy Act, HIPAA.

Sterilization Notes ▶ If contaminated, preclean and disinfect Film Duplicator according to the manufacturer's recommendation.

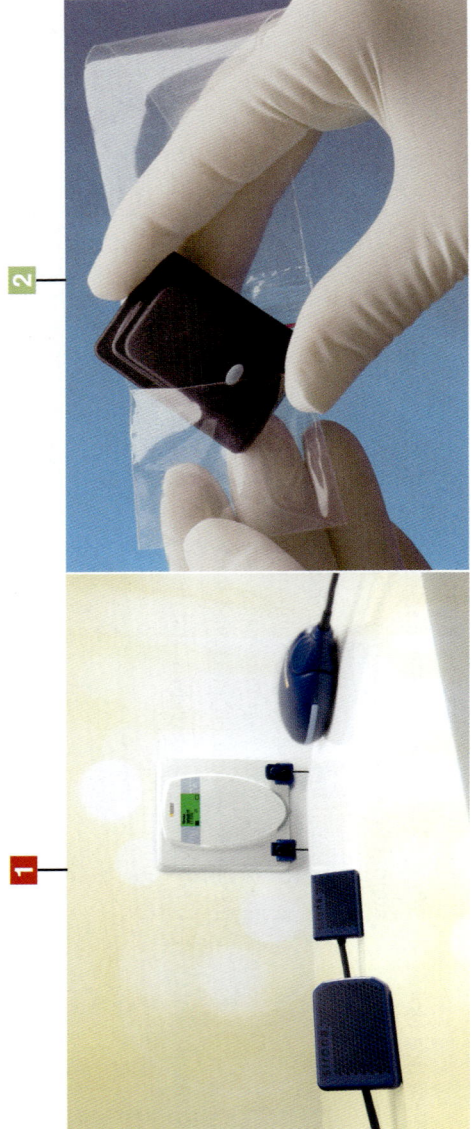

Intraoral Sensors for Digital Images

Functions ▶ To take digital intraoral images without film or without processing the film

To project the image of the teeth by digitally projecting radiation onto an electronic sensor and to computerized imaging system before going to computer storage

Characteristics ▶ Different styles and systems of sensors and digital radiography available

Different size sensors available

1 Some sensors have wire connecting to the computer.

2 Some sensors do not have wire but are put into a specially designed computer after exposure. Picture shows barrier placed on sensor.

Practice Notes ▶ Paperless dental offices store digital images on the computer, along with patient records. Digital image may be printed out on special paper if a copy is required.

Sterilization Notes ▶ Follow standard precautions and cross-contamination protocol when exposing digital film. Barriers must be placed on the sensors. Barriers must be used and the manufacturer's recommendation for disinfection followed. Refer to state regulations for any additional state requirements.

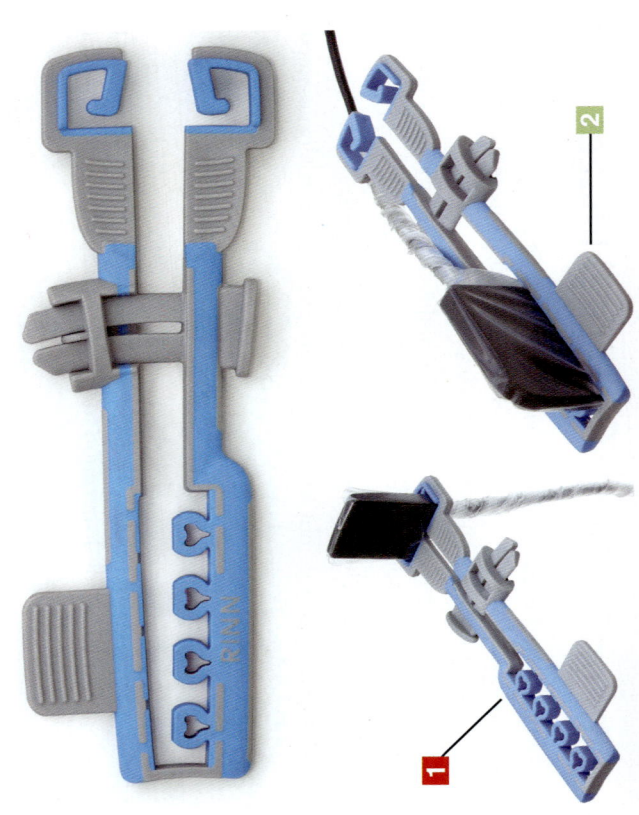

Holder for Digital Sensor (EeZee-Grip)

Function ▶ To position and hold a digital sensor in patient's mouth for periapical images

Characteristics ▶ Double ended:

1 Holds film for anterior teeth projection—Barrier placed on sensor

2 Holds film for posterior teeth projection—Barrier placed on sensor

Designed for snug fit to prevent slipping

Practice Notes ▶ Holder allows room for the wire attached to the sensor

May be used with wireless digital sensor

Sterilization Notes ▶ Follow standard precautions and cross-contamination protocol when taking digital images. Holder must be precleaned, open, and unlocked. Then, place in an open and unlocked position in a sterilizing pouch with an internal process indicator, seal, then sterilize. OR, wrap with an internal process indicator inside and secure on the outside with process indicator tape, then sterilize. Verify appropriate color change has been achieved in external process indicator immediately after removal from sterilizer. Check internal process indicator before treatment. Refer to state regulations for any additional state requirements.

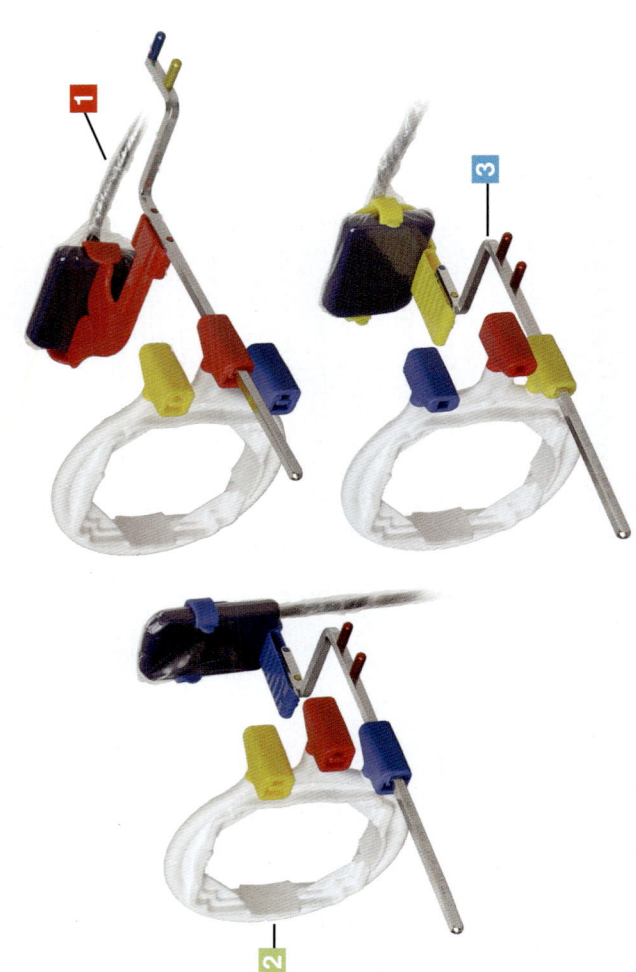

One Ring and Arm Positioning System

■ I N S T R U M E N T

Functions ▶

To position and hold digital sensors or film in patient's mouth for periapical and bite-wing images using parallel technique

To allow patient to bite on holder to keep digital sensor or film in place while positioning the position-indicating device (PID) and exposing the sensor or film

Reduces the number of components needed for positioning—One arm, one ring

Characteristics ▶

1 Holds film for bite-wing projection—Barrier placed on sensor

2 Holds film for anterior and posterior teeth projections—Barrier placed on sensor

3 Holds film for posterior teeth projection—Barrier placed on sensor

Slots on ring are color coded—Blue, anterior; yellow, posterior; red, bite-wing

Allows sufficient amount of space for sensors with wires

Practice Notes ▶

Uses the parallel technique for exposing radiation to the sensor or film

PID is parallel with the ring using a round or square PID

Sterilization Notes ▶

Disassembled Holders must be precleaned. Then, place in a sterilizing pouch with an internal process indicator, seal, then sterilize. OR, wrap with an internal process indicator inside and secure on the outside with process indicator tape, then sterilize. Verify appropriate color change has been achieved in external process indicator immediately after removal from sterilizer. Check internal process indicator before treatment. Refer to state regulations for any additional state requirements.

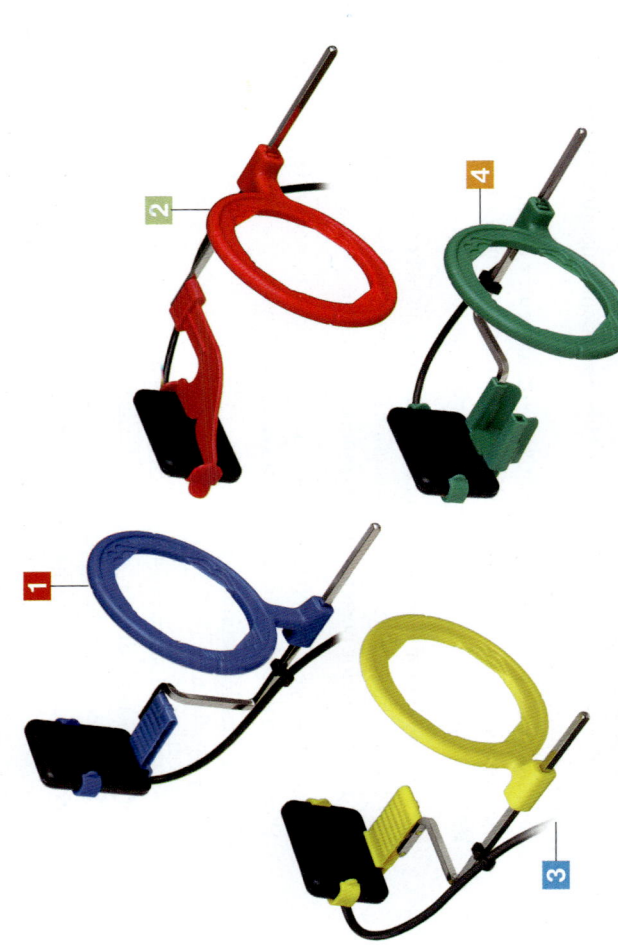

INSTRUMENT

Rinn XCP Holders for Digital Sensors

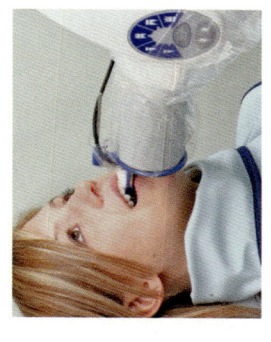

Functions ▶

To position and hold digital sensor in patient's mouth for periapical and bite-wing images, using parallel technique

To allow patient to bite on holder to keep sensor in place while positioning the position-indicating device (PID) and exposing the electronic sensor

Characteristics ▶

1 Blue—Holds film for anterior teeth projection

2 Red—Holds film for bite-wing projection

3 Yellow—Holds film for posterior teeth projection

4 Green—Holds film when taking projections for endodontic procedures

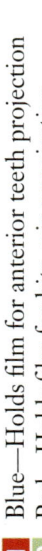

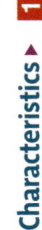

Slots hold electronic sensor in place with barriers placed on sensor and wire.

Several different styles of electronic sensor holders are available.

Practice Note ▶

Sterilization Notes ▶

Dissembled Holders must be precleaned. Then, place in a sterilizing pouch with an internal process indicator, seal, then sterilize. OR, wrap with an internal process indicator inside and secure on the outside with process indicator tape, then sterilize. Verify appropriate color change has been achieved in external process indicator immediately after removal from sterilizer. Check internal process indicator before treatment. Refer to state regulations for any additional state requirements.

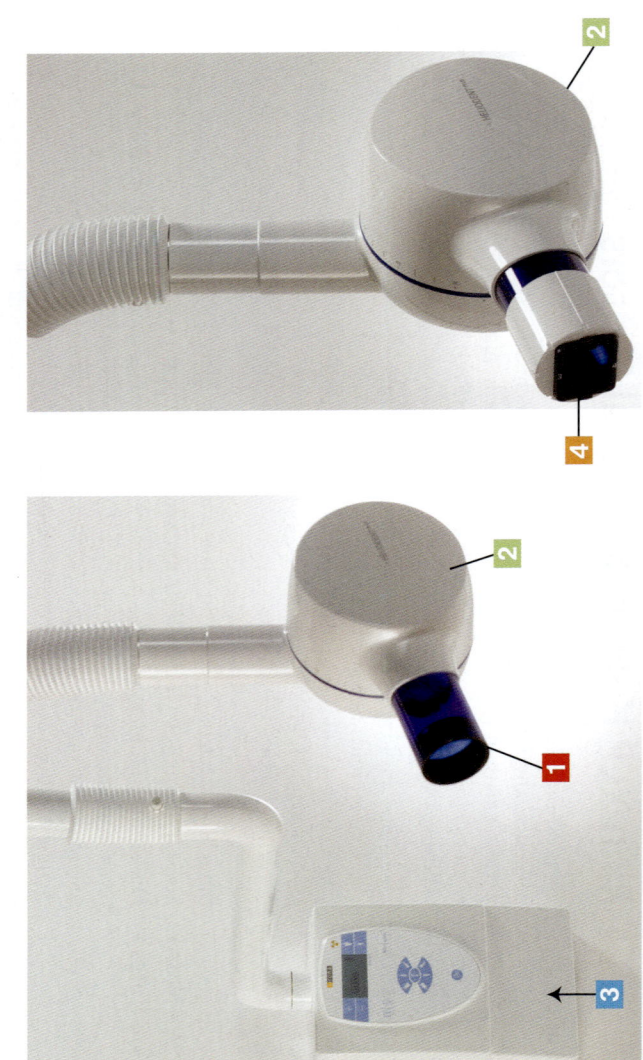

■ INSTRUMENT Digital Intraoral Imaging Unit

Functions ▶ To take digital intraoral images without film or without processing the film
To project the image of the teeth by digitally projecting radiation onto an electronic sensor and then to computerized imaging system

Characteristics ▶
1 Position-indicating device (PID) (round)
2 Tube head
3 X-ray unit with digital panel
4 Rectangular PID

Digital radiographs use less radiation than conventional radiographs.
Networks to computers in all areas of the dental office
Immediate imaging available

Practice Notes ▶ Paperless dental offices store digital images on the computer, along with patient records.
Used in all phases of dentistry, especially endodontics, orthodontics, oral surgery, and implantology.

Sterilization Notes ▶ Follow standard precautions and cross-contamination protocol when exposing and processing film. Barriers should be used on tube head, PID, and panel where x-ray button is pushed. If barriers are not used, follow manufacturer's recommendation for precleaning and disinfecting of the Digital Imaging Unit. Refer to state regulations for any additional state requirements.

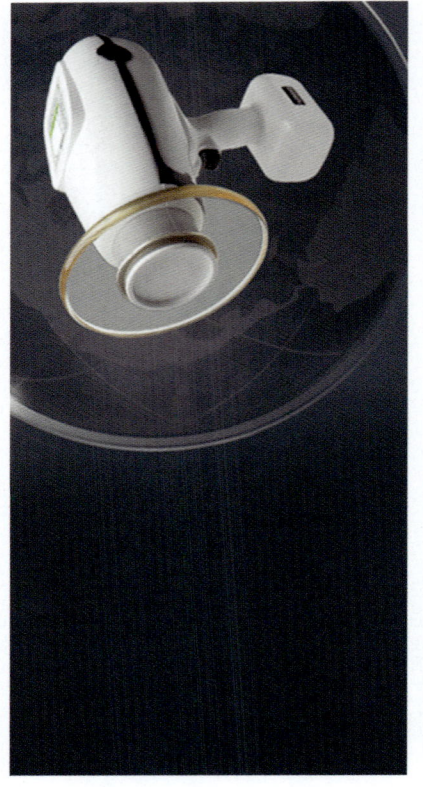

■ INSTRUMENT

Handheld Imaging Unit – KaVo NOMAD™ Pro 2

Functions ▶

To take intraoral images with a portable device

To expose digital sensors or conventional dental radiographic film

Characteristics ▶

Graphical touchpad interface with easy to recognize preset exposure; preset exposure time can be adjusted

Unit has a 2.5-mA current

Features internal shielding and a backscatter shield for operator safety

Easily adhere to ALARA

Can be used in place of wall-mounted units

Captures and displays images to various digital imaging computer systems, film, or PSP.

Practice Notes ▶

Handheld Imaging System is used chairside in dental offices, mobile clinics, humanitarian work, and more.

Sterilization Notes ▶

Follow standard precautions and cross-contamination protocol when images are taken. Barriers can be used on imaging unit. Always follow manufacturer's recommendation for precleaning and disinfection of the Imaging Unit and approved cleaning materials. Refer to local regulations for any additional requirements.

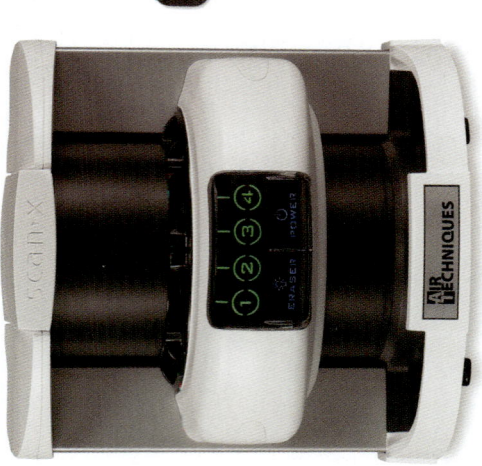

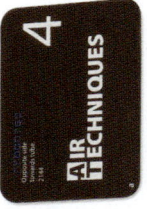

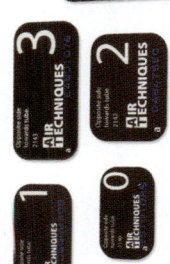

■ INSTRUMENT

SCANX Digital Imaging System

Function ▶ To produce diagnostic intraoral digital images

Characteristics ▶ Uses phosphor storage plates (PSPs)—Plastic plates coated with an x-ray sensitive phosphor material

Plates reused multiple times using one time only plastic barrier for each patient that covers the plates

Plates placed in machine to erase current image taken

Different size plates available for images

Compatible computer software needed for the SCANX digital images

Images appear on computer screen

Computer software compatibility of enhancing digital images to aid in diagnosis

Practice Notes ▶ Use regular intraoral x-ray machines for images

Use requirements—SCANX, computer and practice management software

Can be used in normal room lighting

Sterilization Notes ▶ Follow standard precautions and cross-contamination protocol. Barriers must be used when exposing sensors. Each plastic plate is covered and closed with a plastic barrier. Plastic barrier is removed before placing in SCANX. New plastic barrier is used for each SCANX image. Plastic covers are one time use only and disposed of in garbage after each use. Refer to state regulations for any additional state requirements.

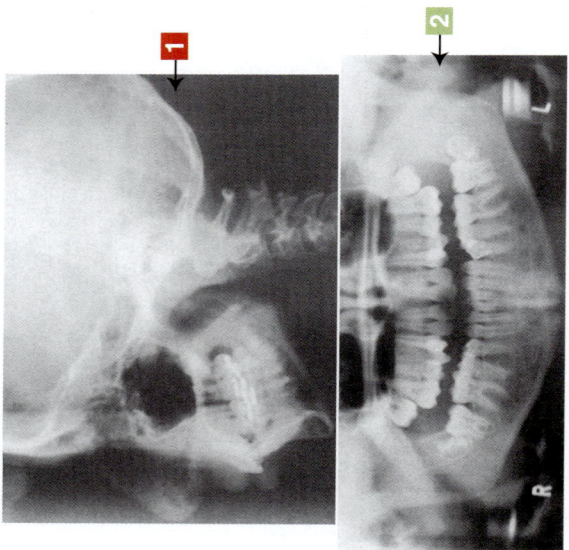

Extraoral Imaging—Cephalometric and Panoramic

■ INSTRUMENT

Functions ▶
To use to project the patient's teeth through images on the radiograph
To use for extraoral projections

Characteristics ▶
Film is placed in a cassette outside the mouth.

1 Cephalometric radiograph—Shows bony and soft-tissue areas of the facial profile

2 Panoramic radiograph—Shows a panoramic view of maxillary and mandibular teeth on one film

Practice Notes ▶
Different styles of extraoral radiograph machines are available.
Cephalometric and panoramic digital radiographs
Cephalometric and panoramic radiographs are used in all phases of dentistry. Panoramic images are used frequently in orthodontics.

Sterilization Notes ▶
Follow standard precautions and cross-contamination protocol when exposing and processing film for developing.

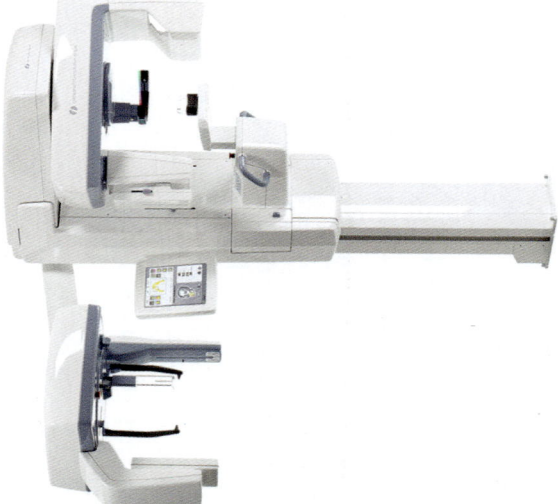

Digital Panoramic/Cephalometric Imaging Unit

■ INSTRUMENT

Functions ▶ To take digital panoramic and cephalometric images without film or without processing the film

To project the image of maxillary and mandibular teeth by digitally projecting radiation onto an electronic sensor and then to computerized imaging system

Characteristics ▶ Unit pictured is a 3-in-1 unit that takes both panoramic and cephalometric images. (It also takes 3D CBCT scans.)

Digital imaging uses less radiation than conventional radiographs.

Networks to computers in all areas of the dental office

Immediate imaging available

Practice Notes ▶ Paperless dental offices store digital panoramic imaging on the computer, along with patient records.

Used in all phases of dentistry, especially orthodontics, oral surgery, and implantology. Panoramic and cephalometric images may also be taken with conventional film.

Sterilization Notes ▶ Follow standard precautions and cross-contamination protocol. Barriers should be used; if not, then follow the manufacturer's recommendation for precleaning and disinfection.

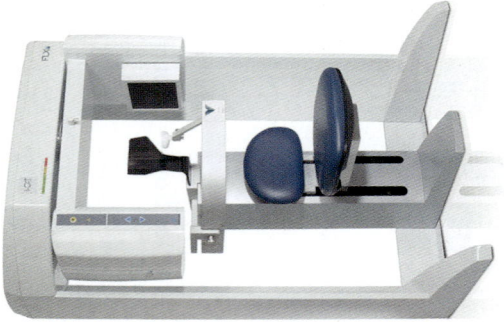

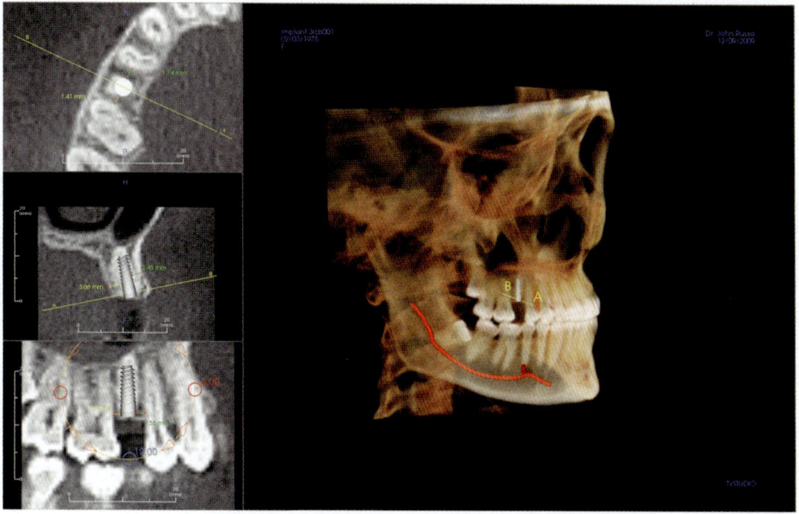

Cone-Beam Three-Dimensional (3D) Imaging System

■ INSTRUMENT

Function ▶ To produce diagnostic 3D images of the head and neck as related to dentistry

Characteristics ▶ High-resolution scans produce images at 0.2–mm voxel size to provide diagnosis for difficult areas to view with conventional radiographs.
Typical scan time of 8.9 seconds
Less radiation and more comfortable for the patient

Practice Notes ▶ Assists in diagnosis for enhanced orthodontic treatment planning, supernumerary teeth, abnormal anomalies, third molars, small root fractures, periodontal conditions, relationship of dentition, and other anatomy requiring detailed visualization.
Assists during treatment with periodontal and oral surgery procedures.

Sterilization Notes ▶ Follow standard precautions and cross-contamination protocol. Barriers should be used; if not, then follow the manufacturer's recommendation for precleaning and disinfection.

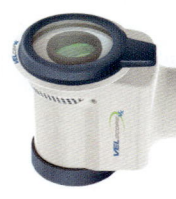

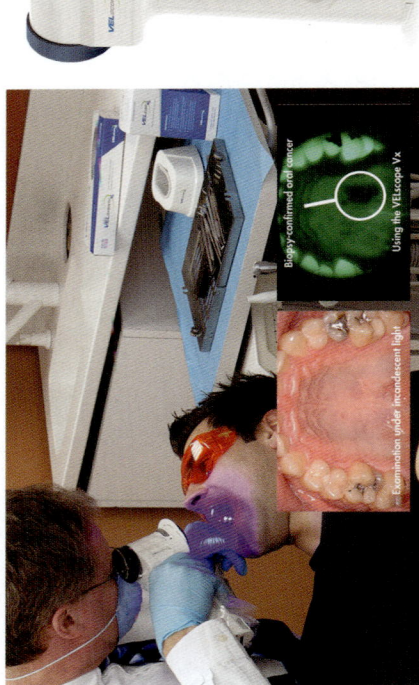

■ INSTRUMENT

Enhanced Oral Assessment System—VELscope Vx

Functions ▶

To aid in the assessment of oral mucosal abnormalities in early visualization of potential oral cancer, precancerous lesions or tissue, infections, and trauma that are not apparent to the naked eye alone

To use as an aid in determining surgical boundaries of oral lesions for excision

To use in conjunction with the traditional intraoral and extraoral examination. Referred to as the comprehensive oral exam (COE)

Characteristics ▶

Technology is based on an imaging modality that is sensitive to tissue changes that illuminates oral cavity to visualize potential abnormalities.

Handheld device emits a harmless ultraviolet (UV) light used to inspect the oral cavity. Device is sensitive to abnormal tissue changes. Distinctive blue-spectrum light causes the soft tissue (oral mucosa) of the mouth to naturally fluoresce.

Imaging adapter with iPod touch attaches to VELscope Vx eyepiece for clinical photographic documentation

Practice Note ▶

Velscope Vx is implemented in general practice as well as periodontal and maxillofacial surgery practices.

Sterilization Notes ▶

Protective barriers should be used on the device for each patient such as VELcap Vx and VELsheath Vx, which is recommended for each patient examination. Manufacturer's recommendation should be followed for precleaning and disinfecting the unit.

21

Patient Assessment and Emergency Equipment

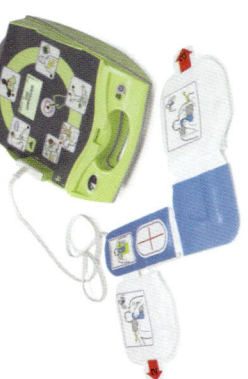

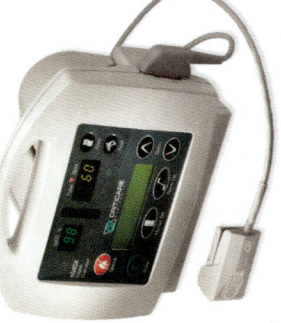

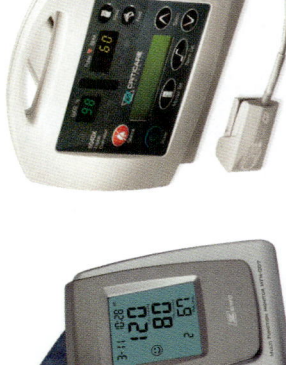

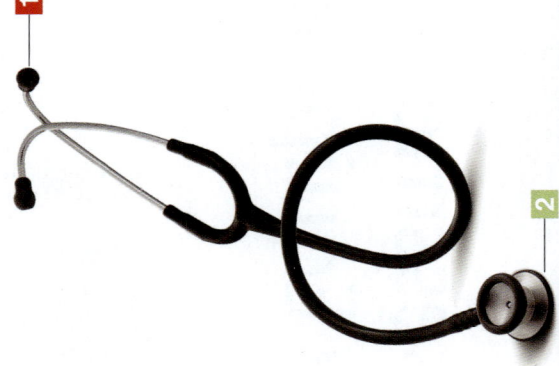

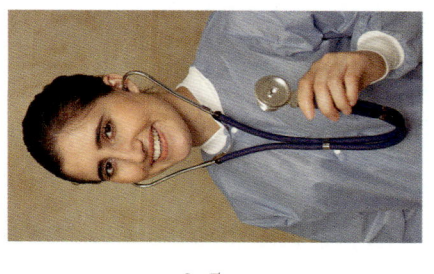

■ INSTRUMENT Stethoscope

Functions ▶ To listen to pulse
To listen to heartbeat
To listen to systolic and diastolic pressure when taking blood pressure

Characteristics ▶
1 Ear pieces to hear pulse, and/or blood pressure
2 Device to place on an artery to hear the sounds from the pulse, systolic and diastolic pressure. Usually, blood pressure is taken at the brachial artery in the arm.

Practice Notes ▶ Stethoscope in dentistry is used in conjunction with blood pressure cuff to hear systolic and diastolic pressure.
Stethoscope is used before dental procedures to hear the pulse, and take blood pressure.

Sterilization Notes ▶ Stethoscope should be precleaned and disinfected according to the manufacturer's recommendation.

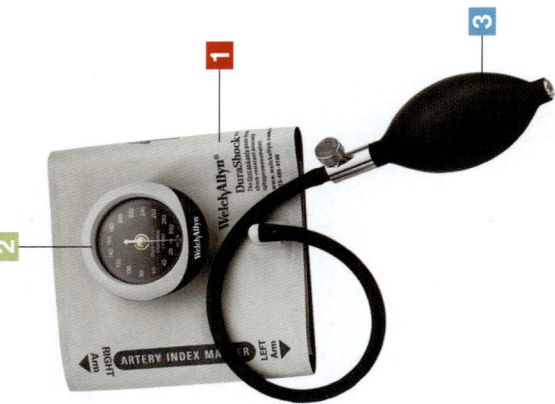

■ INSTRUMENT

Aneroid Blood Pressure Cuff—Sphygmomanometer

Functions ▶

To place pressure on the arteries to hear the systolic and diastolic pressure of the arteries

To place around the part of the arm above the bend in the elbow

Characteristics ▶

1 Blood pressure cuff for the arm

2 Meter—Aneroid dial system (without liquid); the readout for systolic and diastolic blood pressure

3 Rubber bulb—Attached to cuff with rubber tubing

Blood pressure cuff available in regular size, small size, and larger size cuffs to fit various arm sizes

Cuff size should fit properly to obtain accurate blood pressure readings.

Cuff is placed above the bend in the elbow above the brachial artery.

Practice Notes ▶

Blood Pressure Cuff is used in conjunction with the stethoscope to hear the systolic and diastolic pressure at the brachial artery located at the inner side of the bend in the elbow.

Document blood pressure readings in patient's chart.

Sterilization Notes ▶

Blood Pressure Cuff must be precleaned and disinfected according to the manufacturer's recommendation.

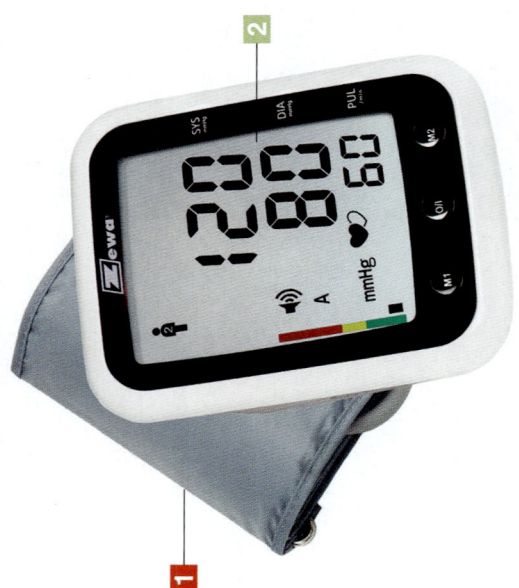

■ INSTRUMENT

Automatic Blood Pressure Monitor

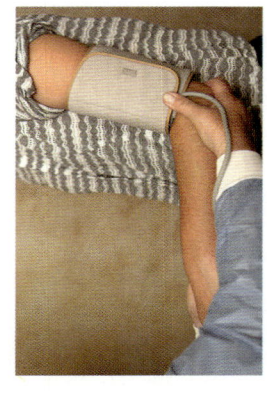

Functions ▸
To measure blood pressure automatically
To display the blood pressure readout on the screen
To measure pulse rate automatically
To display the pulse readout on the screen

Characteristics ▸
1 Blood pressure cuff
2 Readout screen for blood pressure and pulse rate

Blood pressure cuff available in regular size, small size, and larger size cuffs to fit various arms
Correct cuff size important for accurate blood pressure readings
Data from past blood pressure information available on some monitors

Practice Notes ▸
Automatic Blood Pressure Monitor is used before medical and dental procedures.
Document blood pressure readings in patient's chart.

Sterilization Notes ▸
Blood Pressure Cuff must be precleaned and disinfected according to the manufacturer's recommendation.

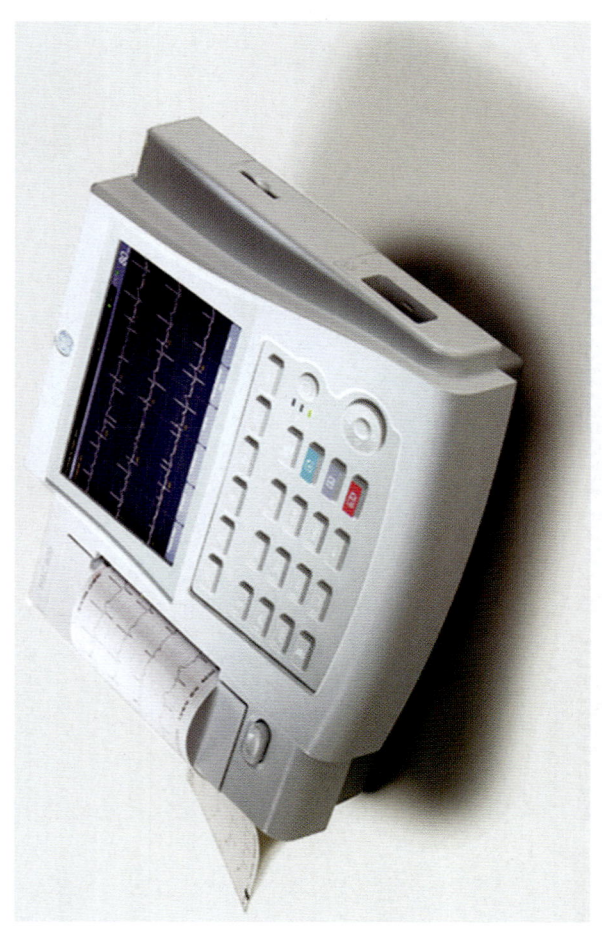

Electrocardiogram (EKG) Machine

INSTRUMENT

Function ▶ To measure the electrical activity of the heartbeat

Characteristics ▶ EKG chest leads; self-adhesive pads with wires attached with electrodes for conductivity and placed in specific locations on the patient which are connected to the EKG machine
A read-out is displayed on the screen.

Practice Note ▶ EKG Machine is used to monitor the patient's heartbeat usually during dental surgical procedures, during intravenous sedation in a dental office (mostly for oral surgeries), and for general anesthesia.

Sterilization Notes ▶ Chest leads are single use only. Chest leads used on the patient are disposable and should be disposed of in garbage. Single use only. Disinfect unit according to manufacturer's recommendation.

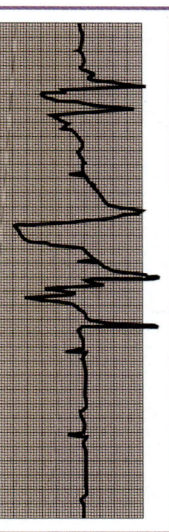

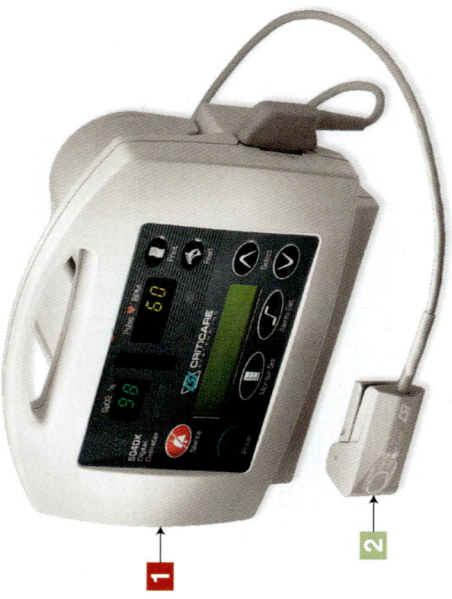

■ INSTRUMENT

Pulse Oximeter

Functions ▶ To measure the concentration of oxygen in the blood
To detect the pulse rate

Characteristics ▶

1 Monitor to display oxygen concentration in the blood and pulse rate

2 Finger device that measures the oxygen concentration and pulse rate that sends information to the monitor

Practice Note ▶ Pulse Oximetry is used to monitor the patient's heart beat as well as oxygen concentration usually during dental surgical procedures, during intravenous sedation in a dental office, and for general anesthesia

Sterilization Notes ▶ Pulse Oximetry should be precleaned and disinfected according to the manufacturer's recommendation.

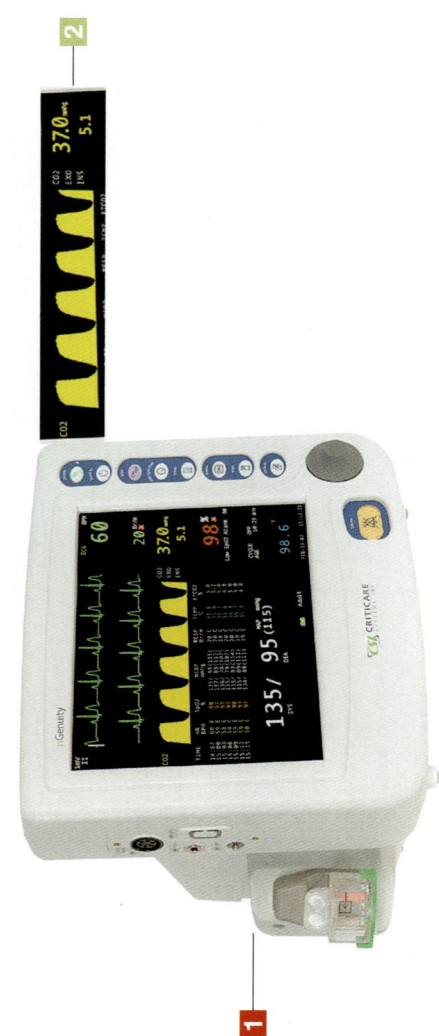

Capnograph

■ INSTRUMENT

Functions ▸
To measure carbon dioxide (CO_2) in exhaled breath
To monitor patient's ventilation

Characteristics ▸
1 Capnograph monitors patient ventilation, providing a breath by breath trend of respirations and an early warning system of impending respiratory crisis.
2 Monitor displays patient carbon dioxide in exhaled breath.

Capnography provides an immediate picture of patient condition.
Example: Holding your breath. Capnograph will show immediate apnea. Pulse oximetry is delayed for several minutes, and the pulse oximeter will show high saturation of oxygen for several minutes with holding your breath.

When a person hyperventilates, their CO_2 decreases.

Practice Note ▸
Used in dental offices for patients who are sedated

Sterilization Notes ▸
Capnograph should be precleaned and disinfected according to the manufacturer's recommendations.

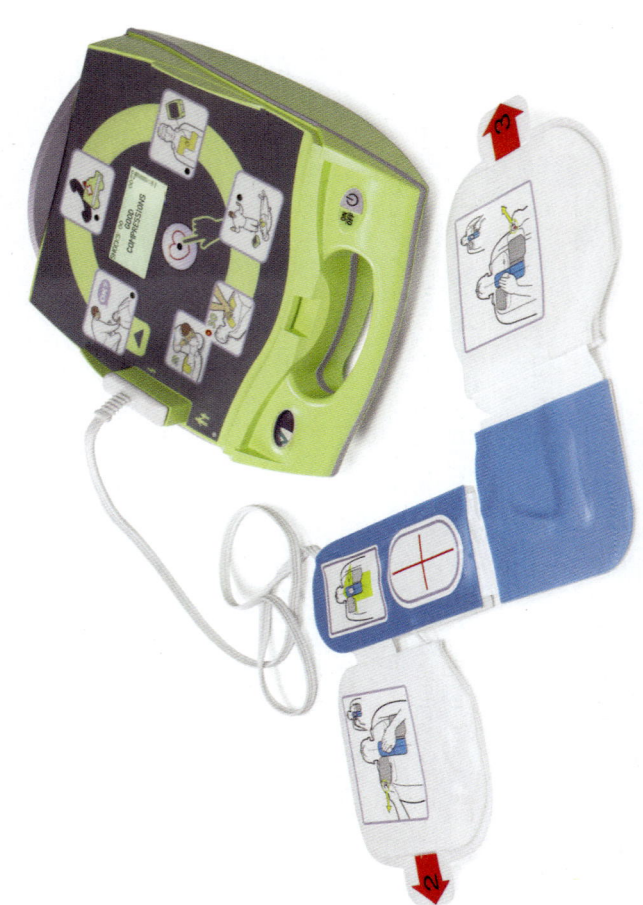

Automated External Defibrillator (AED)

■ **INSTRUMENT**

Functions ▶ To use for emergency situations when a person is unresponsive
To use when a person has no pulse and is not breathing

Characteristic ▶ Place devices correctly on patient and wait
for automated voice directions from AED to
proceed.

Practice Notes ▶ A provider should be trained healthcare provider
with basic life support and using an AED.
Preventive maintenance is required for update
of batteries.

Sterilization Notes ▶ AED should be precleaned and disinfected
according to the manufacturer's recommendations.

Index

Note: Page numbers followed by "f" and "t" indicate figures and tables respectively